Progress in Drug Research
Fortschritte der Arzneimittelforschung
Progrès des recherches pharmaceutiques
Vol. 49

Progress in Drug Research
Fortschritte der Arzneimittelforschung
Progrès des recherches pharmaceutiques
Vol. 49

Edited by / Herausgegeben von / Rédigé par
Ernst Jucker, Basel

Authors / Autoren / Auteurs
Richard M. Eglen · Mont R. Juchau · Gillian Edwards and Arthur H. Weston · Helen Wise · M.D. Murray and D. Craig Brater · Olivier Valdenaire and Philippe Vernier · Annemarie Polak

Springer Basel AG

Editor:

Dr. E. Jucker
Steinweg 28
CH-4107 Ettingen
Switzerland

© 1997 Springer Basel AG
Originally published by Birkhäuser Verlag in 1997
Printed on acid-free paper produced from chlorine-free pulp. TCF ∞

ISBN 978-3-0348-9807-2   ISBN 978-3-0348-8863-9 (eBook)
DOI 10.1007/978-3-0348-8863-9

9 8 7 6 5 4 3 2 1

Contents · Inhalt · Sommaire

Foreword

Volume 49 of „Progress in Drug Research" contains seven reviews and the various indexes which facilitate the use of all the volumes published so far.

The articles in volume 49, all written by experts in the respective fields of their research, deal with 5-hydroxytryptamine (HT)4-receptors and their functions in the central nervous system, with the manifold problems of teratogenesis in humans and with recent advances in potassium channel modulation. The effects of NSAIDs on the kidney are reviewed, the G protein receptors as modules of interacting proteins are presented in a comprehensive way, and the neuronal function of prostacyclin, a rapidly growing and exciting area of research thoroughly dealt with in an article by Helen Wise. Finally, the current situation in the battle against fungal infections in humans is presented in a most interesting chapter by Annemarie Polak. All these reviews contain extensive bibliographies which enable researchers who are interested in the respective subjects to have access to the original literature in a relatively short time and with little effort.

It has always been the aim of the Founder/Editor of PDR to help disseminate information on the vast and fast growing domain of drug research. In particular, it was and still is his goal to supply the active researcher with a tool to facilitate and further their own research work. Those researchers who wish to start a new project will welcome the opportunity of the availability of concise reviews and the corresponding bibliographies. In addition, it was my hope that PDR might help scientists to keep abreast of the latest developments in the field of drug research. The fact that PDR has existed for 38 years demonstrates that at least some of the goals have been achieved. It is, therefore, with great satisfaction that this new volume is presented to the readers. At the same time, feelings of deep gratitude to the authors who are prepared to share their knowledge and experience with our readers are manifest. In addition to the thanks extended to the authors, I would also like to express my gratitude to the readers of PDR and to the reviewers: Their constructive criticism and suggestions helped to maintain the high standard of this monograph series.

My thanks also go to Birkhäuser Publishers for their constant understanding of the problems involved and for their encouragement. It is not possible to mention all those who are involved in the production of PDR here and I have to restrict my thanks to those members of the team with whom I have close contact. They are Mrs. Elizabeth Beckett, Dr. Petra Gerlach and Mssrs. H.-P. Thür, E. Mazenauer and G. Messmer.

Basel, October 1997   DR. E. JUCKER

Vorwort

Der vorliegende 49. Band der Reihe «Fortschritte der Arzneimittelforschung» enthält sieben Übersichtsreferate, die wiederum von anerkannten aktiven Forschern verfasst wurden. Ausserdem finden sich in diesem Band das Stichwortverzeichnis des Bandes, ein Titelverzeichnis aller 49 Bände sowie ein Autoren- und Titelverzeichnis der Bände 1–49. Der Leser hat dadurch die Möglichkeit, nicht nur den vorliegenden Band, sondern auch alle bisher erschienenen Bände zu konsultieren.

Hervorzuheben sind dabei die ausserordentlich umfangreichen Literaturverzeichnisse, die ein Zurückgreifen auf Originalpublikationen gestatten und für den Forscher ein nützliches Arbeitsinstrument darstellen.

Die Artikel des 49. Bandes behandeln 5-Hydroxytryptamin(HT)$_4$-Rezeptoren und ihre Funktionen im Zentralnervensystem, die mannigfaltigen Probleme der Teratogenese und die neuesten Forschungen auf dem Gebiet der Wirkstoffe zur Modulation der Kaliumkanäle. Ausserdem werden die nicht-steroiden Entzündungshemmer im Hinblick auf ihre Wirkung auf die Nieren behandelt, Wechselwirkungen zwischen G-Protein und intrazellulären Proteinen untersucht und die neuesten Entwicklungen auf dem bisher nur wenig erforschten Gebiet der neuronalen Prostacyclin-Rezeptoren übersichtlich dargestellt und ihre physiologische Rolle beleuchtet. Der letzte und längste Beitrag stammt wiederum von Annemarie Polak und behandelt nahezu alle Aspekte von Pilzinfektionen beim Menschen.

Seit der Gründung der Reihe im Jahr 1959 war der Herausgeber stets bemüht, die nicht mehr überschaubare Flut an Informationen über das komplexe und multidisziplinäre Gebiet der Arzneimittelforschung dem interessierten Leser und dem engagierten Forscher näher zu bringen und in Teilgebieten überschaubar zu machen. Diese Zielsetzung habe ich bis heute beibehalten, obwohl es viel schwieriger als vor 38 Jahren ist, mit der Entwicklung auch nur einigermassen Schritt zu halten. Wenn es gelungen ist, das angestrebte Ziel wenigstens teilweise zu erreichen, so ist dies in erster Linie den Autoren zu verdanken. Sie haben mit ihren Übersichtsreferaten eine überaus grosse Arbeit auf sich genommen und ihr umfangreiches Wissen und ihre Erfahrungen mit den Lesern geteilt. Aber auch Leser und Fachkollegen haben mich immer wieder mit Rat unterstützt, und ganz besonders haben die Rezensenten durch ihre wohlgemeinte Kritik und durch ihre Empfehlungen zum Erfolg der «Fortschritte» wesentlich beigetragen. Ihnen allen danke ich auch an dieser Stelle.

Mein Dank gilt auch dem Birkhäuser Verlag, wobei ich ganz besonders die Damen E. Beckett und Dr. P. Gerlach sowie die Herren H.-P. Thür, E. Mazenauer und G. Messmer erwähnen möchte. Sie alle haben durch ihren grossen persönlichen Einsatz den 49. Band mitgestaltet und mitgeprägt.

Basel, Oktober 1997   DR. E. JUCKER

Progress in Drug Research, Voi. 49 (E. Jucker, Ed.)
© 1997 Birkhäuser Verlag, Basel (Switzerland)

5-Hydroxytryptamine (5-HT)$_4$ receptors and central nervous system function: An update

By Richard M. Eglen

Center for Biological Research, Neurobiology Unit, Roche Bioscience, 3401 Hillview Ave., Palo Alto, CA 94304, USA. e-mail: richard.eglen@roche.com

1   Introduction

The 5-hydroxytryptamine (5-HT; serotonin)$_4$ receptor is one of three 5-HT receptor subtypes that couple positively to adenylyl cyclase, the others being the 5-HT$_6$ and 5-HT$_7$ receptors [1]. In terms of sequence homology and pharmacology, these receptors are distinct and have differing distributions and function. In the last 5 years or so, the 5-HT$_4$ receptor has become the focus of much interest in both academia and the pharmaceutical industry. Elucidation of the role of the receptor in the central and peripheral nervous systems is thus emerging, and novel therapeutics with 5-HT$_4$ receptor selectivity are currently in advanced clinical trials.

It is arguable that current understanding of the function of the 5-HT$_4$ receptor in the periphery is more complete than that relating to a central role [2]. In part, this is due to the ease with which experiments on gastrointestinal tissue can be conducted, *in vivo* and *in vitro*. Moreover, the therapeutic potential for 5-HT$_4$ receptor ligands in gastroesophageal reflux disease (agonists) or irritable bowel syndrome (antagonists) favors research in peripheral tissues [2]. Nonetheless, central nervous system studies have played a key role in the discovery of the 5-HT$_4$ receptor. While not recognized as such, the 5-HT$_4$ receptor was initially identified in studies measuring adenylyl cyclase activity in guinea-pig hippocampus [3] and positively identified in cultures of mouse colliculi neurons [4, 5]. Contrary to the later discoveries of the 5-ht$_5$, 5-HT$_6$ and 5-HT$_7$ receptors, cloning of the 5-HT$_4$ receptor [6] was reported after the development of selective agonists and antagonists [7]. Analogues of these compounds were extensively used to characterize the central distribution of the receptor, although it was not until mRNA probes became available for the two splice variants that *intra*receptor heterogeneity was recognized [2, 7, 8]. Collectively, these data, together with neurochemical and behavioral data, using selective agonists and antagonists, are consistent with a role in cognition and anxiety [8].

This update assesses the current understanding of the 5-HT$_4$ receptor and brain function, a subject previously reviewed in 1995 [8]. Several aspects will be covered, divided into sections concerning the distribution, electrophysiology, neurochemistry and behavioral actions of 5-HT$_4$ ligands. To place the data in perspective, a summary of the molecular biology and pharmacology of the 5-HT$_4$ receptor is also included. The role of the receptor in the peripheral nervous system and the medicinal chemistry of 5-HT$_4$ receptor ligands will not be addressed, and the reader is thus referred to extensive reviews published recently [2, 7, 9, 10].

2   Molecular Biology

The 5-HT$_4$ receptor has been cloned from rat [6], mouse [11] and human [12], although only sequences from the first two are publicly available. The sequences are highly homologous and conform to the archetypal G protein-coupled receptor motif. The rat and mouse 5-HT$_4$ receptor exist in two splice variants, a long (5-HT$_{4L}$) and a truncated (5-HT$_{4S}$) form, arising from differences in the length of the carboxy terminus. When isolated from a rat cDNA library, and expressed in *Cos*-7 cells, the pharmacology of the clone is consistent with that of a 5-HT$_4$ receptor [6], and both splice variants positively couple to adenylyl cyclase. The receptor possesses a short, third intracellular loop [45 amino acids] and a long carboxy terminus [6] and is most homologous to the histamine H$_2$ receptor, a receptor that also couples positively to adenylyl cyclase. Radioligand-binding studies at recombinant receptors show that [^{3}H] 5-HT labels two states of the receptor, whereas the antagonist, [^{3}H] GR 113808, labels only one state. Since the states recognized by agonists are sensitive to guanine nucleotides, it is probable that the 5-HT$_4$ receptor exists in high and low affinity conformations, a characteristic of most G protein-coupled receptors [13]. Pharmacologically, both rat isoforms are similar in that they display similar rank orders of agonist potency and antagonist affinity [6]. However, the absolute potencies of agonists differ between the splice variants, possibly due to a differential sensitivity of the isoforms to desensitization. Interestingly, the long form of the receptor possesses four sites for protein kinase C-mediated phosphorylation, while the short form possesses three.

Cloning of the mouse 5-HT$_4$ receptor was undertaken using cDNAs from mouse colliculi neurons [11], a tissue in which the receptor was first defined [4,5]. Sequence analysis reveals an open reading frame of 406 amino acids, with 16 amino acids differing between rat and mouse. Several key residues are conserved, including those responsible for G protein coupling, the cysteines involved in formation of disulfide bridges and the DRY sequence from the N terminal of the second intracellular loop [11]. In contrast to the rat sequence, mouse 5-HT$_{4L}$ receptors carry only two sites for protein kinase phosphorylation, although the carboxy terminus from both rat and mouse sequences contains sites for phosphorylation by G protein receptor kinases. Transfection of the receptor increases basal level of adenylyl cyclase activity, suggesting that at high levels of receptor expression, the receptors precouple. Endogenously expressed 5-HT$_4$ receptors enhance adenylyl cyclase activity in mouse colliculi [14], guinea pig hippocampus [5] and human frontal cortex [15]. It is unclear, however, if precoupling occurs in these tissues at physiologically appropriate expression levels.

Table 1
Potency (pEC_{50}) and affinity (pK_B) of some $5\text{-}HT_4$ receptor agonists and antagonists, respectively

Compound	pEC_{50}	pK_B
Agonists		
5-HT	8.2	
Cisapride	7.3	
BIMU-1	7.9	
BIMU-8	7.6	
ML 10302	8.4	
RS 57639	9.5	
RS 67333	8.7	
RS 67506	8.8	
Antagonists		
DAU 6285		7.6
GR 113808		10.2
GR 125487		10.4
RS 23597		8.4
RS 39604		9.1
RS 67532		8.7
RS 100235		10.0
SB 204070		10.9
SB 207266		10.6
SDZ 205,557		8.6

3   Pharmacology

The $5\text{-}HT_4$ receptor is operationally defined using a range of potent and selective agonists or antagonists (Table 1). Historically, this was undertaken using nonselective agonists, including the benzimidazolones BIMU-1 and BIMU-8, and substituted benzamides such as metaclopramide, cisapride, zacopride and renzapride. Nonselective antagonists with only moderate to low affinity for the receptor included DAU 6285 and tropisetron [7]. Most of these compounds are potent $5\text{-}HT_3$ receptor antagonists, and interpretation of their effects *in vivo* was compromised by this lack of selectivity. The situation improved when antagonists including LY 297524, RS 23597, SC 53606 and SDZ 205,557 were developed [7]. Although they possessed moderate affinity for the $5\text{-}HT_3$ receptor, they exhibited relatively low affinity for the $5\text{-}HT_4$ receptor. This property, as well as poor activity *in vivo*, has limited their use.

The ligands currently available are highly selective and possess high affinity for the receptor. An extensive discussion of the $5\text{-}HT_4$ receptor pharmacophore has recently been published [7]. Potent agonists that preferentially activate the receptor [13] include substituted benzamides and carbazimdamides [7]. Several highly potent agonists, including ML 10302 [16] and analogues [17], contain an ester moiety [14], and are thus unstable *in vivo*. Ketones such as RS 17017, by contrast, exhibit a prolonged time course of action and provide convenient research tools [18]. Analogues of this compound, RS 67333 and RS 67506 [19], exhibit similar pharmacology but possess differential lipophilicity and therefore cross the blood brain-barrier to different degrees. Consequently, they are useful compounds for distinguishing between central and peripheral effects of 5-HT$_4$ receptor activation [19].

Most 5-HT$_4$ receptor agonists have low intrinsic activities and elicit responses dependent upon the tissue receptor reserve. The lack of a response to an agonist thus does not necessarily argue for a lack of 5-HT$_4$ receptor function. Moreover, blockade of agonist response, by a selective 5-HT$_4$ receptor antagonist is critical evidence for invoking participation of a 5-HT$_4$ receptor. Fortunately, several high-affinity, selective antagonists are now available [7]. As is the case for agonists, a major challenge in this area has been to develop compounds that are not esters and thus have significant oral activity [7]. Selective antagonists that undergo rapid metabolism include GR 113808 [20] and, to lesser extent, SB 204070 [21]; a property that accounts for the high doses required for *in vivo* studies. Antagonists with significant oral activity include GR 125487 [22], SB 207266 [23, 24], RS 39604 [25] and RS 100235 [26]. SB 207266, notably, is in advanced clinical trials for beneficial effects in irritable bowel syndrome [7].

Given the identification of a one 5-HT$_4$ receptor gene, it is consistent that the pharmacology of most ligands support a singular form of the 5-HT$_4$ receptor (Table 2). Early studies, particularly with cisapride, hinted at an atypical rank order of agonist potency at 5-HT$_4$ receptors in mouse colliculi when compared to that seen in peripheral tissues [27, 28]. However, recent comparison of the pharmacology of the recombinant receptor with that expressed in guinea pig striatum or human caudate reveals no meaningful differences [14].

4   Distribution

In situ hybridization studies in rat brain have defined abundant expression of receptor mRNA in olfactory system, striatum, medial habenula and hippocampus [20]. Early data suggested that the expression of transcripts for the short form is restricted to the striatum, whereas the long

Table 2
Pharmacology of 5-HT$_4$ receptors in human *post mortem* brain tissue and guinea pig striatum.

Ligand	Putamen	Cortex	Striatum*
GR 113808	10.1	10.1	10.2
SDZ 205,557	8.7	.8.3	8.6
DAU 6285	8.0	8.2	7.6
BIMU-1	7.8	7.8	7.9
DAU 6285	7.4	7.2	–
Tropisetron	7.4	7.4	7.5
5-HT	7.3	7.5	7.5
BIMU-8	7.3	–	–
R-Zacopride	5.8	5.9	6.2

*Guinea pig

form is expressed throughout the brain, except for the cerebellum [6]. By contrast, reverse transcription polymerase chain reaction (RT-PCR) studies in rat and mouse tissue suggest that both isoforms are widely distributed throughout the brain [11]. Comparison of the distribution of oligonucleotide probes for both isoforms reveals similar expression patterns in the olfactory tubercle, basal ganglia, medial habenula and hippocampus. The reasons for the expression of two forms of the receptor in the brain are thus unrelated to regional heterogeneity [30]. It has thus been speculated [1] that differing isoforms enable the receptor to couple to distinct isoforms of adenylyl cyclase in different brain areas.

The tritiated analogue of GR 113808 has been widely used to assess the CNS distribution of 5-HT$_4$ receptors [31], and has provided the basis of a robust radioligand binding assay (Table 3). A second radioligand, [^{125}I] SB 207710, an analogue of SB 204070, has also been used in radioligand binding assays [30, 32], notably in tissues with low receptor density. Both of these radioligands are now available commercially. The distribution of the 5-HT$_4$ receptor has been mapped in human, mouse, rat, pig, cow and primate [33–38]. Collectively, autoradiographical studies demonstrate high levels of receptor density in the olfactory tubercule, islands of Calleja, basal ganglia and substantia nigra, with intermediate to low densities in the hippocampal formation and superior colliculus (Table 2). The distribution of the binding sites, while generally consistent with the mRNA expression data, is not always coincidental [29, 30]. This indicates that in some regions, notably in the substantia nigra and globus pallidus, the receptors are located on axon terminals [30].

Table 3
Regional density of and affinity of [^{3}H] GR 113808 at 5-HT$_4$ receptors in human *post mortem* brain

Brain region	B$_{max}$ (fmol/mg tissue)
Caudate nucleus	8.7
Lateral putamen	8.6
Putamen	5.7
Medial pallidum	3.8
Temporal cortex	2.6
Hippocampus	2.4
Amygdala	2.3
Frontal cortex	1.7
Cerebellar cortex	<1.0

These data are taken from [39].

Generally, the distribution of 5-HT$_4$ receptors can be arranged in two major functional systems, i.e. the septo-hippocampa-habenulo-peduncular and striato-nigro-tectal pathways (Table 3). Minor differences are, nonetheless, apparent between species, such that in most areas more receptors are labeled in guinea pig than in rat, although the converse is true in the interpeduncular nucleus. In primate brain, in contrast, an intermediate level is observed in limbic and sensory regions and not in guinea pig or rat [35]. In adult rat and guinea pig hippocampus, striatum and colliculi, the density of 5-HT$_4$ receptors is low [33, 34, 38]. This raises the possibility that the receptor is developmentally regulated in brain regions such as the colliculi, since the ability of 5-HT to stimulate adenylyl cyclase in this structure declines with age. 5-HT$_4$ receptors, although expressed in low density in rat striatum prenatally, markedly increase during the second and third postnatal week. Conversely, in the brain stem, the high density, present prenatally, declines after birth. In the globus pallidum, expression of 5-HT$_4$ receptors coincides with expression of glutaminergic innervation. Collectively, it has been argued that the ontogeny of 5-HT$_4$ receptors in the rat parallels syntaptogenesis rather than neurogenesis [33].

5   Neurochemistry

Given the distribution of the receptor in the brain, several studies have focused on the regulation of dopamine or acetylcholine transmission [6]. The neuronal location of the receptor has also been addressed by chemical lesion studies [36]. Lesions of the 5-HT system, by injections in 5, 7-

dihydroxytryptamine, cause an increase in 5-HT$_4$ receptor density in several brain regions, excepting the caudal caudate putamen. In contrast, kainic acid lesions of caudate-putamen cause marked decreases in the density of 5-HT$_4$ receptors. This suggests that 5-HT$_4$ receptors are associated with intrinsic γ aminobutyric acid (GABA)ergic and/or cholinergic neurons [36]. Moreover, this hypothesis accords with *post mortem* data [39] in putamen patients with Huntington's disease in whom the density of 5-HT$_4$ receptors is markedly reduced (Table 4). Intranigral injections of 6-hydroxydopamine causes in lesions of dopaminergic neurons yet induces no change in the density of 5-HT$_4$ receptors in the rostral caudate putamen [36].

These data are supported by studies [39] in *post mortem* tissue from Parkinson's disease, in which the density of 5-HT$_4$ receptors remains unchanged in either putamen or substantia nigra (Table 4). These findings strongly suggests the receptor is not localized to dopaminergic neurons. Nonetheless, several *in vitro* and *in vivo* studies demonstrate that 5-HT$_4$ receptor agonists augment the release of dopamine in rat caudate putamen, nucleus accumbens and striatum [40–45]. This effect is not apparent in isolated syntopsomes [44], supporting a process secondary to activation of striatal neurons. Although the nature of this has not been established, an involvement of GABAergic neurons has been postulated [36]. Intranigral injection of 5-HT$_4$ receptor antagonists attenuates dopamine release, but only when augmented by morphine [45]. This could indicate that a basal dopaminergic transmission tone needs to be present to reveal an effect of 5-HT$_4$ receptor activation. However, SB 204070, a selective antagonist with good CNS penetration, does not influence behavioral changes (e.g. hyperactivity) induced by dopaminergic stimulation [46]. Parkinsonian tremor, also related to disorders of dopaminergic transmission, is exacerbated by cisapride therapy in two patients [47]. However, the nonselective action of cisapride, in addition to partial 5-HT$_4$ receptor agonism, complicates interpretation of this finding. Finally, 5-HT$_4$ receptors modulate the release of 5-HT in rat hippocampus *in vivo* [48], the physiological significance of which is unclear. Nonetheless, it is intriguing that peripheral administration of 5-HT$_4$ agonists, such as renzapride, augment hippocampal release of 5-HT [48].

The role of 5-HT$_4$ receptors in regulating cholinergic transmission in the alimentary tract is well established [2, 10, 49]. 5-HT$_4$ receptors also modulate cholinergic transmission in the CNS, since intracerebroventricular injection of BIMU-1 or BIMU-8 increases acetylcholine release in the frontal cortex of freely moving rats [50]. Administration of selective 5-HT$_4$ antagonists alone does not affect acetylcholine levels, suggesting a

Table 4
Levels of [^{3}H] GR 113808 binding in *post mortem* brain tissue in three neurodegenerative diseases

	B$_{max}$ (fmol/mg protein)
Alzheimer's disease	
Hippocampus	
Control	2.3
Patients	0.8
Frontal cortex	
Control	1.8
Patients	1.3
Huntington's disease	
Putamen	
Control	5.3
Patients	2.7
Parkinson's disease	
Putamen	
Control	4.7
Patients	5.9
Substantia nigra	
Control	4.2
Patients	5.6

These data are taken from [39].

low basal 5-HT$_4$ receptor tone [50]. The density of 5-HT$_4$ receptors in *post mortem* hippocampus and frontal cortex taken from patients with Alzheimer's disease is markedly less than in aged matched controls [39; Table 4]. This also implicates the receptor in the regulation of central cholinergic transmission, given the marked attenuation of cholinergic transmission in the disease. This hypothesis accords with the procognitive action of 5-HT$_4$ receptor agonists in rat behavioral studies, in which cognitive function is reduced by disruption of the cholinergic system and aging (see below). This may also explain an early report [51] in which administration of the mixed 5-HT$_4$ agonist/5-HT$_3$ antagonist zacopride reversed the decrements in EEG energy induced by muscarinic receptor antagonism.

6   Electrophysiology

Slow membrane depolarizations induced by 5-HT are associated with a decrease in resting potassium conductance. This includes the responses to 5-HT in rat hippocampal CA1 pyramidal neurons [52]. The reduction in the after-hyperpolarization, observed in the presence of 5-HT$_{1A}$ blockade, is mediated by 5-HT$_4$ receptors, in that the responses are antagonized by selective 5-HT$_4$ receptor antagonists and elicited by 5-HT$_4$ agonists [53]. The inability of phosphodiesterase inhibitors to alter the ability of 5-HT$_4$ receptors to reduce the after-hyperpolarization suggests that other signaling cascades are activated [54]. The lack of effect of protein kinase A inhibitors, however, argues against this contention [54]. 5-HT$_{1A}$ and 5-HT$_4$ receptors are co-localized on rat hippocampal pyramidal cells, where they mediate inhibitory and excitatory effects, respectively [55]. It has been suggested that 5-HT$_4$ receptors exert an excitatory role on rat hippocampus in order to oppose an inhibitory role of 5-HT$_{1A}$ receptors [53, 55]. Chronic treatment with several antidepressant drugs, including fluvoxamine or paroxetine, reduces the potency of zacopride on population spikes in rat CA1 hippocampal neurons [56]. Consequently, the inhibitory tone of the 5-HT$_{1A}$ receptor is "unmasked" under conditions of 5-HT$_4$ receptor desensitization or blockade [56]. Conversely, in NG 108-15 cells, chronic exposure to amitriptyline enhances 5-HT$_4$-induced accumulation of 3'5' cyclic adenosine monophosphate (cAMP) [57].

The regulation of synaptic plasticity is critical in learning and memory and probably involves long-term modulation of ion channel activity [58]. In *Aplysia californica* activation of 5-HT receptors augments adenylyl cyclase activity, inhibits inward potassium currents (via protein kinase A) and facilitates neurotransmitter release [58]. This pathway is involved in a model of elementary learning, the gill withdrawal reflex. In rats a similar mechanism, involving elevations in intracellular cAMP, occurs in the formation of hippocampal long-term memory [59]. Given the ability of 5-HT$_4$ receptors to activate adenylyl cyclase, the *Aplysia* model provides some basis for the procognitive effects of 5-HT$_4$ agonists [2]. Importantly, brief exposures to 5-HT (2–4 s), while initiating homologous desensitization and down-regulation of 5-HT$_4$ receptors [14], causes long-lasting (2 h) inhibition of potassium currents, a loss of after-hyperpolarization and a reduction in spike accommodation [60]. This cascade may facilitate impulse transmission in circuits involved in learning and memory.

7   Behavioral actions

The availability of potent and selective ligands has resulted in a better understanding of the role of the receptor in behavior. Generally, administration of 5-HT$_4$ receptor agonists or antagonists does not induce overt behavioral side effects. To date, *in vivo* studies have centered on a role of the receptor in cognitive processing, anxiogenesis and analgesia.

Preliminary studies using the non-selective 5-HT$_4$ receptor agonists RS 66331 [61] and BIMU-1 [62] showed a reversal of rodent cognitive dysfunction impaired by either cholinergic disruption or hypoxia, respectively. These findings are confirmed by subsequent data using selective agonists and antagonists in two models of cognitive function, the Morris water maze and social olfactory memory [63, 64]. The selective agonist RS 67333 reverses performance deficits in spatial learning and memory in rats, with impaired cognitive function [63]. This effect is abolished by the selective 5-HT$_4$ antagonist RS 67532 [63]. Furthermore, no response is seen to the peripherally acting 5-HT$_4$ agonist RS 67506 [63]. Corticosterone receptors are localized to the hippocampus [65], where they augment the slow after-hyperpolarization induced by 5-HT$_4$ receptor agonists [65]. Consequently, brain function may be influenced by mobilization of steroids induced by an action of 5-HT$_4$ agonists on the adrenal gland [66]. The lack of activity of RS 67506, a 5-HT$_4$ agonist with a predominantly peripheral action, argues against an involvement of this process. 5-HT$_4$ receptor activation is also involved in procognitive effects in rat odorant memory [64]. This paradigm is highly relevant for use in rodent studies, given the high density of 5-HT$_4$ receptors in the olfactory tubercle. In rats, BIMU-1 augments short-term odorant memory, an effect reversed by the selective antagonist GR 125487 [64]. Since the 5-HT$_3$ receptor antagonist ondansetron is inactive, these data support a specific action at 5-HT$_4$ receptors. These findings also accord with preliminary studies in aged primates, in which the non-selective 5-HT$_4$ receptor agonist RS 66331 [61] improves cognitive performance in a delayed match-to-sample paradigm.

Other behavioral effects of 5-HT$_4$ receptor activation include anxiolysis. In mice, the anxiogenic effect induced by elevated 5-HT tone (via 5-hydroxytryptophan) is reversed by 5-HT$_2$ blockade (via ritanserin) [67]. This reversal is inhibited by low doses of the mixed 5-HT$_3$/5-HT$_4$ antagonist SDZ 205,557 [67]. Similar findings have been found with the selective antagonist GR113808 [68]. Administration of the compound alone was without effect, possibly due to the low prevailing 5-HT tone. Paradoxically, the 5-HT$_4$ antagonists RS 23597, GR 113808 and SB 204070 oppose the inhibitory effect of diazepam in mice placed in a light/dark box paradigm [69], supporting previous findings with SDZ 205,557 [70]. Anxiolytic effects of selective 5-HT$_4$ antagonists, alone, have been reported in other paradigms. In an elevated plus maze [71], GR 113808 exhibits an anxiolytic profile in rats at 1 mg/kg s.c. but not at higher doses. This finding is similar to that seen for the 5-HT$_3$ antagonist granisetron [71].

SB 204070 is active at 0.01, 0.1 and 1 mg/kg s.c. in rat social interaction and elevated plus maze paradigms, but inactive in the Geller-Seifter assay [72]. In contrast, chlordiazapoxide is active in all assays [72]. It is possible that, like 5-HT$_3$ antagonists [7], the anxiolytic actions of selective 5-HT$_4$ antagonists are more restricted than the effects of classical anxiolytics. However, other factors may modulate antagonist potency in these assays, including the degree CNS penetration, *in vivo* stability [7] of the antagonists, as well the amount of animal handling prior to the assay [73].

The non-selective 5-HT$_4$ agonists BIMU-1 and BIMU-8 are active as antinociceptive agents in mice [74, 75]. This action is reversed by SDZ 205,557 and the selective 5-HT$_4$ antagonist GR 125487 [74]. Since lesions of the nucleus basalis magnocellularis abolish the antinociceptive effects of BIMU-1 and BIMU-8, the process may involve modulation of central cholinergic transmission [74]. These findings may explain the efficacy of two novel analgesic compounds, SM21 and PG9, although the selectivity of the compounds for the 5-HT$_4$ receptor is not reported [75]. Conversely, in a model of rodent visceral pain, no algesic or analgesic actions of selective 5-HT$_4$ receptor agonists are apparent [24]. Understanding the role of 5-HT$_4$ receptors in sensory processing is important in the context of irritable bowel syndrome, since therapeutic efficacy in this disease necessitates amelioration of enteric nerve sensitivity to intestinal distention. This aspect of selective 5-HT$_4$ receptor antagonism is more fully discussed in a recent review [76].

Finally, role of the 5-HT$_4$ receptor in modulating ethanol intake has been reported, since the effects of morphine on ethanol and water intake are modulated by high doses of the non-selective 5-HT$_3$/5-HT$_4$ antagonist tropisetron [77]. This suggestion is supported by recent data [78] showing that chronic dosing of the selective 5-HT$_4$ receptor antagonist GR113808 also reduces ethanol intake in alcohol-preferring rats.

8   Conclusion

The 5-HT$_4$ receptor is one of seven serotonin receptor families [1, 79] found in the brain, possessing a singular distribution and, presumably, a unique physiological function. The receptor is currently one of the best-characterized serotonin receptor subtypes in terms of primary amino acid sequence, signal transduction mechanism and pharmacology. The emerging data support a role in cognition and anxiety, roles consistent with its distribution, neurochemistry and electrophysiology. The careful use of highly selective agonists and antagonists, possessing good CNS penetration and *in vivo* stability, has facilitated studies on the role of the receptor in animal behavior. The cloning of the mouse gene for the 5-HT$_4$ receptor opens up the possibility of transgenic animals [80] and for potential effects on CNS function to be evaluated. In psychiatric disorders, a future challenge is to define the role(s) of the two splice variants, the prevalence of potential polymorphisms, as well of any naturally occurring mutations Clinical experience with selective agonists and antagonists in advanced evaluation suggest that the central effects are relatively benign. It is possible that 5-HT$_4$ receptor agonists may improve cognitive function [81], while selective 5-HT$_4$ receptor antagonists could act as novel anxiolytics [8]. Nonetheless, unambiguous clinical data are required before the real significance of these behavioral studies, and indeed the role of the 5-HT$_4$ receptor in the human brain, is fully understood.

References

1   T.A. Branchek: Semin. Neurol. *7*, 375–382 (1996).
2   S.S. Hegde and R.M. Eglen: FASEB J. *10*, 1398–1407 (1996).
3   A. Shenker, S. Maayani, H. Weinstein and J.P. Green: Eur. J. Pharmacol. *109*, 427–429 (1985).
4   A. Dumuis, R. Bouhelal, M. Sebben and J. Bockaert: Eur. J. Pharmacol. *146*, 187–188 (1988).
5   A. Dumuis, R. Bouhelal, M. Sebben, R. Cory and J. Bockaert: Mol. Pharmacol. *34*, 880–887 (1988).
6   C. Gerald, N. Adham, H.-T. Kao, M.A. Olsen, T.M. Laz, L.E. Schecter, J.A. Bard, P.J.-J. Vaysse, P.R. Hartig, T.A. Branchek and R.L. Weinshank: EMBO J. *14*, 2806–2815 (1995).
7   L.M. Gaster and F.D. King: Med. Res. Rev. *17*, 163–214 (1997).
8   R.M. Eglen, E.H.F. Wong, A. Dumuis and J. Bockaert: Trends Pharmacol. Sci. *16*, 391–398 (1995).
9   R.M. Eglen and S.S. Hegde: Exp. Opin. Invest. Drugs *5*, 373–388 (1996).
10   A.P.D.W. Ford and D.E. Clarke: Med. Res. Rev. *13*, 633–662 (1993).
11   International patent number WO 94/14957.
12   S. Claeysen, M. Sebben, L. Journot, J. Bockaert and A. Dumuis: FEBS Lett. *398*, 19–25 (1996).
13   N. Adham, C. Gerald, L. Schecter, P. Vaysse, R. Weinshank and T. Branchek: Eur. J. Pharmacol. *304*, 231–235 (1996).
14   H. Ansanay, M. Sebben, J. Bockaert and A. Dumuis: Eur. J. Pharmacol. *298*, 165–174 (1996).
15   E. Monferini, P. Gaetani, R. Rodriguez y Baena, E. Giraldo, M. Parenti, A. Zocchetti and C.A Rizzi: Life Sci. *52*, PL61–65 (1993).
16   M. Langlois, L. Zhang, D. Yang, B. Bremont, S. Shen, L. Manara and T. Croci: Bioorgan. Med. Chem. Lett. *4*, 1433–1436 (1994).
17   D. Yang, J.-L. Soulier, S. Sacsic, M. Mathe-Allainmat, B. Bremont, T. Croci, R. Cardamone, G. Aureggi and M. Langlois: J. Med. Chem. *40*, 608–621 (1997).

18   R.D. Clark, A. Jahangir, J.A. Langston, K.K. Weinhardt, A.B. Miller, E. Leung and R.M. Eglen: Bioorgan. Med. Chem. Lett. *4*, 2477–2480 (1994).

19   R.M. Eglen, D.W. Bonhaus, L.G. Johnson, E. Leung and R.D. Clark: Br. J. Pharmacol. *115*, 1387–1392 (1995).

20   J.D. Gale, C.J. Grossman, J.W. Whitehead, A.W. Oxford, K.T. Bunce and P.P. Humphrey: Br. J. Pharmacol. *111*, 332–338 (1994).

21   K.A. Wardle, E.S. Elliss, G.S. Baxter, G.A. Kennett, L.M. Gaster and G.J. Sanger: Br. J. Pharmacol. *112*, 789–794 (1994).

22   J. Gale, A. Green, R.S. Sargent, N.M. Clayton and K.T. Bunce: Br. J. Pharmacol. *113*, 119P.

23   L.M. Gaster, G.F. Joiner, F.D. King, P.A. Wyman, J.M. Sutton, S. Bingham, E.S. Ellis, G.J. Sanger and K.A. Wardle: J. Med. Chem. *38*, 4760–4763 (1995).

24   K.A. Wardle, S. Bingham, E.S. Ellis, L.M. Gaster, B. Rushant, M.I. Smith and G.J. Sanger: Br. J. Pharmacol. *118*, 665–670 (1996).

25   S.S Hegde, D.W. Bonhaus, L.G. Johnson, E. Leung, R.D. Clark and R.M. Eglen: Br. J. Pharmacol. *115*, 1087–1095 (1995).

26   R.D. Clark, A. Jahangir, L.A. Flippen, A.B. Miller, E. Leung, D.W. Bonhaus, E.H.F. Wong and R.M. Eglen: Bioorgan. Med. Chem. Lett. *5*, 2119–2122 (1995).

27   A.J. Kaumann: Trends Pharmacol. Sci. *15*, 451–455 (1994).

28   E. Leung, M.T. Pulido-Rios, D.W. Bonhaus, L.A. Perkins, K.D. Zeitung, S.A.O. Hsu, R.D. Clark, E.H.F. Wong and R.M. Eglen: Naunyn Schmiedebergs Arch. Pharmacol. *354*, 145–156 (1996).

29   C. Ullmer, P. Engels, S. Abdel'Al and H. Lubbert: Naunyn Schmiedebergs Arch. Pharmacol. *354*, 210–212 (1996).

30   M.T. Vilaro, R. Cortes, C. Gerald, T.A. Branchek, J.M. Palacios and G. Mengod: Mol. Brain Res. *43*, 356–360 (1996).

31   C.J. Grossman, G.J. Kilpatrick and K.T. Bunce: Br. J. Pharmacol. *109*, 618–624 (1993).

32   A.J. Kaumann, J.A. Lynham and A. Brown: Br. J. Pharmacol. *115*, 933–936 (1995).

33   C. Waeber, M. Sebben, A. Nieoullon, J. Bockaert and A. Dumuis: Neuropharmacol. *33*, 527–541 (1994).

34   T. Domenech, J. Beleta, A.G. Fernandez, R.W. Gristwood, F. Cruz Sachez, E. Tolosa and J.M. Palacios: Mol. Brain Res. *21*, 17–180 (1994).

35   L.B. Jakeman, Z.P. To, R.M. Eglen, E.H.F. Wong and D.W. Bonhaus: Neuropharmacol. *33*, 1027–1038 (1994).

36   V. Compan, A. Dazuta, P. Salin, M. Sebben, UJ. Bockaert and A. Dumuis: Eur. J. Neurosci. *8*, 2591–2598 (1996).

37   G.B. Schiavi, S. Brunet, C.A. Rizzi and H. Ladinsky: Neuropharmacol. *33*, 543–549 (1994).

38   Y. Uchiyama-Tsuyuki, M. Saitoh and M. Muramatsu: Life Sci. *59*, 2129–2137 (1996).

39   G.P. Reynolds, S.L. Mason, A. Meldrum, S. De Keczer, H. Parnes, R.M. Eglen and E.H.F. Wong: Br. J. Pharmacol. *114*, 993–998 (1995).

40   S. Benloucif, M.J. Keegan and M.P. Galloway: J. Pharm Exp. Ther. *265*, 373–377 (1993).

41   G.J. Kilpatrick, R.M. Hagan and J.D. Gale: Behav. Brain Res. *73*, 11–13 (1996).

42   N. Bonhomme, P. De Deurwaerdere, M. Le Moal and U. Spampinato: Neuropharmacol. *34*, 269–279 (1995).

43   L.J. Steward, J. Ge, R.L. Stowe, D.C. Brown, R.K. Brunton, P.R. Stokes and N.M. Barnes: Br. J. Pharmacol. *117*, 55–62 (1996).

44   P. De Deurwaerdere, M. Bonhomme, G. Lucas, A. Cheramy and U. Spampinato: J. Neurochem. *68*, 195–203 (1997).

45   L. Pozzi, L. Trabace, R. Invernizzi and R. Samanin: Brain Res. *692*, 265–268 (1995).
46   C. Reavill, J.P. Hatcher, T.S.C. Zetterstrom, V.A. Lewis, G.J. Sanger, J.J. Hagan and S. McKay: Br. J. Pharmacol. *118*, 71P (1996).
47   A.P. Sempere, J. Duarte, C. Cabezas, L.E. Claveria and F. Coria: Clin. Neuropharmacol. *18*, 76–78 (1995).
48   J. Ge and N.M. Barnes: Br. J. Pharmacol. *117*, 1475–1480 (1996).
49   H. Kilbinger, A. Gerbauer, J. Haas, H. Ladinsky and C.A. Rizzi: Naunyn Schmiedebergs Arch. Pharmacol. *351*, 229–236 (1995).
50   S. Consolo, S. Arnaboldi, S. Giorgi, G. Russi and H. Ladinsky: Neuroreport *5*, 1230–1232 (1994).
51   H.G.W.M. Boddeke and H.O. Kakman: Br. J. Pharmacol. *101*, 281–284 (1990).
52   R. Andrade and Y. Chaput: J. Pharmacol. Exp. Ther. *257*, 930–937 (1991).
53   G.E. Torres, I.L. Holt and R. Andrade: J. Pharmacol. Exp. Ther. *271*, 255–261 (1994).
54   G.E. Torres, Y. Chaput and R. Andrade: Mol. Pharmacol. *47*, 191–197 (1995).
55   S. Rowchowdhury, H. Haas and E.G. Anderson: Neuropharmacol. *33*, 551–557 (1994).
56   M. Bijak, K. Tokarski and J. Maj: Naunyn Schmiedebergs Arch. Pharmacol. *355*, 14–19 (1997).
57   M. Simizu, A. Nishida, H. Fukuda, H. Saito and S. Yamawaki: Br. J. Pharmacol. *114*, 1282–1288 (1995).
58   E.R. Kandel and J.H. Schwartz: Science *218*, 433–438 (1982).
59   R. Bourtchuladze, B. Frenguelli, J. Blendy, D. Cioffi, G. Schultz and A. Silva: Cell *79*, 59–68 (1994).
60   H. Ansanay, A. Dumuis, M. Sebben, J. Bockaert and J. Fagni: Proc. Natl. Acad. Sci. USA *92*, 6635–6639 (1995).
61   D.J. Fontana, S. Daniels, C. Henderson, R.M. Eglen and E.H.F. Wong: 3rd IUPHAR Satellite on Serotonin, Chicago, 30 July–3 August, abstract no. 5 (1994).
62   C. Ghelardini, P. Meoni, N. Galeotti, P. Malmberg-Aiello, C.A. Rizzi and A. Bartolini: 3rd IUPHAR Satellite on Serotonin, Chicago, 30 July–3 August, abstract no. 1 (1994).
63   D.J. Fontana, S. Daniels, E.H.F. Wong, R.D. Clark and R.M. Eglen: Neuropharmacol. (in press) (1997).
64   S. Letty, R. Child, A. Dumuis, A. Pantaloni, J. Bockaert and G. Rondouin: Neuropharmacol. (in press) (1997).
65   S. Birstiel and S.G. Beck: J. Pharmacol. Exp. Ther. *273*, 1132–1138 (1995).
66   V. Contesse, C. Hamel, C. Delarue, H. Lefebvre and H. Vaudry: Eur. J. Pharmacol. *265*, 27–33 (1994).
67   C.H. Cheng, B. Costall, M.E. Kelly and R.J. Naylor: Eur. J. Pharmacol. *255*, 39–49 (1994).
68   B. Costall and R.J. Naylor: Br. J. Pharmacol. *119*, 348P (1996).
69   B. Costall and R.J. Naylor: Br. J. Pharmacol. *119*, 352P (1996).
70   B. Costall and R.J. Naylor: Int. Clin. Psychopharmacol. *8*, 11–18 (1993).
71   J.S. Silvestre, A.G. Fernandez and J.M. Palacios: Eur. J. Pharmacol. *309*, 219–222 (1996).
72   G.A. Kennett, F. Bright, B. Trail, T.P. Blackburn and G.J. Sanger: Br. J. Pharmacol. *120*, 138P (1997).
73   N. Andrews and S.E. File: Eur. J. Pharmacol. *235*, 109–112 (1993).
74   C. Ghelardini, N. Galeotti, F. Casamenti, P. Malmberg-Aiello, G. Pepeu, F. Gaultieri and A. Bartolini: Life Sci. *58*, 2297–2309 (1996).
75   M.N. Romanelli, A. Bartolini, C. Bertucci, S. Dei, C. Ghelardini, M.G. Giovannini, F. Gaultieri, G. Pepeu, S. Sepecchi and E. Teodori: Chirality *8*, 225–233 (1996).

76   G.J. Sanger: Neurogastroenterol. Motil. *8*, 319–331 (1996).
77   C.W. Hodge, J.S. Neihus and H.H. Samson: Psychopharmacol. *119*, 186–192 (1995).
78   I. Panocka, R. Ciccocioppo, C. Polodori, P. Pompei and M. Massi: Pharmacol. Biochem. Behav. *52*, 255–259 (1995).
79   C.M. Villalon, J.A. Terron, E. Ramirez-San Juan and P.R. Saxena: Arch. Med. Res., *26*, 331–344 (1995).
80   J.J.Lucas and R. Hen: Trends Pharmacol. Sci. *16*, 246–252 (1995).
81   J. Bockaert, H. Ansanay, C. Waeber, M. Sebben, L. Fagni and A. Dumuis: CNS Drugs *1*, 6–15 (1994).

Progress in Drug Research, Vol. 49 (E. Jucker, Ed.)
© 1997 Birkhäuser Verlag, Basel (Switzerland)

Chemical teratogenesis in humans: Biochemical and molecular mechanisms

By Mont R. Juchau

Department of Pharmacology, School of Medicine, Box 357280, University of Washington, Seattle, WA 98195, USA

1   Introduction: Definitions, scope and focus

In 1993, *Progress in Drug Research* published a review dealing with mechanisms of teratogenic/embryotoxic effects of chemicals on humans and other vertebrates [1] and covering the literature through 1992. Since 1992, significant strides have been made in understanding the biochemical and molecular mechanisms whereby chemicals are capable of eliciting birth defects as the result of prenatal exposure of conceptuses to such chemicals. These strides thus justify this review, which accordingly will focus primarily on research published since 1992 and extending through 1996. Emphasis will be directed toward those chemicals/chemical classes that are frequently regarded at present [1–5] as capable of producing birth defects in humans ("established" or "recognized" human teratogens). Most of the chemicals commonly regarded as established human teratogens (Tables 1 and 2) are xenobiotics, i.e., exogenous chemicals that are not utilized by the reference organism as nutrient materials, are not essential to the reference organism for maintenance of normal physiologic/biochemical function and homeostasis, and do not constitute a part of the conventional array of chemicals synthesized from nutrient chemicals by the reference organism in normal intermediary metabolism. Such xenobiotic chemicals are thus also often classified as "foreign". Exceptions to the generalization that "established" human teratogens are xenobiotics include various endogenous retinoids (e.g. all-*trans*-retinoic acid, all-*trans*-retinol etc.), ethanol (utilizable as an energy source and also generated endogenously in small quantities in various tissues), and certain steroidal androgens (e.g. testosterone). Endogenous chemicals are referred to as endobiotics and, together with exogenously supplied nutrients, represent chemicals that are essential for maintenance of normal homeostasis. Xenobiotic and endobiotic/nutrient chemicals are distinguished here because of the fact that both deficiencies and excesses of endobiotics/nutrients can be significantly damaging to embryos and fetuses, whereas conceptal damage elicited by deficiencies of xenobiotics is not possible. For retinoid and steroid endobiotics, both deficiencies and excesses are reportedly capable of eliciting birth defects in humans. For ethanol, defects resulting from excesses are well established, but deficiency-related defects have not been described in any species and seem highly improbable. Both deficiencies and excesses of many nutrient chemicals have been demonstrated to elicit birth defects in experimental animals [2, 3] and thus would be expected to be capable of doing so in humans. A notable example for which an endobiotic/nutrient chemical deficiency but not (yet) excess is regarded as an "established" human teratogenic factor is folic acid. It is nevertheless quite

Table 1.
Chemicals implicated in the causation of morphologic birth defects in humans

Chemical or chemical class	Characteristic defects
Thalidomide and structural analogs	Phocomelia, amelia, other
Folic acid antagonists	Multiple defects
Alkylating agents	Multiple defects
Purine/pyrimidine analogs	Multiple defects
Retinoids and arotinoids	Craniofacial, cardiovascular
Anticonvulsants	
Phenytoin	Fetal hydantoin syndrome
Trimethadione	Fetal tridione syndrome
Valproic acid	Neural tube defects
Carbamazepine	Neural tube defects
Primidone	Craniofacial, other
Alcohols	Fetal alcohol syndrome
Antithyroid agents	Cretinism, fetal goiter
Aminoglycosides	8th cranial nerve damage
Tetracyclines	Discolored teeth
Organic mercurials	Cerebellar ataxia
Polychlorinated biphenyls	Hyperpigmented skin, other
Hormonal agents	
Androgens	Fetal masculinization
Estrogens	Genital anomalies, neoplasms
Coumarin derivatives	Saddle nose, stippled epiphyses
Angiotensin-converting enzyme inhibitors	Renal, skull defects
Tobacco/tobacco products	Growth retardation, mental deficits
Cocaine	Micro/hydrocephaly, other
Penicillamine	Cutis laxa (lax skin)
Lithium salts	Cardiovascular defects
Toluene*	Craniofacial defects
Methylene blue*	Intestinal atresia

*These agents were recently added by Shepard [2].

probable that, with a sufficiently high exposure level, route of administration, correct timing and appropriate genetic background, excesses of folic acid would also serve as a teratogenic stimulus. For example, concern has been expressed that excess folate may decrease absorption of dietary zinc and thereby increase birth defect incidence. This review deals with both endobiotic/nutrient and xenobiotic chemicals as teratogens and embryotoxins, but the focus is on excesses (toxicity) rather than deficiencies. (It should be noted, however, that certain xenobiotics appear to act via elicitation of endobiotic deficiencies – prime examples of such are the folic acid antagonists, base analogs, angiotensin-converting enzyme inhib-

Table 2.
Chemicals implicated in the causation of neurobehavioral defects in humans

Chemical or chemical class	References*
Ethanol	Schardein, Adams
Methyl mercury	Schardein, Adams
Lead	Schardein, Adams
Retinoids	Schardein, Adams
Phenytoin	Schardein, Adams
Valproic Acid	Schardein, Adams
Narcotics	Adams, Schardein[P]
Polychlorinated biphenyls	Adams, Schardein[P]
Cocaine	Adams
Cigarette smoking	Schardein[P]
Nicotine	Schardein[P]
Progestins	Schardein[P]
Tranquilizers	Schardein[s]
Antidepresssants	Schardein[s]
General anesthetics	Schardein[s]
Aspirin	Schardein[s]
Marijuana	Schardein[s]
Neuroleptics (e.g. chlorpromazine)	Schardein[s]
Thalidomide	Schardein[s]

* Schardein refers to reference [3] and Adams to reference [5].
[P] Listed by Schardein [3] as probable human neurobehavioral teratogens.
[s] Listed by Schardein [3] as suspected human neurobehavioral teratogens.
General agreement appears to exist pertaining to ethanol, methyl mercury, lead, retinoids, phenytoin and valproic acid, and these agents may be regarded as "established" neurobehavioral teratogens for humans. All except lead are also listed in Table 1. It should be noted that androgens and many of the other agents listed in Table 1 also appear capable of eliciting neurobehavioral and other functional deficits.

itors and the antithyroidals.) Also the review will be directed primarily to mammalian species with special attention given to studies shedding light on mechanisms in humans.

Definitions of a number of other terms at the outset of this discussion seem essential to optimal communication. These include conceptus, embryo, embryotoxicity, fetus, fetotoxicity, teratogen, teratogenicity, teratology, teratogenesis, birth defects, organogenesis, dysmorphogenesis and dysmorphology. "Conceptus" refers to the prenatal organism, including associated membranes of nonmaternal origin, from the time of fertilization to parturition, i.e. during the entire prenatal period. "Embryo" refers to the embryo proper (excluding associated membranes) from the time of fertilization to the end of organogenesis. "Embryotoxicity" refers to any type of toxic or deleterious effect on the embryo elicited by excess exposure to an endobiotic or xenobiotic chemical(s). This includes transient as well as persistent (teratogenic) toxicity and includes both direct and indirect (e.g. maternally mediated, membrane-mediated or other indirect) effects. "Fetus" refers to the fetus proper (excluding associated membranes) with reference to the period of development extending from the end of organogenesis until parturition. (After parturition, the organism is referred to as a neonate.) "Fetotoxicity", like embryotoxicity, is a general term and refers to any kind of damage or deleterious effect on the fetus elicited by excess exposure to an endobiotic or xenobiotic chemical(s). The term includes both transient and persistent (teratogenic) toxic effects and both direct and indirect effects. The term "teratogen" refers broadly to any agent (chemical, microbe, radiation, traumatic physical injury etc.) capable of directly or indirectly causing – via either excess or deficiency – germ cell, embryonic or fetal damage to the extent that permanent or semipermanent (persistent) damaging or undesirable sequelae are evident after parturition. The terms "teratogenicity" and "teratogenesis" refer to the process just described; "teratology" is the science that investigates such processes and, in broadest and simplest terms, is the science that deals with abnormal development.

Although many still prefer to think of the terms "teratogenicity", "teratology" etc. solely in terms of morphologic defects ("teras", the root form, taken from the Greek and meaning "monster" or "marvel"), such terms as "behavioral teratology" and "functional teratology" have become sufficiently commonplace and embedded in the literature that to exclude those types of clearly nonmorphologic abnormalities or defects would seem a disservice. Thus, for this discussion, the terms "teratogen", "teratogenesis", "teratogenicity", "teratology" and so on will refer to both morphological and nonmorphological defects of a persistent nature, i.e. permanent or semipermanent. Defects not observable as morphologic or anatomic are often referred to as "functional" defects, even though functional defects are also almost always associated with observed morphologic abnormalities and are commonly more severe when accompanied by morphologic defects. A "birth defect" refers to a persistent (i.e. long-lasting, non-transient, permanent or semipermanent) damaging abnormality in anatomic structure or biochemical/physiologic function of an organism irrespective of cause; the abnormality is present at the time of birth but may not be detectable immediately, or even much later, after parturition (i.e. may be covert or latent). (Note that, by the above definitions, the terms "birth defect" and "teratogenic defect" are equivalent in all respects.) It is also important to re-emphasize that morphologic defects are nearly always accompanied by defects in function of the morphologically affected organ or tissue. Structure or function would be regarded as "abnormal" if deviant or variant to the extent that the organism is disadvantaged in terms of survival, function or appearance outside the normal range. Severity and persistence, of course, both occur as a continuum rather than as binomial (all or none, yes or no) phenomena, and thus certain deformations, deviancies or variances may or may not be regarded as birth defects, depending upon judgment and opinion rather than upon preformulated descriptions.

"Organogenesis" refers to conceptal development during the period of gestation between implantation of the fertilized ovum and (arbitrarily) to complete palatal closure [2, 3]. Time periods of organogenesis for humans and species most often studied are given in Table 3. The terms "dysmorphogenesis" and "dysmorphology" refer strictly to grossly observable (with the naked eye or low-power light microscope) structural or anatomical defects and abnormalities. These abnormalities may be persistent or transient, are not dependent upon the developmental stage, e.g. need not be manifest after parturition, and do not depend upon the nature of the cause, i.e. need not be caused by chemicals. In 1973, Wilson [6] classified developmental defects as manifest under four categories: (1) intrauterine death, (2) morphologic abnormalities, (3) functional abnormalities and (4) growth retardation. Although this system of classification has been very useful and has been widely employed for many years, it seems well at this point to extend the categorization to include a differentiation between persistent and transient effects, both of which clearly should be includable as developmental (intrauterine) abnormalities. Seven categories are proposed:

1) Intrauterine death
2) Persistent malformations
3) Transient malformations
4) Persistent functional defects
5) Transient functional defects
6) Persistent growth retardation
7) Transient growth retardation

Persistent malformations, persistent functional defects and persistent growth retardation (categories 2, 4 and 6, above) are the developmental abnormalities classifiable as birth defects. Persistence, transience and severity each are parameters measured on a smooth, uninterrupted scale (continuum) and are thus subject to considerable interpretation. A possible implication of the above classification is that morphologic, functional

Table 3.
Periods of organogenesis in the more common experimental animals and humans

Species	Average length of gestation (days)	Approximate period of of organogenesis[a] (days)
Human	270	18–58
Rhesus monkey	165	20–45
Guinea pig	68	14–30
Rabbit	32	7–20
Rat	22	9–17
Chick[b]	21	1–13
Mouse	19	8–15
Hamster	16	7–12

[a] The approximate period of organogenesis is designated arbitrarily as the time between the appearance of the neural plate and complete palatal closure.
[b] For the chick, times are in days after the egg is laid; eyelid closure rather than palatal closure is indicated as the marker for the end of organogenesis.

and growth deficiencies occur independently, and it should be re-emphasized that this is not the case. Malformations, as discussed above, are frequently accompanied by conceptal demise, functional deficits and/or growth retardation, and each of the latter two can occur independently as well as concomitantly.

2   Exposure of embryos and fetuses to chemicals

Research during recent years has demonstrated amply that exposure-time parameters are crucial determinants of the nature, observable incidence and severity of birth defects [7, 8]. Route, frequency and duration of exposure, exposure quantity (dosage, including total exposure as well as exposure quantity per unit of time) and stage of gestation at which exposures (at different levels occur) are exposure parameters that all can be extremely important determinants of the qualitative nature or kind of defect observed, incidence (percentage of individuals exhibiting) and severity (degree of malfeasance) of defects elicited. It has become increasingly apparent that classical pharmacokinetic analyses, in which maternal plasma levels of the parent offending toxic agent are measured as a function of time, are frequently of far lesser relevance to assessments of teratogenic potential and mechanisms of teratogenesis than measurements of tissue levels, particularly in the tissues and cells affected (targets) by the teratogenic agent(s). It is also increasingly appreciated that peak (maximal) tissue concentrations (at the critical times of gestation), rather than total areas under the tissue concentration-time curve, are often the most important determining parameter. From these perspectives, initial identification of the proximate or ultimate teratogenic agent assumes paramount importance. If a metabolite(s) of the parent compound rather than the parent compound *per se* is acting as the ultimate causative agent(s), ascertainment of tissue levels of the ultimately causative metabolite(s) is clearly of far greater importance than measurements of tissue levels of the parent compound. Unfortunately, the identities of ultimately acting metabolites of teratogenic chemicals are very frequently unknown, and even when known, such metabolites are often unstable. Therefore, in the large majority of cases, it is very difficult to assess quantities of ultimate chemical teratogens in conceptal tissues and thereby perform mechanistically meaningful pharmacokinetic investigations. In many cases, the small quantities of conceptal tissues available for study also present a further impediment to these kinds of investigations.

Sources of exposure of pregnant women to teratogenic agents and the general principles governing access of contacted chemicals to conceptal target tissues have not experienced significant changes as the result of research during the past 5 years. These two topics were treated in the previous review [1] and have been discussed in various other reviews. The interested reader should consult such reviews for details. The critical importance of pharmacokinetic parameters as determinants of the nature, incidence and severity of teratogenic effects elicited by chemicals during the period of gestation has been emphasized and treated extensively in monographs edited by Nau and Scott [7] and in a more recent review by Clarke [8]. An important additional issue relative to the exposures of embryos and fetuses to chemicals deals with the question of recent trends in the exposure of pregnant women to chemicals with teratogenic potential and whether such trends are significantly correlated with trends in birth defect incidence and/or severity. It would appear that no major trend changes in either exposure to chemicals or birth defect incidence and severity have occurred during the past 4–5 years, although one would expect such changes to be very gradual and difficult to detect statistically. A notable exception is with respect to exposures to newly marketed drugs because of the continual appearance of new drugs. An example is the concern for newer and highly popular antidepressant drugs such as fluoxetine [9]. As of this writing, legally marketed newer drugs do not appear to have produced significant problems in terms of the causation of birth defects. Chronic low-level exposures to environmental contaminants appear to present minimal overall birth defect problems or to cause increases in incidence of birth defects that are often extremely difficult to detect statistically. The most obvious exception to this generalization is with respect to lead (see Sec. 6.8, below). A perusal of several epidemiologic studies reported at the meetings of the International Clearinghouse for Birth Defects Monitoring Systems [10] tends to persuade one that, in general, the low-level exposures to environmental and industrial chemicals commonly encountered are not causally associated with significant increases in birth defect incidence and that acute, high-level exposure to such chemicals by handlers and distributors or via accidents or abuse (e.g. toluene) present a much more important problem. However, experience with lead dictates that much more careful and extensive investigations of overall chronic, low-level exposure trends as well as of trends in acute, higher-level exposure related to trends in specific birth defect incidence and severity appear to be warranted at present. Logic dictates that pregnant women avoid all types of chemical exposures to the extent possible unless the benefits of exposure clearly outweigh the potential risks. At present, information on risk/benefit ratios for the large majority of chemicals in terms of teratogenic potential is scanty at best. A review of trends in drug usage by pregnant women in the United States between 1979 and 1990 is given in reference [11].

3   Role of chemicals in the etiology of birth defects

Both the scientific as well as the public perceptions of the role of chemicals as causative factors for birth defects appear to be in the process of undergoing healthy changes toward a more enlightened view. It is becoming increasingly recognized that causes of birth defects are most frequently multifactorial in nature and that individual chemicals as sole causative agents represent only an exceedingly small part (estimated 1–3%; see [1–6] of the etiology picture. Genetic factors, nutritional factors, disease pathologies (especially endocrine-related diseases and diseases elicited by certain microbial organisms), physical factors (e.g. trauma), radiation, temperature extremes, hormonal imbalances, placental failure, hypoxia, stochastic errors in protein synthesis, signaling and so on, each have been shown to be capable of eliciting birth defects as individual causative factors but are probably much more important in terms of contributory interactions with one or probably more of the other etiologic factors, including other chemicals. Although it appears to have been quite difficult for many to make the transition from viewing causation in terms of individual factors to a combination of causative factors, encouraging progress (as judged from communications from both the lay press as well as the scientific community) has been evident. This is, of course, a non-objective evaluation but, if true, mimics the gradual change in perception of the causality of malignant tumors and is extremely important in helping to lay the foundation for more informed approaches toward the needed research related to causation and prevention. Unfortunately, many (including some otherwise knowledgeable scientists) are of the view that, since chemicals as individual agents appear to play a relatively minor role in the causation of birth defects, the problem of chemically elicited birth defects should not merit a high research priority. In fact, nothing could be further from the truth – both from the viewpoint of practical and clinical considerations as well as from the viewpoint of achieving a solid and basic understanding of the more basic and fundamental aspects of birth defect causation. Now critically needed is an understanding of the interactive and contributory roles of all known causative factors in the increasingly appreciated multifactorial causation of birth defects. Clearly, the multifactorial nature of causation renders research into evaluation of the roles of individual chemicals as participants in the etiology of individual birth defects a highly complex venture, but one that nevertheless merits a very high priority.

4 Classes of chemicals with high teratogenic potential

Research performed during the past 5 years appears not to have markedly changed our capacity to predict the potential of a given chemical (of known structure but unknown teratogenicity) to elicit teratogenic effects – either alone or in combination with other causative factors. Such change expectedly will be gradual in light of the enormous complexity of developmental processes and their regulation, in the multifactorial nature of causation and in the context of current funding for studies of abnormal development. Nevertheless, it is appreciated that certain chemicals and chemical classes exhibit a particularly high propensity to elicit or contribute to the elicitation of developmental abnormalities, and, at least in many cases, closely related structural analogs may be expected to elicit (or contribute to elicitation of) qualitatively similar defects. Quantitative potential (incidence, severity), of course, is dependent on a great many factors and is often much more difficult to predict. Classes of chemicals for which teratogenic potential is at least to some degree predictable from chemical structure include androgenic steroids, retinoids, estrogens, alkylating agents, thalidomide/congeners, folic acid antagonists, base analogs, polyhalogenated biphenyls, coumarin derivatives and angiotensin-converting enzyme inhibitors. These are each discussed in greater detail below. Although very minor structural changes can result in profound changes in the teratogenic potential within these (and other) groups of chemicals, it is recognized that many structural analogs produce terata that are qualitatively very similar when compared with other agents within the same group. For androgenic steroids, for example, the androgenicity *per se* appears to be the crucial criterion rather than structure *per se*, but of course there is a very strong relationship between chemical structure and androgenic activity. Thus, the capacity of androgenic chemicals to elicit malformations of masculinization in female genital organs is highly predictable from previously acquired and extensive knowledge of chemical structure-androgenicity relationships. The capacity of chemicals to elicit the type of defects produced by exposure to all-*trans*-retinoic acid are also, at least to a certain extent, predictable from investigations of the relationships between biologic activity and retinoid structure ([12] and cited references). The other examples listed above are further discussed below.

Teratogenic activity is also to some degree predictable from a knowledge of non-receptor-mediated biologic activity. For example, if it is known that a chemical possesses high clastogenic, mutagenic, cytotoxic or carcinogenic potential, it may reasonably be expected that the same chemical will also exhibit a relatively high teratogenic potential. However, this is somewhat more difficult to predict quantitatively because of confounding and potentially confounding dispositional factors and poorly understood conceptal defense mechanisms. For example, many chemicals exhibiting such biological and toxicological properties produce the aforenamed effects only following bioactivation catalyzed by biotransforming enzymes. Bioactivation results in the generation of certain reactive intermediary metabolites which are frequently the species ultimately responsible for the observed biologic activity (ultimate reactive metabolites). The maternal liver is the major site for generation of these reactive intermediary metabolites, but since many reactive intermediates are chemically unstable, they are not transported to conceptal target tissues from the liver in sufficient quantities to effect significant damage. Thus, bioactivation in conceptal target tissues, as opposed to maternal hepatic tissues, would seem far more likely to result in damage, and this is an area of research that is now under investigation. Studies indicate that although overall conceptal bioactivation capacity appears in general to be very low in comparison with that in adult hepatic tissues, capacity for conceptal inactivation of reactive intermediates may be even lower – such that the overall balance of bioactivation/bioinactivation appears relatively higher in conceptal tissues than in hepatic tissues, at least for certain chemicals. This topic has been reviewed recently [13–15]. Clearly, other pharmacokinetic considerations such as absorption of the chemical(s) from maternal sites of exposure or entry, distribution to conceptal target tissues and elimination via excretion, biodegradation and redistribution must also be taken into account in predicting teratogenic activity. If other factors are equal, those chemicals with the lowest clearance rates, longest half-lives, highest lipid solubility and most rapid transmembranal flux rates (or various combinations of these properties) will be those with the highest teratogenic potential.

It is of interest that for the chemicals listed in Tables 1 and 2, both receptor-mediated mechanisms (using a very broad definition of the term "receptor") involving specific, high-affinity interactions of teratogens with specific proteins (e.g. for retinoids, steroids, folic acid antagonists, angiotensin-converting enzyme inhibitors and possibly polychlorinated biphenyls and receptor-independent mechanisms (e.g. for alkylating agents, ethanol, toluene, tetracyclines) have been implicated. For most of the chemicals in the tables, however, it is not known whether receptor-dependent, receptor-independent or a combination of the two mechanisms are applicable. It would seem that a very early step in elucidation of mechanisms should be to address that issue. It is also of interest that cell-surface receptors, which account for the large majority of biological receptor proteins, do not appear (with the possible exception of thalidomide, see Sec. 6.1, below) at present to be important mediators of teratogenic effects. This is very probably because the ligands for such receptors are ordinarily substances with high clearance rates, short half-lives, low lipid solubility, variable transmembrane flux rates and various combinations of these properties. They would not be expected to reach conceptal target sites readily following maternal exposure from the outside environment. Chemicals capable of interacting with cell-surface receptors also appear to be very infrequently present in significant concentrations in the external environment. Thus, maternal exposure from the outside environment to chemicals capable of interacting with cell-surface receptors would expectedly be very uncommon, and there are few examples (thalidomide?) of effective teratogens acting via interactions with cell-surface receptors. One near example appears to be cocaine (discussed below), which appears to produce teratogenic effects at least in part by interacting with fast sodium ion channels – transmembranal proteins that may also be regarded as receptors by the broader definition – but these are not regarded as cell-surface receptors. By contrast, there are several examples of teratogens which appear to elicit their primary teratogenic effects via interactions with intracellular receptors (androgens, estrogens, retinoids etc.). Classes of chemicals with relatively high teratogenic potential also include those that are capable of disrupting nutritional balance (e.g. folic acid antagonists), those capable of disrupting hormonal balance (e.g. thyroid, androgen, estrogen hormone) and those capable of acting as overall general depressants of cellular metabolism (e.g. heavy metals, antithyroidals etc.). Certain agents are highly notorious teratogens, even though not potent, because of high levels of exposure in human populations (e.g. ethanol, tobacco smoke, lead, cocaine). For these agents (which currently are leading causes of chemical teratogenicity in humans), the exposure parameter in the risk equation (exposure × potency × susceptibility = risk) is unquestionably a highly dominant factor.

Among current therapeutic agents (most of the chemicals listed as "established" human teratogens are/were therapeutic agents), those that are specifically designed to kill cells or to act as cytotoxins might be expected to be among those most problematic in terms of birth defect causation. Such agents include chemotherapeutic chemicals, in particular anticancer agents, but also antiviral antimicrobials as well as certain other antimicrobials. Even though this expectation is largely valid, many chemicals not regarded as highly cytotoxic, including thalidomide, retinoids, steroids, anticonvulsants, antithyroidals, penicillamine and lithium salts are regarded as effective teratogens. These chemicals illustrate forcibly that effective teratogenic chemicals need not be potent from a general or overall toxicologic (cytotoxic) perspective. Because they appear to be selectively toxic to certain developmental processes, this immediately calls to mind the importance of a consideration of maternotoxicity/conceptotoxicity dose ratios. A great lesson of the thalidomide tragedy is that the predicability of teratogenicity based on either structural considerations or biologic activity is often quite tenuous with the exceptions discussed above

5   Evaluation of chemicals for teratogenic activity

A significant problem in evaluations of teratogenicity in the past has been the persistence of a binomial categorization of chemicals as either teratogenic or nonteratogenic. Even though a more scientific or quantitative perspective is now rapidly evolving, the binomial mentality is still evident in textbooks, journal literature and even in oral presentations and conversations. It is vexatious because it implies that some chemicals have no teratogenic potential at all, when in fact all chemicals have at least some potential, including water, oxygen, carbon dioxide, glucose, sodium chloride and sucrose [1–3]. This very basic and fundamental principle of toxicology was recognized early in the 16th century by Paracelsus [4, 16], is a recognized tenet of the science of modern toxicology and was re-emphasized specifically for teratogenesis by Karnofsky [17] in the 20th century. Such a simplistic binomial categorization provides no clues as to the relative teratogenic potential of drugs and other chemicals. Unfortunately, the binomial mentality is giving way to an almost equally fallacious "pigeonholing mentality" in which the desire to place chemicals (and other agents) into specific, designated quantal categories in terms of their teratogenicity appears overwhelming. For example, the Food and Drug Administration has provided five pigeonholes designated as A, B, C, D and X into which therapeutic chemicals may be placed [4]. Although these categories, by definition, provide more information pertaining to the degree of ignorance concerning the teratogenic potential of drugs (yet do represent a significant advance over the very crude binomial approach), they are often misinterpreted to indicate the degree of teratogenic potential per se. Internalization of the idea that chemicals do not elicit teratogenic effects as all-or-none or quantal phenomena, but rather as dose-related, smoothly graded effects measurable on a continuum, will lead to more rational approaches toward evaluation of teratogenic potential. Clearly of greatest interest and value is information pertaining to the probability of the occurrence of one or more of the seven possible adverse outcomes (discussed in Sec. 1, above) relative to a particular exposure(s) scenario. More information on individual susceptibility and predisposing factors would, of course, also be of great value. More mechanistic information is clearly (and desperately) needed. Rational approaches toward quantitative evaluation of teratogenic potential of chemicals relative to exposure levels and times remain one of the most challenging aspects of modern teratology. Again, the multifactorial nature of the causation of birth defects demands that chemicals be evaluated as contributory factors in the context of a large number of other known causative factors.

6   Chemicals recognized as teratogenic in humans

The extensive practice of placing (or not placing) chemicals on lists of "recognized" human teratogens is an example of the binomial mentality discussed above. It should be appreciated from the outset that chemicals are placed on such lists because of compelling correlative evidence that those chemicals have caused, or at least have significantly contributed to the causation of birth defects in humans. Placement on such lists implies that these chemicals have definitive potential to cause birth defects in the event of future exposures. One should also realize that the appearance of chemicals on such lists is primarily an expression of the degree of confidence that exposures to such chemicals have resulted in the occurrence of birth defects in humans in the past. With these caveats, we also present such lists (Tables 1 and 2), realizing that this practice has distinct problems. For purposes of this review, it serves to restrict the agents discussed to a manageable number and provides for a focus on those agents regarded as most likely to have been causative factors for birth defects in humans in the past. The ensuing discussion will deal with mechanisms whereby the chemicals placed on those lists (lists from different sources will vary) may be capable of eliciting teratogenic effects in humans.

6.1   Thalidomide and congeners

Thalidomide (α-phthalimidoglutarimide), once sold in 48 countries as a sedative-hypnotic and as a treatment for the morning sickness of pregnancy after introduction to the market in 1956, was banned worldwide in 1962 after thousands of infants were born with missing or defective limbs and abnormalities involving a variety of other organs and structures. It is considered by many to be the world's most infamous drug, and the dramatic sequelae of its earlier usage served as a major impetus for implementation of much stricter drug regulations in the United States and other countries. In subsequent decades (1960–1980), thalidomide was regarded as an extremely interesting, prototypic human teratogen with an unusually high potency in humans and a highly mysterious mechanism(s) of action on developmental processes, but with muted concern because of lack of availability and exposure. Relatively recent discoveries of several important therapeutic uses of thalidomide for a variety of clinical conditions, however, have markedly changed the picture pertaining to availability and potential exposure. On 13 November 1996, newspapers throughout the United States published an Associated Press report that Celgene, a company based in Warren, New Jersey, would seek FDA approval to market thalidomide for treatment of the painful, inflamed lesions of leprosy (erythema nodosum leprosum) and that a competitive company, Andrulis Inc., based in Beltsville, Maryland, would seek FDA approval for marketing of thalidomide for treatment of the excruciating aphthous ulcers that afflict patients with human immunodeficiency virus (HIV) infections. Applications for treatments of numerous other conditions (e.g. a multitude of acquired immunodeficiency syndrome (AIDS)-related conditions, lupus erythematosus, chronic graft-versus-host disease, chronic actinic prurigo, diabetic retinopathy, macular degeneration, and several others – often involving chronic inflammatory diseases and other disorders of the immune system) would be expected to follow shortly. In 1994 it was reported [18] that 46 malformed babies had been born to thalidomide-exposed mothers in Brazil where (among other developing countries) the drug is already sold over the counter for treatment of leprosy. These and related developments are likely to stimulate a greatly increased interest in investigations of biochemical and molecular mechanisms whereby thalidomide and related compounds elicit teratogenic effects.

In the previous review [1], it was stated that, in terms of a mechanistic understanding, thalidomide appeared to be the least understood of all "established" human teratogens. A review of 24 mechanisms proposed prior to 1988 and discussed in detail by Stephens in an extensive 1988 review [19] suggested quite strongly that none of the proposed mechanisms was based on a solid foundation of research-supported evidence. Since the writing of that review, a number of research findings have appeared in the literature which provide exciting encouragement for future elucidation of mechanisms. Possibly one of the most striking findings was reported by D'Amato and co-workers in 1994 [20]. They found that orally administered thalidomide inhibited angiogenesis induced by basic fibroblast growth factor (bFGF) in a rabbit cornea micropocket assay. The anti-angiogenic activity of a series of thalidomide analogs – including supididimide, phthaloyl glutamic acid, phthaloyl glutamic anhydride and EM-12 – correlated with the teratogenic effectiveness but not with the sedative-hypnotic or immunomodulating properties of the analogs. Furthermore, electron microscopic examination of the corneal neovascularization of thalidomide-treated rabbits indicated ultrastructural changes similar to those observed in the deformed limb bud vasculature of thalidomide-treated embryos. The proposed mechanism is logical and appealing inasmuch as the limb bud requires a complex interaction of both angiogenesis and vasculogenesis during limb development, and the limbs also represent a characteristic target of thalidomide dysmorphogenesis. Interestingly, thalidomide exhibited no effect on bFGF-induced proliferation of endothelial cells in culture. The inhibition of angiogenesis was observed after only two doses of thalidomide, and the rabbits exhibited no obvious sedation or other toxicity, including weight loss. Cyclosporin A, an immunosupressant, failed to inhibit angiogenesis, and immunosuppressed rabbits (given maximally tolerated doses of total body irradiation) responded equally well to the antiangiogenic effects of thalidomide, suggesting that the now well-known (but poorly understood) immunomodulating properties of thalidomide were not related to its antiangiogenic effects. Also the now widely known capacity of thalidomide to suppress the production of tumor necrosis factor α (TNF-α) did not appear to be related to the antiangiogenic effect. Several other angiogenesis inhibitors (e.g. antimitotic agents, 13-*cis*-retinoic acid, tamoxifen) were reported as not orally effective.

Neubert et al. [21] have postulated a highly interesting potential mechanism for thalidomide teratogenicity that involves the downregulation of adhesion receptors on cell surfaces of primate embryos. They hypothesized that the teratogenicity of thalidomide may be linked to alterations in the expression of adhesion molecules. They provided evidence for the expression of a variety of adhesion receptors (β1, β2 and β3-integrins and selectin) on cells of essentially all primordia of marmoset embryos during early organogenesis and showed that treatment with relatively low doses (1–20 mg/kg) of a highly teratogenic thalidomide derivative (α-EM12) triggered a dramatic down-regulation of several surface adhesion receptors (e.g. CD11a/CD18, CD49d/CD29, CD61 and others) on early limb bud cells and cells of other primordia during early organogenesis of marmoset embryos. The investigators suggested that these profound downregulations might be expected to alter cell-cell and cell-extracellular matrix interactions and could be the long-sought primary mechanism of the teratogenic action of thalidomide and thalidomide-type substances. This suggestion, touted as a "probable mechanism" [21] certainly appears meritorious and worthy of further research along these lines, particularly in view of the more recently reported findings [22] that two thalidomide derivatives with very low teratogenic potential (β-EM12 and phthalimidophthalimide) were not detectably able to produce the downregulation of cell-surface adhesion receptors elicited by the teratogenically potent thalidomide derivatives as described above.

In yet another interesting investigation, Arlen and Wells [23] found that acetylsalicylic acid, an irreversible inhibitor of prostaglandin H synthase, could decrease thalidomide-initiated limb abnormalities and fetal lethality in rabbits by approximately 61%. The authors suggested that the results provided evidence that thalidomide could undergo bioactivation by embryonic prostaglandin H synthase to a teratogenic reactive intermediate (free radical). As further support for this idea, the authors pointed to observations of thalidomide-initiated oxidation of reduced glutathione [24] and DNA [25] and to the studies of Parman et al. [26] indicating catalysis of the generation of a free radical metabolite of thalidomide by prostaglandin H synthase. While the results obtained in Wells's laboratory are consistent with the authors' proposed hypothesis, several additional studies would be desirable to provide convincing evidence that prostaglandin H synthase-catalyzed generation of a free radical metabolite of thalidomide represents a major mechanism for thalidomide-elicited teratogenesis. Further pursuit of this line of investigation does appear merited, however, and will be of considerable interest.

It was recently pointed out by Vaisman [27] that thalidomide was earlier shown capable of depleting ascorbate levels in tissues of guinea pigs and that thalidomide appeared capable of acting as a potent teratogen primarily only in species incapable of ascorbate synthesis. He postulated that thalidomide would produce its characteristic teratogenic effects mainly in such species (e.g. humans, subhuman primates, guinea pigs) and that the/a mechanism of thalidomide teratogenicity involves depletion of embryonic tissue ascorbate, resulting in decreased collagen synthesis. Reluctance to accept these ideas may be related to the lack of a "thalidomide-like" effect on conceptuses produced by ascorbate deficiencies [2, 3]. Nevertheless, it should be conceded that such an effect could be significantly contributory and that pursuit of mechanistic interpretations should certainly consider such a possibility. Pursuit of mechanisms should also consider the apparent lack of mutagenic activity of thalidomide, a characteristic recently discussed and referenced by Ashby and Tinwell [28].

In view of the current spate of investigative efforts pertaining to the unique immunomodulatory effects of thalidomide, it is tempting to speculate that one or more of the immunomodulating effects may contribute significantly to the teratogenic effects of thalidomide. It seems reasonable to speculate that research during the next few years will shed considerable additional light upon this mechanistic question.

In the previous review [1] it was suggested that the bulk of investigative reports dealing with thalidomide through the middle of 1992 tended to indicate a receptor-mediated mechanism(s) for its teratogenicity. Such a view is based on the following considerations: (1) a high degree of effectiveness at very low tissue levels (especially in humans), (2) strict requirements in terms of structure-activity relationships, (3) a very characteristic syndrome – the most striking of which involves limb reduction defects and (4) extremely striking species differences in potency as well as the qualitative nature of the effects elicited. Each of these characteristics would be consistent with and tend to argue for a receptor-dependent mechanism rather than a mechanism involving non-specific cytotoxic effects elicited by chemical electrophiles or free radicals. Of course, the various mechanisms under consideration need not be mutually exclusive, a single mechanism seems quite improbable, numerous mechanisms could be significantly contributory and it is clear at the moment that few should be ruled out entirely. As stated above, it is tempting to speculate, particularly in view of the recent work produced in the laboratories of Neubert and colleagues ([21, 22] and references therein), that some of the unique immunomodulating properties of thalidomide are responsible (at least in part) for the teratogenicity of thalidomide. If their hypothesis is correct, it would constitute the first documented example of a chemical teratogen acting via interactions with cell-surface receptors. It is anticipated that research during the next few years also will provide considerable additional information pertaining to this potential mechanism.

6.2   Cancer chemotherapeutic agents

In general terms, cancer chemotherapeutic agents have been developed for the purpose of killing populations of more rapidly dividing cells (malignant tumor cells) and are not uncommonly referred to as "cytotoxic agents". Because the developing embryo or fetus consists largely of rapidly dividing cells, it would automatically appear to be a prime target for cytotoxic and teratogenic effects of the majority of cancer chemotherapeutic agents currently marketed as well as for other environmental cytotoxic agents to which pregnant women may be exposed. In light of these considerations, it seems somewhat surprising that the offspring of pregnant women who have undergone cancer chemotherapy during gestation with clearly toxic doses (usually maximally tolerated doses) of highly potent cancer chemotherapeutic agents have exhibited an incidence of adverse embryotoxic or fetotoxic effects that seems far lower than one might expect in view of the exposure conditions and the potent cytotoxic effects of the chemicals in question [2, 29–33]. Estimates for incidence of malformations associated with chemotherapy during pregnancy and observable at birth have been in the neighborhood of 10–17% for first trimester exposures [34] – considerably above the 3–5% basal background incidence normally reported for human populations [2, 3, 6] but nevertheless indicative that greater than 80–90% of exposures to cancer chemotherapeutic regimens result in no causation of detectable malformations at birth. Even aminopterin, probably the best-established human teratogen of all cancer chemotherapeutic agents, elicited reported teratogenic effects in only approximately 50% of exposed infants [2]. (Later and/or more subtle [e.g. functional] defects, however, are clearly possible as has been demonstrated for radiation exposures [35] but apparently have not been reported in the literature.)

It seems likely that this apparent resistance to the teratogenic effects of these and other frankly cytotoxic chemicals (virtually all cancer chemo-

therapeutic agents are regarded [2–6] as potent cytotoxins and teratogens
in experimental animals) is related to as yet poorly defined embryonic/fetal
defense mechanisms, a subject desperately in need of additional research
for understanding of teratogenic mechanisms and risk. Such conceptal
defense and resistance mechanisms are very likely to be under significant
genetic control as is evidenced from several case reports involving dizy-
gotic twins (e.g. [2, 36, 37]). These kinds of observations also have substantial precedent in studies of the littermates of experimental animals;
that is, it is commonly observed that, within litters, certain members of
the litter are highly susceptible and markedly affected, whereas others
are highly resistant and not observably affected. Such observations are
commonly regarded as evidence for differences in genetic susceptibility
to chemical teratogenesis, and there would seem to be little reason to suspect that humans would not exhibit such differences. The biochemical,
cellular and molecular basis for such genetic differences, however, is at
present poorly understood. In terms of the resistance of human conceptuses to the embryotoxic or fetotoxic effects of cytotoxic agents, it would
seem likely that certain pregnancies (perhaps 7–10%) are deficient (genetically or by other means) in one or more maternal or conceptal systems
that otherwise provide adequate protection against chemically-elicited
cytotoxic effects directed against conceptal cells. In terms of electrophilic
chemicals or metabolites (e.g. alkylating agents), it has already been shown
in numerous experiments [38, 39 and therein cited references] that reduced
glutathione (GSH) and associated systems involved in the regulation of
this critically important endogenous nucleophile serve as highly important protection against the embryo/fetotoxicity of chemical electrophiles.
Genetic deficiencies in GSH-related systems could feasibly play an important role in observed embryotoxic or teratogenic effects of cancer chemotherapeutic regimens which usually employ at least one alkylating agent
as a part of the treatment regimen. Genetic differences in the activities
of bioactivation and/or bioinactivation systems could also be involved.
Numerous other possibilities as determinants of genetic susceptibility can
also be envisioned. In any event, it seems logical to presume that cytotoxic agents will elicit teratogenic effects primarily in genetically susceptible individuals. Of course, susceptibility may also be modified by non-
genetic (environmental) factors as well.

In the last review [1] only three classes of cancer chemotherapeutic agents
were considered: folic acid antagonists, alkylating agents and base (purine
and pyrimidine) analogs. Other classes of cancer chemotherapeutic agents
(e.g. antimitotic agents such as vincristine, vinblastine and paclitaxel, epi-
podophyllotoxins such as teniposide and etoposide, antibiotics such as dac-

tinomycin, anthracyclines, bleomycins and plicamycin and miscellaneous agents such as L-asparaginase, platinum complexes, hydroxyurea procarbazine and mitotane-hormonal and antihormonal agents are considered separately) were not considered because no individual agent within those classes has yet been identified as an "established" human teratogen. Most have substantial teratogenic activity in several species of experimental animals [2, 3], and lack of definitive data for humans rather than lack of intrinsic teratogenic potential *per se* is probably the primary reason why most of those agents are not included on lists of established human teratogens. Nor, since the last review, have any additional cancer chemotherapeutic agents been added to the lists; thus, discussion is again restricted to the same three groups. In general terms, it would seem probable that differences in teratogenic potency and effectiveness of cancer chemotherapeutic agents could be due in large measure to pharmacokinetic differences rather than to differences in intrinsic teratogenic activity, since all are potent cytotoxic agents which act in a relatively selective fashion upon populations of rapidly dividing cells. Capacity to cross cell membranes (especially the placenta) might be expected to be a major determinant of and positively correlated with the relative teratogenic potential of systematically administered cancer chemotherapeutic agents. It is thus of interest that the nitrosourea alkylating agents (e.g. carmustine, lomustine), which are known to be capable of readily crossing the blood-brain barrier, have not yet been included on lists of established human teratogens. In contrast, folic acid antagonists, which are among the best established of human teratogens (present on all lists of established human teratogens) are polar and cross poorly. Clearly, other factors must also be considered. Capacity to undergo rapid maternal or conceptal bioinactivation also should expectedly be a major determinant of but negatively correlated with teratogenic potential. For cancer chemotherapeutic agents, no concrete examples of this idea have yet been published to my knowledge.

Advances in our knowledge of mechanisms whereby frankly cytotoxic agents elicit teratogenic effects have not increased dramatically during the past 4 years. It now seems more likely than ever that mechanisms for the teratogenic effects of this group of chemicals are closely linked with mechanisms for their capacity to elicit necrotic cell death. Virtually all cytotoxic chemicals will also stimulate increases in apoptotic cell death at lower concentrations and at earlier time periods than are required to produce necrotic cell death; but the doses required to elicit teratogenic effects seem more consistent with necrotic than apoptotic mechanisms, although the latter may certainly play some role. In terms of mechanistic understanding, the relationship(s) and linkage(s) between induced conceptal cell death and the specific embryo/fetotoxic effects observed (pathogenesis) are at present extremely vague and will require considerable additional study. This may represent the greatest investigative challenge for this group of agents.

6.2.1 The folic acid antagonists

Although numerous other mechanisms may also play some role, it now seems dogmatic that the primary mechanism whereby amethopterin (Methotrexate), aminopterin and other folic acid (pteroylglutamic acid) antagonists elicit teratogenic effects is via an extremely high affinity binding to and correspondingly effective inhibition of dihydrofolate reductase. Inhibition of dihydrofolate reductase leads to cytotoxic effects and thus presumably also the pertinent teratogenic effects through partial depletion of the tetrahydrofolate cofactors that are required for the synthesis of purines and thymidylate [40], as well as through direct inhibition of the folate-dependent enzymes of purine and thymidylate metabolism by the polyglutamates and dihydrofolate polyglutamates that accumulate with dihydrofolate reductase inhibition. To function as a cofactor in one-carbon transfer reactions, folate must first be reduced to tetrahydrofolate in a reaction catalyzed by dihydrofolate reductase. Single-carbon fragments are added enzymatically to tetrahydrofolate in various configurations and may then be transferred in specific synthetic reactions. Possibly the most important metabolic event involved is disruption of the thymidylate synthase-catalyzed synthesis of thymidylate, an essential component of DNA. In this reaction, the synthase catalyzes the transfer of a one-carbon group (methyl) from 5,10-methylene tetrahydrofolate to 2'-deoxyuridylate (dUMP) to produce thymidylate. In the process, the tetrahydrofolate is oxidized to dihydrofolate. In order to function again as a cofactor, the dihydrofolate must be reduced to tetrahydrofolate, and the reaction requires dihydrofolate reductase as a catalyst. Aminopterin, amethopterin (Methotrexate) and other folic acid antagonists are capable of inhibiting the reductase with differing relative potencies – amethopterin exhibits a K_i of approximately 0.02 nM – that are also correlated with teratogenic potency. Inhibition of the formation of tetrahydrofolate results in an acute intracellular deficiency of certain folate coenzymes and a vast accumulation of the toxic inhibitory substrate, dihydrofolate polyglutamate. The one-carbon transfer reactions crucial for the *de novo* synthesis of purine nucleotides and thymidylate are strongly inhibited, resulting in interruption of the synthesis of DNA and RNA as well as the disruption of other vital metabolic reactions. The cytotoxic as well as the teratogenic effects [41, 42] of folate antagonists can be reversed by admin-istration of tetrahydrofolate derivatives, providing persuasive evidence that the teratogenic effects of these agents are closely linked to the cyto-toxic effects. Again, subsequent (linking) mechanistic factors involved as pathogenic determinants of specific teratogenic defects (a wide variety of defects can be elicited) are not yet understood and represent a major investigative challenge for this group of agents.

6.2.2   Alkylating agents

These chemicals are substances that bear an electrophilic charge of suf-ficient strength to result in covalent bond formation as the result of inter-action with nucleophilic groups present in biological systems. Those agents implicated most strongly as human teratogens include cyclophosphamide, chlorambucil, busulfan and mechlorethamine [1-6], all of which are ther-apeutically utilized, bifunctional alkylating agents that become strongly electrophilic via the formation of carbonium ion intermediates. For cyclo-phosphamide, P450-dependent monooxygenation is required for gener-ation of the electrophilic species as well as for elicitation of teratogenic effects [43], providing additional strong supporting evidence for a xeno-biotic electrophile-endobiotic nucleophile interaction as the primary mechanism of teratogenicity. Several nucleophilic moieties are present in proteins and nucleic acids and include phosphate, amino, sulfhydryl, hydroxyl, carboxyl and imidazole groups. Nucleophilic groups in nucleic acids tend to have more localized (hard) positive charges, whereas nucle-ophilic groups in protein molecules tend to be delocalized (soft). The gen-erated electrophilic positive charges on the alkylating agents regarded as established human teratogens are relatively localized (hard), providing for preferential SN1 interactions with the localized (hard) negative nucle-ophilic charges on nucleic acids (DNA, RNA). These considerations are important from a mechanistic point of view because soft electrophiles, which interact preferentially with proteins rather than nucleic acids and are generated from such chemicals as acetaminophen, tend to be much less teratogenic than hard electrophiles, and this implicates nucleic acid interactions and disruptions rather than protein disruptions much more heavily in the mechanistic process. For monofunctional alkylating agents, hard electrophiles tend to have a relatively higher mutagenicity/cytotox-icity ratio than soft electrophiles by virtue of preferential interactions with nucleic acids. For bifunctional alkylating agents, however, cross-linking of nucleic acid chains appears to result preferentially in cell killing as opposed to mutagenesis. Since the teratogenically most effective alkylat-ing agents are bifunctional in nature, the importance of somatic cell mutagenesis as a possible mechanism for alkylating agent-elicited teratogenesis is diminished relative to the importance of cell death *per se*. The relative importance of apoptotic cell death versus necrotic cell death remains to be more firmly delineated, but in view of the relatively high dosages required to elicit readily detectable defects, one would surmise that necrotic cell death would be most heavily although probably not exclusively involved.

6.2.3   Base analogs

Of the three base analogs that are currently listed as established human teratogens, 6-azauridine, cytosine arabinoside (Ara C) and 5-fluorouracil, all are pyrimidine analogs; no purine analogs have yet been listed. Reasons for this are as yet unclear, as both pyrimidine and purine analogs are potent cytotoxic and chemotherapeutic agents and are clearly effective teratogens in experimental animals [1–6], but are probably related to a lack of definitive exposure-outcome data in humans for purine analogs. It seems logical to expect that all of the therapeutically employed cancer chemotherapeutic base analogs possess significant teratogenic potential in humans based on knowledge of mechanisms of cytotoxic effects and potency as well as on studies in experimental animals where all exhibit significant and potent teratogenicity [1–6]. Again, mechanisms whereby base analogs elicit cytotoxic effects are in all probability the same mechanisms responsible for initiation of teratogenic effects.

Base analogs appear to produce cytotoxic effects primarily via two principal mechanisms: (1) inhibition of the synthesis of nucleic acids by inhibition of key enzymes that catalyze the synthesis of key intermediates and (2) "fraudulent" incorporation into DNA molecules in place of the corresponding endogenous base following metabolic conversion to the nucleotide derivative – incorporation of the incorrect base results in normal base mispairings with ensuing disrupted structure and function, ultimately followed by resultant death of the cell. 5-Fluorouracil requires enzymatic conversion via both ribosylation and phosphorylation to the nucleotide in order to exhibit significant incorporation; cytosine arabinoside and 6-azauridine are administered as the sugar derivatives and require only phosphorylation. For cytosine arabinoside, arabinose has replaced the ribose of cytidine, the naturally occurring base, and after phosphorylation the metabolite competes with deoxycytidine phosphate for incorporation into DNA [44], where it blocks elongation of the DNA strand and its template function. Currently, cytosine arabinoside and 5-fluorouracil are the most extensively utilized pyrimidine analogs and serve as prototypes; 6-azauridine is no longer used extensively.

All pyrimidine analogs have in common the capacity to inhibit the synthesis of DNA via inhibition of various enzymes in the synthetic pathway. 5-Fluorouracil is an exceptionally effective inhibitor of thymidylate synthase and thus could be expected to produce at least some teratogenic effects similar to those produced by the folic acid antagonists, discussed above. It is also incorporated into both DNA and RNA, but the total significance of the DNA incorporation is not yet clear. Presumably, DNA incorporation activates the excision-repair process, which could ultimately result in strand breakage. Incorporation of 5-fluorouracil into RNA results in major deleterious effects on both the processing and function of RNA. Cytosine arabinoside is an analog of 2'-deoxycytidine with its 2'-hydroxyl group in a position trans to the 3'-hydroxyl of the sugar moiety. The 2'-hydroxyl causes steric hindrance to the rotation of the pyrimidine base around the nucleosidic bond, resulting in abnormal stacking of the bases. Incorporation into the DNA chain also results in potent inhibition of chain elongation [45] and slowing of DNA template function.

During the past 4 years, 5-fluorouracil has been utilized extensively as an experimental tool in investigations of normal embryonic and fetal development. Such investigations inevitably also shed light on teratogenic mechanisms applicable to 5-fluorouracil as well as other base analogs. For example, Zucker et al. ([46] and cited references) have studied fetal erythropoiesis with 5-fluorouracil employed to block or inhibit yolk sac, hepatic and splenic erythropoiesis at varying stages of gestation. Studies were designed to investigate conceptal response to anemia which would be an expected effect of compromised erythropoiesis and thus also of exposure to 5-fluorouracil (and other hematotoxic cancer chemotherapeutic agents). Such effects might be expected to contribute significantly to the embryo/fetotoxic and teratogenic effects of these agents, particularly during the later stages of gestation when the conceptus is more dependent upon conceptal hematopoiesis.

Investigations reported by Shuey et al. ([47] and cited references) have provided evidence that a rapid, dose-dependent inhibition of thymidylate synthase and cell cycle alterations are in large measure responsible for many of the teratogenic effects of 5-fluorouracil. The investigators utilized a combination of *in utero* exposure and explant culture of embryonic craniofacial tissue and hind limbs to examine early events in embryonic target tissues. Results indicated that events occurring within 3 h of maternal administration of 5-fluorouracil were sufficient to produce both growth retardation and dysmorphogenesis of embryonic palates and hind limbs. Tissues dissected 6 h after exposure were, if anything, less affected than tissues dissected after 3 h. The results are important because they provide a much more solid basis for the supposition that mechanisms for teratogenesis are very similar if not identical to mechanisms for cytotoxicity and for antitumorigenicity.

Other pyrimidine analogs as well as purine analogs are not considered further here because they are not included on lists of established human teratogens. Until more careful studies provide a basis for thinking otherwise, however, it seems prudent to regard these other base analogs as effective as 5-fluorouracil and cytosine arabinoside in terms of teratogenicity.

6.3   Retinoids and arotinoids

Retinoids constitute a class of chemicals with structures and (often, but not always) biological properties similar to those of vitamin A_1 (all-trans-retinol). When metabolites are included, endobiotic retinoids number well into the hundreds, and in addition, thousands of xenobiotic analogs (including arotinoids – derivatives with aromatic ring structures – have been synthesized by chemists in an attempt to better understand the biochemistry, physiology, pharmacology and toxicology of this class of chemicals. A literal renaissance of investigative effort in this area has been termed "the retinoid revolution" [48]. It has become clear that, among other important biologic processes, the retinoids are intimately and importantly involved in both normal and abnormal development. Both deficiencies and excesses of retinoids can result in abnormal morphogenesis as well as a host of persistent functional defects [1–6], indicating the need for tight regulatory control of conceptal tissue levels of endobiotic retinoids. For this review, discussion is limited to teratogenic effects elicited by excess exposure to retinoids (toxicity) and the mechanisms whereby such exposures to retinoids and retinoid analogs elicit persistent developmental defects.

Several very recent review articles dealing in detail with retinoid-elicited teratogenesis have appeared [12, 49–51]. Each tends to persuade that the principal, heavily dominant mechanisms whereby excess retinoids produce teratogenic effects are intimately connected to interactions of high-affinity retinoid receptor ligands to retinoid nuclear receptor proteins of the steroid/thyroid/retinoid/D_3 superfamily.

Although many investigators in the field of retinoid research have accepted this view as dogma, both in the past and at present, it seems clear from a careful review of the literature that significant participation of several other proposed mechanisms has not been ruled out and also merits important consideration. Some of these potential mechanisms were mentioned in the previous review [1] and included altered prostaglandin metabolism, retinoylation of biologically important macromolecules, labilization of lysosomal membranes, altered cell-cell communication, induction of protein glycosylation, generation of free radicals, increased apoptosis and so forth. While it is true that some of these mechanisms need not be mutually exclusive of receptor-dependent processes, others clearly seem to be, yet should still be seriously considered as possible significant, participating, contributory mechanisms for teratogenic effects. The narrow view that all biological effects of retinoids are mediated through interactions with either retinoic acid receptors (RARs) or with retinoid X receptors (RXRs) clearly represents nonobjective science that borders on the naive.

Evidence is accumulating, however, to indicate that a great many (perhaps the majority) of the biological, pharmacological and toxicological (including teratogenic) effects of retinoids are mediated via interactions with RARs, RXRs or perhaps certain other (e.g. "orphan") receptors. Chambon [52] has recently provided an excellent summary of the status of research pertaining to retinoid receptors, providing clear insights into current, commonly held views of biological mechanisms of retinoid actions. It is well established that retinoids, particularly retinoic acids, can control the expression of numerous genes including several genes deemed crucial insofar as normal development is concerned (homeobox genes). The homeobox genes are a retinoid-responsive gene family that is known to control embryonic development and cellular differentiation. Evidence for a role of homeobox genes in retinoid teratogenesis includes observations that retinoids modify the patterns of normal homeobox gene expression in developing embryos and that transgenic mice with altered homeobox gene expression exhibit malformations reminiscent of retinoid-elicited terata. In his review of retinoid receptors, Chambon [52] has strongly emphasized the extremely complex nature of retinoid-related gene regulation, making it apparent that simple explanations of mechanisms of receptor-mediated retinoid teratogenicity should not be invoked at present and may not be feasible even for the foreseeable future.

For retinoid-elicited teratogenic effects, several lines of research suggest strongly that retinoid receptor interactions play a major, predominant (perhaps sometimes exclusive, depending upon the specific defect under consideration) mechanistic role. These include investigations of structure-activity relationships in which it can be shown that a terminal carboxylic acid group (or similar group) as well as several other structural features are commonly needed for both high-affinity receptor binding and potent dysmorphogenic effects (see [12] for a recent review). Studies of retinoid metabolism also indicate ([52] and cited references) that those metabolites exhibiting high affinities for retinoid receptors are also those that appear to behave as ultimate teratogens. This is, of course, highly important, because if thoroughly proven, it would indicate that retinoid metabolites such as 13-*cis*-retinoic acid (an established human teratogen), 9,13-di-*cis*-retinoic acid, retinoyl and retinyl glucuronides retinyl esters, retinaldehydes and a host of other metabolites as well as parent all-*trans*-retinol (vitamin A1) have little or no intrinsic teratogenic activity *per se* but must first be converted to receptor-active forms in order to produce teratogenic effects. Enzymatic control of such conversions then would be expected to play a highly significant mechanistic role.

A wide variety of approaches have been utilized in attempts to determine which of the six known retinoid receptor proteins (RARs α, β, γ and RXRs α, β, γ – several subtypes of these receptors are also known) is most important in mediating retinoid-elicited teratogenic effects [12, 49–53]. These include the use of transgenic animals for studies of overexpressed or underexpressed genes, targeted mutagenesis with null and double-null mutations, transgenic promoter analyses, antisense technology and investigations with receptor-selective agonists and antagonists (e.g. [53]). Agonists selective for RXRs appear to be far less capable of producing teratogenic effects than agonists that are selective for RARs [12]. Null mutants lacking single genes coding for retinol-binding proteins or for any of a number of retinoid receptors have exhibited surprising normality of development, and double-null mutations involving deletions of combinations of RAR and RXR receptors have been needed to demonstrate significant disruptions in embryogenesis. At this writing it appears that RARβ2 and RARγ1 may be the receptors most heavily involved in retinoid-elicited teratogenesis, although much more research in this area is clearly indicated. Advances in this area of research have been highly impressive, but very important questions remain to be answered.

6.4   Anticonvulsant drugs

Although most anticonvulsant agents have been implicated to some degree as causes of teratogenic effects in humans, only phenytoin, trimethadione, valproic acid, carbamazepine and primidone have been listed with other established human teratogens (Tables 1 and 2). No additional anticonvulsants have been added to the list since the previous review [1]. Phenytoin and valproic acid each are currently regarded both as established dysmorphogenic human teratogens (Table 1) and also as established functional (neurobehavioral) teratogens (Table 2). They share this distinction with only the retinoids, ethyl alcohol and methyl mercury. Considerable additional mechanistic information concerning the teratogenic effects of phenytoin, valproic acid and carbamazepine has been published since the previous review, but only minimal information concerning trimethadione and primidone has appeared and has not significantly advanced our understanding of mechanisms for the two latter agents (this understanding is currently minimal). Thus, the ensuing discussion will focus primarily upon phenytoin, valproic acid and carbamazepine.

Although apparently now losing favor, the idea still persists that the epileptic condition *per se* (rather than the anticonvulsant medications) is significantly or even solely responsible for the observed increases in incidence of birth defects associated with epilepsy. The idea has lost credibility primarily due to observations that the same chemicals will elicit similar kinds of malformations in a wide variety of experimental animals that are free of seizure conditions or of predisposal to seizures. Also, some epidemiologic investigations have provided evidence that the epileptic condition *per se* contributes only minimally if at all to the increased incidence of malformations associated with epilepsy; that is, children born to epileptic women who are not treated with anticonvulsant medications during pregnancy appear to exhibit only minor increases in incidence of morphologic abnormalities when compared with seizure-free controls [3]. This area of research, however, is still controversial, and further studies are needed to completely resolve this issue. The possibility of interactive contributing effects of the epileptic condition and anticonvulsant medications also remains to be satisfactorily resolved.

6.4.1   *Phenytoin*

Phenytoin (diphenylhydantoin) has been extensively investigated in terms of its status as an established human teratogen with much consideration of exposure, risk, of the kinds and patterns of defects elicited (both morphological and functional), and in terms of mechanisms whereby teratogenic effects are elicited. Of the anticonvulsant medications, it is probably the best-established human teratogen and is found on virtually all recent lists of established human teratogens. Investigations of mechanisms during the past 4 years have demonstrated interest in three possibilities:

1) the connection between low levels of epoxide hydrolase (<35% of a control) in cultured amniocytes from pregnancies in which infants were exposed to phenytoin *in utero*, and the increased incidence of malformations exhibited in the same infants. This correlation is still being investigated ([54] and cited references) even though a cause-effect relationship now seems highly improbable theoretically, for reasons

detailed in the previous review [1]. Further investigations will be needed to firmly establish that a significant correlation is consistent. Beyond that, it would be of mechanistic interest to determine why such a correlation exists and, particularly, whether it would be anything more than simply coincidental;

2) the idea that conceptal peroxidases – in particular, embryonic/fetal prostaglandin synthases – catalyze the conversion of phenytoin to free-radical intermediates that are capable of eliciting cytotoxic effects in embryonic and fetal tissues to the extent that malformations are produced. Details of these ideas have appeared in a recent review of research emanating primarily from the laboratory of Wells [55]. Support for this idea includes observations of enhancement of phenytoin teratogenicity by inhibition of glutathione peroxidase or glutathione reductase, reduction of phenytoin-elicited teratogenicity by antioxidants such as the tocopherols and caffeic acid, by free-radical spin-trapping agents and by desferrioxamine. Also, additions of exogenous superoxide dismutase or catalase to the medium of cultured rodent embryos reduced the molecular damage and embryopathy initiated by phenytoin. Mice lacking p53, important for DNA repair, were also much more susceptible to the teratogenic effects of phenytoin. While each of these observations is consistent with the "free-radical hypothesis", positive results from critical experiments that would provide convincing substantive underpinning are still lacking;

3) the idea that phenytoin produces embryotoxicity, including malformations, by virtue of its capacity to induce hypoxia/ischemia in conceptal tissues by reducing blood flow through the placenta and other conceptal tissues. This seemingly logical idea, proposed by D.R. Danielsson, has been discussed extensively in a recent research article [56]. A stabilizing effect of phenytoin on excitable membranes in cardiac myocytes and an inhibitory action on Na^+, Ca^{++} and K^+ channels would represent the basic, primary biochemical and cellular mechanisms responsible for cardiac toxicity which, in turn, would produce reduced blood flow, ultimately leading to the teratogenic effect. Support for this idea is provided by observations of very similar kinds of defects produced by clamping of uterine blood vessels, by exposure of embryos to subnormal concentrations of oxygen and by a variety of other factors (e.g. vasodilators, K^+-channel inhibitors etc.) that reduce blood flow or produce hypoxia. Furthermore, placing of mice in a hyperoxic chamber [50% O_2) resulted in a large decrease in incidence of phenytoin-elicited malformations. This mechanism proposed by Danielsson is similar to one proposed for cocaine (see Sec. 6.13, below).

Numerous other ideas and hypotheses have been promulgated in the past; several were mentioned in the previous review [1], but most lack experimental support and have not received substantial additional experimental support during the past 4–5 years. It may be of importance to emphasize that the mechanisms postulated need not be mutually exclusive and that several could be substantially contributory. Resolution of these aspects will require considerable additional investigation.

6.4.2   Valproic acid

This anticonvulsant [2-propyl-pentanoic acid] is a more recently established human teratogen but has attracted considerable investigative attention. It is a simple, branched-chain fatty acid now used to treat a wide variety of seizure disorders and is one of the most widely used anticonvulsant drugs. It is known to be capable of producing dysmorphic teratogenic effects in several species of experimental animals and is believed capable of causing an increased rate of neural tube defects, specifically spina bifida, in humans. In addition, valproic acid appears capable of causing delayed neurological development in both experimental animals and humans and is currently regarded as an established human neurobehavioral teratogen (Table 2). As with phenytoin, numerous suggestions, ideas and hypotheses have been proposed as mechanisms for valproate-elicited teratogenicity, but on the same note, few of these ideas have enjoyed the support of high-quality research findings and have not been given substantial additional credibility based on solid research findings during the past 5 years. Some of the earlier suggestions and hypotheses were noted in the previous review [1].

In relatively recent studies, Sato et al. [57] showed that pantothenic acid not only decreased the incidence of neural tube defects caused by valproic acid in mice but also prevented valproic acid from causing a profound reduction in acetyl coenzyme A in developing animals. They suggested the possibility that valproic acid might cause teratogenic effects via reduction of acetyl coenzyme A, a crucial metabolic intermediate for several important biochemical reactions. Further pursuit of these investigations and their mechanistic implications will be of substantial interest.

Evidence for a highly interesting potential mechanism for elicitation of the skeletal and craniofacial malformations produced by valproic acid has been presented very recently by Barnes and co-workers [58]. With early developmental stage chick embryos, they showed that treatment with valproic acid produced dose-dependent malformations in somite development as well as a decreased level of *Pax-1* gene expression and that somite anomalies correlated spatially with regions of decreased Pax-1 gene expression. In addition, specific antisense oligonucleotides directed against *Pax-1* and used to block *Pax-1* gene expression produced somite abnormalities very similar to those produced by valproic acid. These included discrete somite fusions and areas of somites with disrupted patterning and/or loss of boundaries. *Pax-1* is an established member of the *Pax* family of pattern-forming genes and is an important regulator of axial skeletal patterning at the somite level. It is specifically implicated in the formation of the distinct somitic sclerotome, which subsequently gives rise to the axial skeleton, including the vertebrae, intervertebral discs, ribs and neural arches. Follow-up studies of this highly interesting and promising research seem strongly indicated.

Because valproic acid is believed to increase the frequency of neural tube defects (especially spina bifida) and because increased intake of folic acid is believed to reduce the incidence of neural tube defects (especially spina bifida) in humans, there has been considerable interest in the idea that valproic acid might act as a folic acid antagonist and that this may constitute a mechanism for its teratogenic effects. This has also been a hypothesized mechanism for the teratogenic effects of phenytoin. Several problems with this hypothesis were mentioned in the earlier review [1], and recent studies [59 and cited references) have provided strong evidence to counter the hypothesis, at least insofar as mice are concerned. The question of species differences in mechanisms involving folate, however, remains.

6.4.3 Carbamazepine

In the past it was common practice to switch pregnant epileptic women from phenytoin to carbamazepine because of a perceived lack of teratogenic potential of carbamazepine. Currently, it is regarded not only as an effective teratogen in experimental animals but also as an established (although perhaps somewhat more controversially established) human teratogen [1–6]. Major mechanistic interest evident in the literature has been in whether parent carbamazepine or one or more of its metabolites acts as the proximate or ultimate teratogen. Interest in this aspect was spurred by observations of an apparent synergistic teratogenicity of carbamazepine and other drugs, notably other anticonvulsant agents known to have definitive effects on P450-dependent biotransforming systems. These ideas have been reviewed recently by Finnell et al. [60], who also provided evidence that a reactive metabolite (unidentified), rather than the parent carbamazepine, was responsible for teratogenic effects in Swiss Webster (SWV) mice. Support for this idea was based on investigations of covalent binding and incidences of malformations when phenobarbital, a P450 inducer, and stiripentol, a P450 inhibitor, were used to modulate these parameters and, simultaneously, rates of P450-dependent biotransformation and bioactivation of carbamazepine. Results were consistent with, but not yet compelling evidence for, the hypothesis. Results reported recently by Hansen et al. [61] from investigations with cultured mouse and rat embryos suggest quite strongly that, if a metabolite is responsible, it is not carbamazepine-10,11-epoxide, a stable epoxide metabolite often implicated in the past. The possibility that peroxidase-catalyzed generation of free-radical intermediates or other metabolites [55] has not yet been intensively investigated. Clearly, our knowledge of mechanisms of carbamazepine-elicited teratogenesis are presently at a primitive stage and will require much further study.

6.5   Alcohols

Several members of this category of agents, as well as glycols and glycol ethers, have demonstrated effective teratogenic potential in experimental animals. However, only one agent, ethyl alcohol (ethanol), is currently regarded as an established human teratogen (Tables 1 and 2), and the ensuing discussion will be limited primarily to this compound. Among all chemical teratogens, ethanol produces by far the highest number of defects in human populations. Thus it is of interest that it also appears to be the least potent of all established human teratogens, producing defects only when plasma/tissue concentrations are in the millimolar range. Of course, it should be remembered that such concentrations are not uncommon in individuals who drink alcoholic beverages recreationally. Thus, heavy and largely unregulated exposure to ethanol appears to be responsible in large measure for what is perhaps the greatest societal problem connected with developmental toxicology.

From a mechanistic point of view, it is rapidly becoming obvious that mechanisms for a large number of different developmental defects and anomalies require consideration, and that mechanisms could differ for each defect. A large number of ethanol-elicited defects have been described; the morphologic craniofacial defects classically listed are those that characterize the fetal alcohol syndrome (FAS), but effects on the central nervous system that are not readily detected morphologically are now usually regarded as the most serious manifestation of *in utero* exposure to ethanol – resulting in mental retardation and various behavioral abnormalities (hyperactivity, decreased social interaction etc.). Many other morphologic and functional defects have also been reported, and it can be expected that several additional effects will be reported in the future.

It also seems highly likely that several mechanistic factors may be involved for any defect described. A likely predominant primary mechanism appears not to have emerged. Probable significantly contributing mechanistic factors include:

1) Reduction of blood flow to the conceptus. This appears to be largely a function of the well-known capacity of ethanol to produce profound peripheral cutaneous vasodilatation, thus increasing blood flow to the periphery and concomitantly reducing flow to internal organs and structures. Hypoxic damage to the conceptus would not be unexpected. Of interest in this regard is the reported [62] apparent synergistic embryolethality with cocaine (a chemical that also reduces blood flow to the conceptus) but lack of interactive effect on brain growth.

2) Generation of acetaldehyde as a major, intermediary, reactive ethanol metabolite that is known to be highly cytotoxic, clastogenic, mutagenic, genotoxic and carcinogenic. This metabolite has been implicated in various other toxicities elicited by ethanol, notably hepatotoxicity. In cell cultures it is also known to be capable of inhibiting cell division and cell migration. Fatty acid ester metabolites of ethanol are also known to be toxic and could possibly contribute.

3) Increases in the fluidity of lipid membranes. Ethanol produces this well-established, well-known effect in common with volatile general anesthetic agents. A large number of different toxic (including embryo/fetotoxic) sequelae resulting from this effect can be envisioned.

4) Nutritional deficiency – especially of thiamine – which is common in alcoholics because ethanol provides significant caloric intake, is known to contribute to toxic effects of chronic ethanol ingestion (e.g. cerebellar degeneration, peripheral neuropathies, myopathies etc.) and would seem likely to contribute significantly to embryo/fetotoxicity as well. Damage to the gastric mucosa (gastritis with gastric bleeding), commonly observed in chronic ethanol users, may also contribute to nutritional deficiencies.

5) Depletion of NAD^+. NAD^+ is consumed in dehydrogenase-catalyzed reactions in which ethanol is oxidized to acetaldehyde and acetaldehyde is oxidized to acetic acid. For each mole of ethanol oxidized to acetic acid, 0.75 kg of NAD^+ is consumed via conversion to NADH. NAD^+ is required for a large number of important biochemical reactions, notably the citric acid cycle but also several others. Depletion of NAD^+ results in concomitant increases in tissue lactate and decreased

metabolism through the Kreb's cycle. Any or all of these effects could contribute to embryo/fetotoxicity and teratogenesis.

Various other well-established effects of ethanol may also possibly contribute to mechanisms of teratogenicity of ethanol, particularly to the serious and persistent developmental neurotoxicity. These include: (1) Effects on γ-aminobutyric acid (GABA) receptors. Ethanol enhances the action of GABA acting on GABA receptors and also can decrease the density of $GABA_A$ receptors. (2) Inhibition of calcium entry through voltage-gated Ca^{++} channels (inhibits the opening of the channels). Ethanol also increases the density of voltage-gated Ca^{++} channels. (3) Inhibition of glutamate receptor function – ethanol inhibits the excitatory effects of glutamate, apparently by inhibition of N-methyl-D-aspartate receptor activation. Various other associated pathogenic mechanisms including increased embryonic cell death, altered hormonal status, impaired protein synthesis, altered prostaglandin metabolism and so forth have been discussed in a relatively recent review by Kotch and Sulik [63].

Two possible mechanisms that have received more recent attention appear meritorious of discussion. One mechanism involves the generation of reactive oxygen species (ROS). Kotch et al. [64] reported that exposure of day 8 mouse embryos to ethanol for 6 h in a whole-embryo culture system resulted in increased superoxide anion generation, increased lipid peroxidation, excess cell death and dysmorphogenesis, all of which were diminished by addition of superoxide dismutase to the culture system. The results strongly suggested at least a participatory role for ROS generation in the dysmorphogenic effect (failure of anterior neural tube closure) monitored. They are of particular interest in view of the recently reported expression of P4502E1 in cephalic tissues of human embryos during the late stages of organogenesis [65] and in human hepatic tissues during fetal development [66]. P4502E1 not only catalyzes the conversion of ethanol to reactive acetaldehyde but in the process releases electrons which reduce molecular oxygen (O_2) to superoxide anion which may be converted to more reactive ROS species such as hydroxyl radicals. P4502E1 also is capable of catalyzing the conversion of ethanol to a hydroxyethyl radical, also known to be highly toxic. In addition, P4502E1 will catalyze the conversion of lipid hydroperoxides (generated during free radical-initiated lipid peroxidation) to highly toxic aldehydes such as 4-hydroxynonenal. Generation of these reactive species in target tissues themselves might be expected to be highly cytotoxic and contribute significantly to ethanol's teratogenic effects. Further research along these lines seems to merit a very high priority.

The second is with reference to the hypothesis promoted by Duester [67] that ethanol produces embryotoxic effects by virtue of its capacity to inhibit competitively the alcohol dehydrogenase that catalyzes the rate-limiting conversion of retinol to morphogenic retinoic acid. This would result in an effective deficiency of the active retinoid acid in embryonic and fetal tissues and thereby elicit dysmorphogenesis and perhaps other embryo/fetotoxic effects. Recent results from this laboratory [68, 69] argue against Duester's hypothesis, although the question of species differences again remains. Further research along these lines also will be of high interest.

6.6   Antithyroid agents

Thyroid hormone provides an additional example for which both excess and deficiency will elicit significant teratogenic effects, at least in experimental animals [1–6, 70]. Thus far, only antithyroidal agents – which mimic thyroid deficiency – are regarded as established human teratogens (Table 1) even though thyroxine, triiodothyronine and triiodothyroacetic acid produce a variety of defects (involving the thyroid, eye, limbs, CNS and heart) and are well-established teratogens in animal experiments. In humans, excess exposure to thyroid hormone is relatively rare because thyroid hormone as a drug is normally administered only in quantities sufficient to replace thyroid hormone deficiencies in hypothyroid states, and for pathologic hyperthyroidism such as thyrotoxicosis, antithyroid agents are usually administered for therapy of the condition. In either case, the pathologic condition *per se* (as well as the therapeutic agent used to treat the condition) may feasibly contribute to the abnormalities observed, and with respect to studies in humans, this fact appears too frequently not to be taken into serious consideration. Experiments with euthyroid animals do indicate that the drugs themselves are capable of producing defects. In view of the extremely important role of thyroid hormone in developmental processes as well as the demonstrated teratogenicity of administered thyroid hormones in experimental animals, there seems little reason to doubt that excess exposure to thyroid hormone is capable of producing birth defects in humans, although this remains to be demonstrated. Experiments demonstrating greater than additive and apparently synergistic dysmorphogenic effects of triiodothyronine plus all-*trans*-retinoic acid or 9-*cis*-retinoic acid [71] create additional interest in this aspect.

Treatment of hyperthyroid pregnant women with antithyroidal (goitrogenic) agents results in birth defect problems due to a relatively facile

placental transfer of such agents to the conceptus and the resultant inhibition of conceptal thyroid function. As might be expected, the predominant morphologic effects of prenatal antithyroid hormone exposure
appear related to the thyroid gland itself; enlarged fetal thyroid glands
have been reported for numerous human cases as well as in animal experiments [2,3]. Various investigators (e.g. [70]), however, have observed that
both thyroid hormone (triiodothyronine) and antithyroid (propylthiouracil) can also produce persistent effects on the development of other
organs, in the case cited, on the heart and kidney. Effects of antithyroidal
agents on the developing nervous system are of greatly increasing concern because it is known that an imbalance of thyroid hormone can cause
irreversible damage to neuronal cells in the developing nervous system;
such damage can occur even if levels are corrected. Observations of persistent mental retardation in individuals exposed *in utero* to antithyroidal
agents would seem to bear heavily on these considerations. It is thus of
interest that antithyroidal agents appear to have lacked consideration as
neurobehavioral teratogens (Table 2), even though evidence suggests
strongly that effects on the developing CNS may be the most serious complication of prenatal exposure to these agents (morphologic defects such
as enlarged thyroid glands are usually reversible within a relatively short
period of time after parturition). Experience with cretinism resulting from
congenital lack of or deficiency in thyroid tissue/function and the resultant mental retardation associated with this condition should teach us that
antithyroid agents could produce very similar effects on mentation, and
an examination of the literature indicates that they in fact do. It seems
surprising that these effects have not been considered more seriously.

Specific antithyroid agents implicated in human birth defects have included iodine (excess is antithyroidal), which is converted to iodides in
the body, iodides (sodium, potassium, ammonium), radioactive iodine
(I^{131}) and thioureylenes such as thiouracil, propylthiouracil, methimazole
and carbimazole. Currently, all except non-radioactive iodine are regarded
as established human teratogens, but little doubt remains that all goitrogenic agents have qualitatively similar teratogenic potential. Radioactive
iodine is used for treatment of thyroid tumors, iodides are used as expec-
torants in asthmatic conditions and thioureylenes are used for treatment
of hyperthyroid conditions, primarily thyrotoxicosis. Lithium, discussed
further below (Sec. 6.14) also exhibits antithyroidal properties and is used
extensively in the treatment of bipolar depressive disorders. Propylthiouracil is regarded as the prototype of the thioureylenes, which are usually considered the most important antithyroid agents in terms of clinical usage.

In terms of mechanisms, radioiodine is selectively taken up by the thyroid gland by mechanisms identical to those for unlabeled iodine. The radiolabelled compound emits β-rays which are cytotoxic to the thyroid follicle cells. The conceptal thyroid gland is affected in the same way. Iodine, as mentioned above, is converted to iodides in the body. It will decrease the vascularity of the thyroid gland by poorly defined mechanisms. Iodides depress the secretion of thyroid hormone by mechanisms that also are not entirely clear but appear to be due to inhibition of iodination of thyroglobulin, possibly by inhibiting the hydrogen peroxide generation required for iodination. Perchlorate and thiocyanate, goitrogenic agents no longer employed extensively in therapy, compete with iodide for the iodide transport system in the membranes of the thyroid follicle cells. The thioureylenes, also referred to as thioamides, also decrease the output of thyroid hormone from the gland. Like the iodides, they inhibit the iodination of tyrosyl residues in thyroglobulin, an oxidation reaction that is catalyzed by thyroperoxidase. The thioureylenes apparently inhibit the thyroperoxidase-catalyzed reaction by acting as alternate substrates for the postulated peroxidase-iodinium complex, thus competitively inhibiting interaction with tyrosine. Propylthiouracil also inhibits the deiodination of thyroxine (which is three-to-fourfold less active than triiodothyronine) to triiodothyronine and is somewhat more effective than other agents by virtue of this inhibitory capacity. In terms of teratogenicity, inhibition of these activities in the conceptal thyroid glands appears to be much more important than inhibition in the maternal thyroid glands.

6.7   Antimicrobial agents

Antitumor antibiotics are normally regarded as fairly potent teratogenic agents (although none are currently listed as established human teratogens). With respect to antimicrobial antibiotics, only two classes have been placed on lists of established human teratogens – the aminoglycosides and the tetracyclines. With the possible exceptions of chloramphenicol and vancomycin, virtually all other currently employed antimicrobial antibiotics are regarded as chemicals with very low teratogenic potential that have extremely little danger of producing teratogenic effects in humans under most expected exposure conditions. Only the aminoglycosides and tetracyclines are discussed.

6.7.1   Aminoglycosides
As of this writing, aminoglycoside antibiotics used to a significant degree in the United States as therapeutic agents include streptomycin, neomy-

cin, gentamicin, tobramycin, amikacin, netilmicin and kanamycin. They are widely used and important agents for the treatment of infections caused by aerobic gram-negative bacteria and, in the case of streptomycin, for tuberculosis. Toxicity is a major limitation of their usefulness, and important for this discussion, they all share the same qualitative spectrum of toxicity when given to adult patients. The most notable toxicities are nephrotoxicity and ototoxicity. Ototoxicity, which occurs both in adults and during early development (including prenatally), is often largely irreversible [72] and can involve both the auditory and vestibular functions of the eighth cranial nerve. Streptomycin and gentamicin appear more likely to interfere with vestibular function; kanamycin, neomycin and amikacin preferentially affect auditory (cochlear) function. Other ototoxic drugs such as the loop diuretics (ethacrynic acid, furosemide) will potentiate the ototoxicity of the aminoglycosides.

Aminoglycosides are highly polar polycations, poorly absorbed from the gastrointestinal tract, cross the blood-brain barrier very poorly and would thus also be expected to exhibit poor transplacental transfer. Nevertheless, they do cross the placenta in sufficient quantities to produce toxicity and also accumulate on the fetal side [72]. At least 50 cases of ototoxicity have been attributed to *in utero* exposures to streptomycin and dihydrostreptomycin, another 10 to kanamycin and some possible cases to gentamicin [2, 3]. Cochlear damage results in varying degrees of hearing loss (usually permanent), and vestibular damage results in abnormal vertigo, ataxia and loss of balance.

The mechanism(s) whereby aminoglycoside antibiotics produce cochlear and vestibular damage *in utero* appear at present to be the same mechanism(s) by which these antibiotics produce ototoxicity in adults. Progressive destruction of vestibular and cochlear sensory cells is observed. Degeneration of type I sensory hair cells in the central part of the crista ampullaris (vestibular organ) and fusion of individual sensory hairs into giant hairs has been demonstrated in studies with guinea pigs. Loss of hair cells in the cochlea of the organ of Corti in the inner ear has also been demonstrated. Damage proceeds from the base of the cochlea, where high-frequency sounds are processed (loss of hearing of high-frequency tones occurs earliest), to the apex, which is necessary for the perception of low-frequency sounds. Aminoglycosides will accumulate in the perilymph and endolymph of the inner ear, but the precise biochemical and molecular mechanism(s) by which they are cytotoxic to the specific cells affected are not yet understood. Early changes appear to be reversible by Ca^{++}, and it has been suggested that aminoglycosides interfere with the active transport system essential for maintenance of the ionic balance of the endolymph [73]. This could lead to alterations in the normal concentrations of ions in the labyrinthine fluids, with impairment of electrical activity and nerve conduction, and such changes could lead ultimately to irreversible damage to the hair cells. It has also been suggested that aminoglycosides interact with membrane phospholipids, particularly phosphatidyl inositol and its phosphorylated derivatives, which are precursors of intracellular second messengers (inositol 1,4,5-triphosphate and diacylglycerol). In terms of ototoxicity *in utero*, it is interesting that exposure to aminoglycosides during early gestation is implicated more heavily than exposure during later gestation after the inner ear structures have become more fully developed. Nephrotoxicity, a major complication in adults, has not emerged as a major embryotoxic effect. It is clear that much further research will be required to elucidate mechanisms.

6.7.2   Tetracyclines

These are orally active, bacteriostatic, broad-spectrum antibiotics that are capable of chelating calcium and are thereby deposited in growing bones and teeth. Commonly used tetracyclines have included chlortetracycline, oxytetracycline, demeclocycline, tetracycline, methacycline, doxycycline and minocycline. Capacity to inhibit protein synthesis in prokaryotic cells does not extend significantly to eukaryotic cells. Tetracyclines chelate a variety of metal ions including calcium, magnesium, iron and aluminum, thereby forming complexes that do not transfer readily across biological membranes – thus, absorption from the gastrointestinal tract is greatly impeded by the presence of milk. Uncomplexed tetracyclines cross placental membranes at significant rates and gain access to all conceptal tissues, including bones and teeth. Virtually all of the commonly described teratogenic effects of tetracyclines appear to be referable to the chelation of calcium in developing conceptal bones and teeth. These antibiotics are known to be capable of causing staining of bones and teeth and sometimes also dental hypoplasia and bone deformities. They are contraindicated in children, pregnant women and nursing mothers. In pregnant women, hepatotoxicity is not an uncommon side effect.

It would sometimes appear from the literature [2, 3] that the only significant problem pertaining to prenatal exposures to tetracyclines in humans is the staining of deciduous teeth. For commonly utilized dosage regimens and expected exposures, this may well be the only significant concern. In experimental animals, higher doses/exposures are known to be capable of eliciting skeletal abnormalities, and in view of mechanistic considerations as well as commonplace occurrence in experimental animals, there seems little reason to suspect that the same effect could not occur in humans. Also, Cohlan et al. [74] reported a 40% depression of bone growth, as determined by measurement of fibulas, in premature infants treated with tetracyclines (bones begin calcification at approximately 2 months' gestation in humans).

In terms of mechanisms of tooth staining, the tetracyclines deposit as fluorescent compounds, primarily in calcifying teeth and bones. The period of greatest danger to the teeth appears to be from midpregnancy to about 4–6 months postpartum for deciduous teeth and from about 2 months postpartum to 5 years of age for permanent teeth. First trimester exposures appear to produce no detectable effects. Chelation in bones and teeth results in the formation of a fluorescent, yellow, tetracycline-orthophosphate complex. As time progresses, the yellow fluorescence is replaced by a nonfluorescent brown to brownish-gray color that may represent an oxidation product (oxidized tetracycline/calcium complex). Formation of the oxidized product is hastened by light, and the discoloration is permanent.

6.8   Heavy metals and organometals

Heavy metals have the reputation of being highly toxic substances and are thus automatically suspect in terms of capability of eliciting developmental defects. Exposures of humans to heavy metals are most frequently of the chronic, low-level type that would not be expected to produce a high incidence of morphologic abnormalities. Of course, there are numerous exceptions to this generality, and acute, high-level exposures during pregnancy do appear to present a far greater hazard to the developing conceptus. Although numerous metals and organometals have been shown to act as relatively effective teratogenic agents in experimental animals [2, 3], only two, methyl mercury and lead, are currently regarded as established human teratogens. Methyl mercury is listed in both Tables 1 and 2; that is, it is deemed capable of producing both morphologic abnormalities as well as neurobehavioral abnormalities in humans. Lead, on the other hand, is listed only in Table 2, because morphologic abnormalities resulting from lead exposure in humans have been more difficult to document adequately. It is, however, a very well established neurobehavioral teratogen.

6.8.1   Methyl mercury

On the basis of chemical speciation, there are three forms of mercury: elemental, inorganic and organic compounds. Each of the three forms exhibits characteristic toxic effects. Methyl mercury is regarded as the most important form of mercury in terms of toxicity and health effects from

environmental exposure [75]. Neurotoxic effects are regarded as the major
human health effect in adults, and the brain is believed to be the critical
target organ. Investigations of the effects of methyl mercury exposure *in
utero* likewise point to the brain as a primary target [76], and many/most
investigators believe that the developing brain is more sensitive to methyl
mercury toxicity than the adult brain. Studies in experimental animals [76]
definitely support that viewpoint. Exposure of conceptuses *in utero* to elevated levels of methyl mercury result in abnormal neuronal migration and
deranged organization of brain nuclei (clusters of neurons) with layering
of neurons in the cortex [75]. Infants born to women exposed to high concentrations of methyl mercury (in a number of well-publicized exposure
incidents) exhibited an increased incidence of microcephaly and a syndrome resembling cerebral palsy as the most frequent defects. A variety
of other malformations and defects were observed, but the CNS and eyes
appeared to be particularly affected. The cerebrum and cerebellum appear
to be prime CNS targets for methyl mercury-elicited toxicity. In the cerebellar hemispheres, methyl mercury produced a diffuse neuronal disin-
tegration with gliosis, particularly evident in the granular layer of *in utero*-
exposed offspring [3]. In the cerebral cortex, degeneration and loss of neuronal cells with astrocytosis and glial fiber proliferation were found.
Numerous other CNS lesions were also found in the offspring of women
exposed to methylmercuric sulfide and methylmercuric chloride in the
area around Minamata Bay in Japan. Reported excessive prenatal exposures [3] have occurred in Japan (Minimata and Niigata areas), Sweden,
Bakulina (former Soviet Union), New Mexico and Iraq and were consistently associated with symptoms resembling cerebral palsy and with severe
mental retardation as well as with numerous other defects, but particularly neurologic lesions and deficits.

Reasons for the apparently highly selective effects on the CNS and the
precise mechanisms whereby methyl mercury compounds elicit such serious CNS defects are not understood at present. It is known that methyl
mercury crosses membranes (including the blood-brain barrier) readily
and gains ready access to CNS tissues. Studies in mice have demonstrated
disruptive effects on neuronal microtubules [75], and this seems logically
related. It is also known that mercury compounds readily form covalent
bonds with the sulfur atoms of sulfhydryl groups, and it is commonly
believed that this property accounts for most of the biological effects of
the metal. Organic mercurials form mercaptides of the type RHg-SR', and
even at very low concentrations, mercurials are capable of inactivating
enzymes that depend on sulfhydryl groups for enzymatic activity. Disruption of these enzymic activities thereby compromises cellular metabolism

and function. Mercurials also combine with other ligands of physiologic importance, including phosphoryl, carboxyl, amide and amine groups. These interactions may be of importance in terms of interactions with nucleic acids, changes in the secondary structure of DNA and RNA, and in biosynthesis of DNA and RNA. Which of the specific biochemical effects are causally accountable for elicitation of specific defects, however, remains to be elucidated, and it is clear that much remains to be learned in terms of mechanistic aspects.

6.8.2   Lead and lead compounds

In a relatively recent review, Bellinger [77] provided an update on the capacity of lead-lead compounds to produce birth defects in experimental animals and humans. He pointed out the weaknesses of various epidemiologic investigations and the difficulties in providing information of sufficient quality to definitively establish the >1000-year old concept that lead exposure is strongly associated with significant increases in the incidence of morphological abnormalities and growth retardation. Isolated outbreaks of lead poisoning that would lead to markedly increased levels of lead compounds in conceptal tissues (analogous to those described above for methyl mercury) appear not to have been available for analyses in terms of birth defects. Bellinger also pointed out, however, that in terms of neurobehavioral defects, the data are in sufficiently good general agreement to indicate that lead has elicited such defects. Retarded mental development in early life following *in utero* exposure to lead has been a relatively consistent correlation in the studies available. It has been argued that such mental deficits are somewhat transient – no longer statistically significant by the time of school age. It does appear, however, that persistence of the effect can be related to exposure levels and that higher levels can result in more persistent impairment.

Based on investigative data available from epidemiological studies in humans, the profound effects of *in utero* exposure to lead compounds in experimental animals and the well–established capacity of lead compounds to produce neurotoxic effects (particularly on the developing CNS) in both animals and humans, there seems very little reason to doubt that prenatal lead exposures, at least at relatively high exposure levels, are capable of producing defective human offspring. It also seems evident that such high exposure levels can be encountered in the environment, although questions pertaining to "safe" exposure levels apparently will be debated for some time. Nevertheless, it seems prudent to concede that lead is capable of producing teratogenic effects in humans (particularly functional teratogenicity) and that, as with methyl mercury, the developing brain is a principal target. Once this concession is made, a primary question of importance is, By what mechanism(s)?

Silbergeld [78, 79] summarized possible mechanisms whereby lead might elicit neurotoxic effects in relatively recent reviews. The complexity of neurodevelopment points to almost innumerable possibilities for contribution to interference with normal brain development, and the question then becomes one of which of such potential mechanisms is significantly contributory in terms of birth defects. One of the more likely possibilities appears (at present) to include the capacity of lead to impair the timed programming of cell-to-cell connections, leading to disrupted neuronal circuitry. Induction of the precocious differentiation of glial cells, resulting in inappropriate positioning of neuronal cells during structuring of the CNS has also been reported. Lead can cause numerous effects on biochemical and neurotransmitter systems including interference with the release of several neurotransmitters, activation of protein kinase C in brain microvessels, interference with the mitochondrial release of Ca^{++} with resultant compromised energy metabolism, inhibition of membrane-bound Na^+,K^+-ATPase, inhibition of heme biosynthesis and inhibition of numerous sulfhydryl-dependent enzymes. Again, considerable research will be needed for provision of a clear understanding of lead-elicited teratogenicity in spite of indications that substantial progress is now evident in this area.

6.9   Polyhalogenated aromatics

A class of chemicals referred to collectively as polyhalogenated aromatic hydrocarbons and, in particular, the planar polyhalogenated aromatic hydrocarbons (PPAHs) are persistent environmental contaminants that are now known to be extremely toxic to early stages of vertebrate development. This topic has been reviewed relatively recently by Peterson et al. [80]. The member of this class of chemicals that exhibits the highest toxicologic potency and that is regarded as prototypic is 2,3,7,8-tetrachlorodibenzo-p-dioxin (TCDD). TCDD itself is not currently regarded as an established human teratogen, but a group of structurally related chemicals, the planar polychlorinated biphenyls (PPCBs) appear to have caused sufficient teratogenic damage in humans to be included (Table 1). Several accidental exposures to mixtures of planar and nonplanar polychlorinated biphenyls (PCBs) followed by large numbers of characteristic defects have provided the evidence necessary for PCBs to be placed on such lists of established human teratogens [2, 3]. TCDD, regarded as a prototype, is currently under very intensive investigation in terms of its potent capacity to elicit a variety of toxicologic effects including teratogenicity, and it is widely presumed that the mechanism(s) whereby planar PCBs elicit toxicologic damage occur via the same mechanism(s). Current dogma indicates that the diverse consequences of TCDD exposure for vertebrate reproduction and development are principally mediated through a multicomponent cytosolic receptor complex which includes the Ah (arylhydrocarbon) receptor, also referred to as the dioxin receptor [81]. TCDD binds with extremely high affinity to this cytosolic receptor, and the bound complex translocates to the nucleus where, in heteromeric combination with another protein referred to as Arnt, the complex binds to specific regions on 5'-upstream regions of various genes, resulting in marked changes in gene expression. The best characterized genes that are affected encode enzymes that catalyze xenobiotic biotransformation and include cytochrome P4501A1, P4501A2, P4501B1, NAD(P)H:quinone oxidoreductase (NQO1], a class 3 aldehyde dehydrogenase (ALDH3c), one of the glucuronosyl transferases (UGT1*6) and one of the subunits (Ya) of the glutathione transferases. These enzymes are markedly upregulated after exposure to TCDD or any of a number of other chemicals that likewise bind with high affinity to the Ah receptor. Such chemicals include the PPCBs mentioned above as well as the closely related planar polybrominated biphenyls (PPBBs) and other polyhalogenated dibenzodioxins, dibenzofurans, azobenzenes, azoxybenzenes and naphthalenes, collectively referred to as halogenated aromatic hydrocarbons (HAHs). In addition, however, chemicals less structurally related but which also bind the Ah receptor with high affinity and induce the same spectrum of enzymes include the notoriously carcinogenic polycyclic aromatic hydrocarbons (PAHs) of which benzo(a)pyrene and 3-methylcholanthrene are prototypes, certain dietary flavones of which β-naphthoflavone is a prototype, certain dietary indoles of which indole-3-carbinol is a prototype and xanthines of which caffeine is a (weakly binding) prototype. If the hypothesis for mechanism of elicitation of teratogenic effects by PPCBs is correct, one would expect all Ah receptor-binding ligands to produce at least some of the same kinds of teratogenic effects as TCDD, the prototype ligand. Such a generalization, however, does not appear to apply to the PAHs, flavones, indoles and xanthines for reasons that are not yet understood. The generalization does appear to apply for the other mentioned (structurally closely related) ligands, however.

The coplanar HAHs appear to produce very similar toxicologic effects in experimental animals, including a characteristic "wasting syndrome" (progressive anorexia with body fat/weight loss), involution of lymphoid tissues (e.g. thymus) with concomitant immunosuppression, hepatotoxicity (e.g. hepatoporphyria), epidermal pathologies (chloracne in humans), gastric lesions, urinary tract hyperplasia and tumor promotion. Dysmorphogenic effects observable in animal experiments are also similar and include cleft palate, hydronephrosis, thymic hypoplasia, genital malformations, polydactyly and so on. As mentioned above, the PCBs are now on most lists of established human teratogens [1–6]. "Cola-colored" infants (hyperpigmented skin, gingivae and nails) with low birth weights, hypoplastic nails, abnormal hair, teeth and gums and enlarged eyelid sebaceous glands were born to mothers in Kyushu, Japan, who had ingested cooking oil contaminated with mixtures of both planar and nonplanar polyhalogenated biphenyls (Kanechlor). Adults who ingested the contaminated cooking oil developed chloracne, a skin condition also known to be caused by TCDD. A more recent outbreak in Taiwan resulted in 39 cases with similar birth anomalies. Importantly, the exposed children exhibited deficits in cognitive development and behavioral abnormalities, again implicating the human conceptal brain as an important target [82].

It appears at present that the only seriously considered mechanistic hypothesis (as a primary mechanism) for the teratogenic effects of PPCBs involves interaction with the Ah receptor as described above. Relatively recent observations that tend to support this idea include detection of Ah receptors in embryonic tissues ([83] and cited references) and inducibility of P4501A1 and 1B1 in human embryonic tissues [65]. Such results tend to satisfy the question of expression and function of the Ah receptor in embryonic target tissues and are consistent with the hypothesis but leave open questions pertaining to the relationships between the regulation of specific genes and observable effects (pathogenesis). Of particular interest in this regard is the observed capacity of Ah receptor ligands to induce genes coding for a number of growth factors including c-fos, c-jun, jun-D, jun-B, transforming growth factors α, β, c-erbA and others (expression of more than 30 genes is known to be affected by TCDD exposure). Elucidation of the events that occur between receptor binding and appearance of specific birth defects will undoubtedly occupy the energies of investigators for several years to come.

6.10   Steroidal and nonsteroidal sex hormones

Chemicals with biological effects mimicking hormonal activities can be either endobiotics or synthetic xenobiotics; thus both excesses and deficiencies can be expected to result in developmental abnormalities. Only excess exposures are considered here, although it should be noted that deficiencies, particularly of steroidal androgens, are well known to cause birth defects (pseudohermaphroditic femininization of male conceptuses) experimentally, and chemical antiandrogens such as cyproterone acetate, an androgen receptor antagonist, produce such effects predictably and consistently. Of hormonal chemicals, only androgens and estrogens and their synthetic analogs are currently regarded as established human teratogens (not considering the retinoids), even though several others are known to exhibit effective teratogenicity in experimental animals. Discussion will be focused on the androgenic and estrogenic agents.

6.10.1   Androgens

Of all chemical teratogens, androgenic steroids may be the best established and are also some of the best understood, at least from the viewpoint of primary causative mechanisms. They elicit teratogenic effects in all species that have been investigated, and do so in a highly predictive and consistent fashion. In humans, frank effects on the morphology of the external genitalia (clitoromegaly, labial enlargement, labioscrotoal fusion etc.) are usually observed in fetal/infant females only after maternal exposure to relatively high doses of potent androgens such as testosterone, methyltestosterone, danazol and so on. However, cases of female masculinization *in utero* have also been reported after exposures to norethindrone and ethisterone [2, 3], progestins with relatively weak androgenic potency. Norethindrone and ethisterone have been heavily used in oral contraceptive preparations; ethisterone has been largely replaced. Concern for the capacity of oral contraceptives containing progestins with androgenic activity was once high but has now largely abated, apparently due to lack of reported cases in the context of very heavily used drugs by women of child-bearing age.

The morphologic defects elicited by androgens are very heavily selective for the developing external genitalia (pseudohemaphroditic masculinization of female conceptuses) with very few other morphologic abnormalities (limb defects etc., quite probably non-causally related) reported for humans. Exposure between the 8th and 13th weeks of gestation is regarded as the critical period, although certain manifestations of masculinization (e.g. phallic enlargement) can occur with later exposures. The ovaries appear normally not be affected, but the uterus may be small or, in extreme cases, absent. The masculinizing effects described for humans are very similar to those obtained experimentally in animals. A full description has been given by Wilkins et al. [84]. For mild cases of androgen-induced masculinization or virilization, regression of the anomaly can be "almost total", and many of those affected appear to mature as fertile females [3, 84]. For severe cases, corrective surgery is often of great benefit. Severity, as expected, has been shown to be dose-related, resulting in varying degrees of masculinization.

In experimental animals, excess prenatal exposures to androgenic agents also appear capable of causing behavioral changes via changes in programming in the CNS. These are usually manifest as increased aggressiveness and "masculinized" behavior. Currently, there is no good literature documentation for such an effect having been produced by administered androgenic agents in humans. Evidence for the capability of excess prenatal androgen exposure to produce a "hypermasculinizing" effect on male conceptuses and offspring has precedent in animal experimentation as well as in experience with the adrenogenital syndrome in humans. Again, such effects elicited by androgenic chemicals administered to humans appear not to have been reported. From a theoretical viewpoint, such effects would not be unexpected.

In terms of mechanisms, androgens exert their effects via binding to an intracellular (nuclear) protein receptor; the steroid-receptor complex then binds to specific hormonal regulatory elements that are 5'-upstream from the transcription start site of various genes. This binding can result in increased transcription of the gene, and increased quantities of enzymes and other proteins required for the masculinization process are thereby elaborated. The androgen receptor is a typical member of the superfamily of steroid/thyroid/retinoid/D_3 (zinc-finger) receptors. It is encoded by a gene on the X chromosome and contains androgen-binding, DNA-binding and functional domains [85]. Mutations of this receptor impair virilization of male conceptuses, resulting in feminization. Thus, the initiating mechanism for virilizing effects of administered androgenic chemicals is very well understood, but subsequent events occurring between receptor binding and specific morphologic changes (pathogenesis) are not yet well understood and will require considerable further research.

6.10.2   Estrogens

The dysmorphic teratogenic effects of estrogens, like the androgens, also appear confined largely to the external genitalia, although cardiac anomalies, cleft palate, eyelid defects, mammary gland abnormalities and other extragenital defects have been reported in association with estrogen exposures. The degree to which estrogen exposure is actually causal for such defects, however, has not been definitively established. Pseudohermaphroditic feminization of male conceptuses of experimental animals has been reported on numerous occasions as might be expected, but paradoxical masculinization of female conceptuses has also been reported on several occasions in both experimental animals and humans [2, 3]. Administration of estriol reportedly produced feminized males and masculinized females in the same rat litters [3]. In humans, eight cases of masculinization (regarded as "paradoxical", since estrogens have no androgenic properties) of female fetuses and offspring following exposures *in utero* to estrogenic substances have been reported. Thus, the transplacental effects of estrogens on genital development appear to be far less straightforward than the effects of androgens, and mechanistic explanations are far more difficult.

For cases in which feminization of male conceptuses and offspring are observed in association with exposure to estrogens *in utero*, the external genitalia as well as the gonads are underdeveloped. The Wolfian ducts, epididymes, seminal vesicles and prostate gland are also underdeveloped; cryptorchidism, hypospadias, ambiguous genitalia and various testicular changes also have been reported. For cases of masculinization of female conceptuses and offspring, the effects described above for androgen-induced masculinization appear generally to apply.

By far the most publicized effect resulting from prenatal exposure to estrogens was the 1970s epidemic of clear cell vaginal and cervical adenocarcinomas appearing in human female offspring of mothers given diethylstilbestrol (or similar synthetic, non-steroidal estrogens) during their pregnancies, particularly prior to the 18th week of gestation. This topic, together with an updated and complete account of associated abnormalities, has been reviewed recently by Mittendorf [86]. The average age for appearance of the carcinomas was 19, but they appeared as early as age 7 and as late as age 42 (91% were between the ages of 15 and 27]. Apparently, no abnormalities were obvious at the time of parturition or even several years thereafter; thus this represents an excellent example of a covert, delayed defect. Malignant adenocarcinomas were relatively rare, occurring in an estimated less than 0.1% of known exposures; however, exposures initiated after the 18th week of gestation appeared not to result in any increase in incidence of adenocarcinomas. Numerous other, perhaps in many cases less serious, effects, however, have also been reported. In females, these include vaginal adenosis occurring in a high percentage (>30%; ~73% if during the first 2 months of gestation) of exposures, irregular menses, decreased fertility, gestational bleeding, cervicovaginal abnormalities including cervical erosions, ridges, hoods and cocks combs, squamous cell dysplasias, carcinoma *in situ*, T-shaped uteri with a variety of uterine lesions, premature deliveries (with associated concomitant increase in perinatal mortality), increased spontaneous abortions and ectopic pregnancies, and other indices of poor pregnancy outcome. Diethylstilbestrol has been described as a "mullerian tract teratogen" [86].

In the male offspring of diethylstilbestrol-exposed women, no cases of genital cancer appear to be causally associated (as was earlier feared and expected), but numerous other genital-related and reproductive effects have been reported. These include epididymal cysts, hypoplastic penis, hypotrophic testes and capsular induration of the testes as the most common and appearing in approximately 25% of exposed cases. Also reported have been decreased semen volume, decreased sperm density and motility, "seriously pathologic semen", decreased fertility, infertility and penile urethral abnormalities. Thus, the estrogens offer an excellent example of covert, delayed functional teratogenicity in which the reproductive function can be markedly affected in both males and females. It seems likely that all potent estrogens, including closely related structural stilbene (nonsteroidal estrogen) analogs as well as steroidal estrogens, would exhibit the same kinds of defects, but the best documentation for such at present is with diethylstilbestrol.

By what mechanisms do estrogens elicit their teratogenic effects? In terms of their feminizing effects on male conceptuses, it seems most reasonable to presume that this is due to an antiandrogen effect. Pharmacologically, it is well known that estrogens will antagonize many of the effects of androgens. The precise mechanisms by which this antagonism occurs in terms of male conceptal genital development are not completely understood, but part of the effect may be due to suppression of the release of luteinizing hormone from the anterior pituitary gland. Interactions may also occur via interactions at the receptor level. In terms of mechanisms for their "paradoxical" masculinizing effects on female conceptuses, an even more puzzling scenario is encountered. It seems possible that a masculinizing effect could be due to alterations in androgen metabolism in conceptal target tissues (inhibited breakdown?) or/and to possible interactions at the receptor/gene level. The fact that the masculinizing effect has been termed "paradoxical" reveals the current lack of understanding pertaining to a mechanism(s) for the effect.

In terms of transplacental carcinogenesis, it has been suggested [3] that "the chemical may act to sensitize the proliferating stroma of the lower mullerian duct so that it is incapable of fostering upgrowth of urogenital sinus epithelium covering the vagina and cervical portico by 18 weeks when this event should occur. The drug may also preferentially affect the stroma of the developing cervix". The fact that the nature of the time course for appearance of the carcinoma resembles a regimen for tumor initiation and promotion has led to the idea [86] that a diethylstilbestrol metabolite may act as an electrophilic tumor initiator *in utero* with the promoting influence being later provided by estrogens secreted at and after the menarche. *In utero*, diethylstilbestrol would tend to accumulate (and thus produce its most significant effects) in uterine and cervical tissues by virtue of high-affinity receptor binding. The merit of this suggestion is presently unknown. Biotransformation/bioactivation of diethylstilbestrol to reactive, electrophilic intermediates is known to occur and can also occur in embryonic tissues [14], thus supporting the idea that diethylstilbestrol could act as a tumor-initiating agent during the early stages of gestation. Investigations of the dysmorphogenic effects of estrogens in cultured rodent embryos have indicated a highly important role for biotransformation/bioactivation of the estrogens studied [87]. It would appear at present, however, that our understanding of mechanisms whereby estrogens elicit untoward effects on developing conceptuses is very primitive and requires much further investigation.

6.11   Coumarin derivatives

Coumarin derivatives, sometimes also referred to as coumadin derivatives, are used quite extensively as oral anticoagulants and include the following substances: bishydroxycoumarin (dicoumarol), warfarin – regarded as the prototype and by far the most frequently prescribed of the group, phenprocoumon, ethyl biscoumacetate and acenocoumarol. The latter three agents are not generally available in the United States but are prescribed in Europe and other parts of the world. All are effective anticoagulants that inhibit coagulation via actions as antagonists of vitamin K. Only warfarin is regarded as an established human teratogen among this group of chemicals. However, the data available to date suggest that all of these coumarin derivatives produce very similar pharmacological and toxicological (including teratogenic) effects that now appear, for the most part, to be generally dependent on antagonism of vitamin K. Thus, they are considered together, but with emphasis on warfarin.

Exposure of humans to warfarin during the first trimester of gestation, particularly during organogenesis, can result in a birth defect syndrome characterized by nasal hypoplasia and stippled epiphyseal calcifications of the bone that resemble chondrodysplasia punctata. Skeletal defects and abnormalities of the ears also have been commonly reported, and together these abnormalities constitute the "classical" set of defects referred to as "warfarin embryopathy". Exposure during the second and third trimesters can elicit abnormalities in the CNS that include microcephaly, cerebral agenesis, ventricular dilatation, Dandy-Walker malformation, midline cerebellar atrophy and others [2, 3]. Administered late in gestation, warfarin can produce fetal and/or neonatal hemorrhage as a natural consequence of its anticoagulant effect. Hemorrhaging can result in intrauterine death even when plasma levels of warfarin (or other oral anticoagulants) are within the therapeutic range. Thus, it appears that three separate types of defects can be elicited – these are subsequently referred to as (1) "classical" defects, (2) CNS defects and (3) hemorrhagic defects. In terms of mechanisms, evidence is increasing that the "classical" defects (especially the stippled epiphyses and skeletal abnormalities) and the hemorrhagic defects occur via a similar mechanism. The earliest proposals for mechanisms of the classical defects were via inhibition of blood clotting resulting in microhemorrhages in the immature cartilage with subsequent scarring and calcification [88]. It was observed, however, that the critical period of exposure for classical defects was approximately 6–9 weeks of gestation, prior to the appearance of warfarin-sensitive clotting factors [89 and cited references). Hall et al. [89] theorized that warfarin produced the early (classical) defects by virtue of its capacity to inhibit the vitamin K-dependent carboxylation of a protein then referred to as "bone Gla protein" (BGP). The protein, secreted by osteoblasts, binds to hydroxyapatite in the extracellular bone matrix. In the absence of vitamin K, BGP remains in a decarboxylated form which has a very low affinity for hydroxyapatite, and it was suggested that warfarin, by virtue of inhibition of carboxylation of BGP, caused disordered ossification in the embryo. Similar theories were later proposed involving the carboxylation of other bone/bone matrix proteins. For example, Howe and Webster [90] proposed that inhibition of carboxylation of a matrix protein (MGP) was the critical biochemical lesion. At present, it is recognized that a relatively large number of proteins involved in bone development require vitamin K-dependent carboxylation in order to perform that function. The vitamin K-dependent carboxylation (and warfarin inhibition) of these bone/bone matrix proteins (osteopontin, sialoprotein, osteocalcin, osteonectin etc.) does not appear to affect adult bone but may well play an important role in cartilage and bone formation during prenatal development – differentiation and mineralization [91, 92]. Thus, inhibition by warfarin of the carboxylation of important bone proteins appears to occur by the same general mechanism as inhibition of the carboxylation and function of several proteins crucial to blood clotting, including coagulation factors II, VII, IX and X and anticoagulant proteins C and S. It is known that the gamma-carboxyglutamate (Gla) residues confer Ca^{++}-binding properties and functionality on these proteins. Warfarin does not directly inhibit the carboxylase-catalyzed carboxylation reaction *per se*, but the carboxylation is directly coupled to the oxidation of vitamin K to the corresponding epoxide. Warfarin inhibits the reduction of the epoxide back to the reduced hydroquinone (KH2) form, and the carboxylation reaction fails to occur in the absence of KH2. This results in undercarboxylation of proteins required for the normal function of both the coagulation proteins as well as the proteins intimately involved in bone formation and provides a coherent mechanistic explanation for both the classical and hemorrhagic defects elicitable by the coumarin class of agents. The mechanism whereby warfarin inhibits reduction of vitamin K epoxide remains to be elucidated, as do also several other aspects of the carboxylation reactions. Precisely how carboxylation is related to function also requires further research, as does the extent to which undercarboxylation of proteins may play a role in the CNS defects elicited by coumarin derivatives. A recent report that a vitamin K-dependent bone Gla protein is undercarboxylated in humans [93] is of interest with reference to the higher susceptibility of humans to the classical warfarin embryopathy.

6.12   Angiotensin-converting enzyme inhibitors

Angiotensin-converting enzyme inhibitors (ACEIs) as well as angiotensin II receptor antagonists (ATRAs) both are now regarded as agents with established fetopathic/teratogenic potential in humans, even though there are no rigorous epidemiological evidences to assist in the substantiation of this concept. Members of both classes of these agents are currently marketed as drugs used for the treatment of hypertension and are widely prescribed. Captopril (Capoten), the first ACEI to be marketed, is the prototype of the ACEIs and is a very potent inhibitor of the enzymic conversion of angiotension I to angiotensin II catalyzed by angiotensin-converting enzyme, a zinc metalloprotease. This enzyme catalyzes the hydrolysis of polypeptides to yield carboxy terminal dipeptides; angiotensin I and bradykinin appear to be principal substrates, but other polypeptides also undergo hydrolysis catalyzed by this enzyme. Captopril exhibits competitive inhibition with a Ki of approximately 1.7 nM. Inhibition of the enzyme prevents the synthesis of angiotensin II, a highly potent vasopressor agent. Several other ACEIs (some are esterified prodrugs) with very similar biochemical, pharmacologic and toxicologic effects are also used to treat hypertension and include enalapril, lisinopril, benazepril, fosinopril, quinapril, ramipril, spirapril and moexipril. Differences in teratogenic potency would likely be attributable to differences in transplacental transfer as well as to differences in enzyme affinity.

Losartan is the prototype of the ATRAs, which also include several other chemicals (e.g. candesartan, irbesartan, volsartan, telmisartan, eprosartan, zolasartan etc.). Losartan and most other clinically used ATRAs are selective AT1 receptor antagonists. These agents inhibit the contractile effects of angiotensin II on vascular smooth muscle by blocking the binding of angiotensin II to AT1 receptors in the vasculature. All of the known effects of angiotensin II are blocked *in vivo* by these agents. Thus, both ACEIs and ATRAs produce biologic effects and act as antihypertensive agents by effectively preventing the actions of angiotensin II. This also appears to be the primary mechanism whereby the fetopathic/teratogenic effects are elicited. These effects have been the subject of a relatively recent and thorough, detailed review of the teratogenicity of ACEIs by Barr [94]. *In utero* exposure to ACEIs or ATRAs is capable of causing oligohydramnios, fetal calvarial hypoplasia, fetal pulmonary hypoplasia, fetal growth retardation, fetal death, prolonged neonatal hypotension, neonatal anuria and neonatal death. Histological examinations consistently indicate renal tubular dysgenesis. Of special interest is the fact that such effects appear to be produced almost exclusively after the first trimester, of pregnancy, the period when most chemicals produce their most profound teratogenic and conceptotoxic effects. The principal underlying pathogenetic mechanism for such effects appears to be fetal hypotension, which, from a theoretical point of view, would be capable of causing each of the described effects and which in turn is caused by blockade of the highly potent hypertensive effects of angiotensin II. The structures affected are highly dependent upon an adequate supply of blood and oxygen. This mechanistic scenario suggests that any agent capable of inducing fetal hypotension should also be capable of eliciting the same spectrum of fetotoxic and teratogenic effects (described above) elicited by ACEIs and ATRAs. While there currently appears to be no rigorous experimental evidence in the open literature to support this idea, it seems very likely that such could be the case. Other contributing mechanisms such as inhibition of bradykinin synthesis or altered prostaglandin metabolism [94, 95] remain a possibility, but thus far there appear to have been no data published in the open literature that would convincingly support the involvement of other contributing mechanisms. Recent studies of the teratogenic effects of losartan ([96] and cited references) support the inherently logical idea that ACEIs and ATRAs produce fetotoxicity via the same basic mechanism – prevention of the potent vasopressor effects of angiotensin II. Thus, the basic underlying mechanisms whereby these chemicals produce teratogenic effects appear to be reasonably well (although certainly not completely) understood at present. Much remains to be learned in terms of pathogenesis as well of other possible contributory mechanisms. As with several other established human teratogens (e.g. alcohols, antithyroidal agents, tetracyclines, aminoglycoside antibiotics, coumarin derivatives, cocaine, methylene blue), the period of greatest danger of exposure to these agents appears to be during the latter part – second and third trimesters – of pregnancy.

6.13   Recreational agents

Chemicals and agents often self-administered by members of the populace to induce pleasurable responses are commonly referred to as "recreational" agents and drugs or sometimes as drugs of abuse. Substances so utilized that have been particularly implicated in the causation of birth defects in humans include ethyl alcohol, tobacco products (e.g. cigarette smoking) and cocaine. Rigorous evaluation of the teratogenic potential of individual chemicals among these and other recreational agents in human populations is particularly difficult because of the possible involvement and interactions of numerous other risk factors. For example, concomitant exposure to various combinations of ethanol, cigarette smoke, cocaine and other recreational chemicals is the rule rather than the exception. For the same reason, elucidation of mechanisms whereby such agents elicit birth defects in humans is also very difficult. In this section, tobacco and tobacco products and cocaine will be considered. Ethyl alcohol was discussed in Section 6.5, above.

6.13.1   *Tobacco and tobacco products*
Increasingly it is accepted that tobacco and tobacco products are capable of eliciting serious birth defects in human populations [1–6] – the notable exceptions to this generalization being those who derive financial profit from sales of tobacco and tobacco products. It has been estimated that, after eliminating all other contributing variables, maternal smoking accounts for an annual toll in the United States of somewhere between 19,000 and 141,000 deaths *in utero* and between 1900 and 4800 deaths during or immediately after parturition [97]. Increased incidences of prematurity, growth retardation with varying degrees of persistency, mental retardation and behavioral deficits also have been the most frequently implicated non-fatal sequelae, but numerous other defects have also been associated. These include increased cancer risk, reduced reproductive function upon achievement of reproductive age, anencephaly, cardiovascular abnormalities and urogenital anomalies. Recent studies (e.g. [98] and cited references) have provided additional evidence that risks are increased in cases of combined paternal and maternal smoking.
Smoking of tobacco results in exposure of the pregnant female and her conceptus to a very large number (>500) of chemicals, many of which have

been studied as potent toxic agents. Agents in cigarette smoke that have been most heavily implicated as embryotoxic and fetotoxic agents include cadmium, nicotine, carbon monoxide, polynuclear aromatic hydrocarbons, nitrosamines, anabasine (a potent animal teratogen), cyanides, organic aldehydes, acids and bases as well as others. It must be appreciated that each of such chemicals or classes of chemicals could feasibly contribute to birth defect causation via a separate set of mechanisms that could be complexly interactive. Thus, attempts to define "a mechanism" for the teratogenic effects of tobacco and tobacco products is not realistic. At present, attempts to define mechanisms of embryotoxic and fetotoxic effects of individual components are progressing (albeit slowly), and a number of mechanistic factors can be tentatively invoked. Nicotine, for example, appears capable of eliciting conceptal hypoxia and ischemia by virtue of its ability to produce uterine vasoconstriction, resulting in decreased perfusion of conceptal tissues. Tolson et al. [99] have recently shown that postnatal but not prenatal nicotine exposure combined with neonatal hypoxia can interact to produce cardiac cell damage. Carbon monoxide could contribute to hypoxic effects via competition with molecular oxygen for binding to hemoglobin. Carbon monoxide binds with roughly 200 times the affinity of molecular oxygen and thus effectively prevents the hemoglobin-mediated transport of oxygen to conceptal tissues. Cyanides could further contribute by virtue of their capacity to inhibit electron transport through the mitochondrial electron transport system. Cigarette smoking is also known to result in marked increases in rates of conversion of polynuclear aromatic hydrocarbons (present in cigarette smoke) to reactive electrophilic intermediates via induction of Family 1 P450 cytochromes, and this feasibly also could contribute significantly to conceptotoxic and teratogenic effects [100]. It is clear, however, that in spite of advances in knowledge concerning biologic and toxicologic effects of tobacco and cigarette smoke components, an enormous amount of research remains to be accomplished before we will have a definitive understanding of the principal mechanisms whereby tobacco and tobacco products elicit teratogenic effects. A scenario involving interactions of multiple contributory mechanisms by several toxic chemicals seems highly likely at present.

6.13.2 Cocaine

Although the teratogenicity of cocaine in humans has long been regarded as controversial, it appears that most of the controversy lies in definitions of the term "teratogenicity". With the definitions presented at the beginning of this review, there now seems little doubt that cocaine should be regarded as an established human teratogen, and it is so regarded by most experts in the field [1–5]. As a result of recent investigations [101] it was concluded that if a recognizable "cocaine syndrome" exists that could be characterized dysmorphologically or anthropometrically, its occurrence would seem infrequent. Nevertheless, it was agreed that fetal growth retardation – especially reduced growth in head circumference with altered prosencephalic development – now appears to be a consistent finding in cocaine users. Also, with respect to morphologic abnormalities, a meta-analysis of 23 studies indicated a significant risk of genitourinary defects [102]. The greatest concern at present, however, appears to lie in a consideration of functional deficits, particularly functional deficits involving the CNS. A neonatal neurological syndrome that includes abnormal sleep, tremor, poor feeding, irritability and occasional seizures has been reported to the extent that it seems probable that a cause-effect relationship involving prenatal cocaine exposure is involved. A concern for persistent effects on mentation and behavior is also prevalent, and more and better studies of this aspect are clearly needed. Animal studies also indicate that functional defects may be of greater concern than morphologic abnormalities elicitable by cocaine. It is of both mechanistic and clinical interest and importance that the conceptotoxic effects of cocaine appear to be greatest during the second and third rather than the first trimester of pregnancy. With respect to mechanisms whereby cocaine may be capable of causing birth defects, its capacity to inhibit neuronal uptake of norepinephrine has been the most frequently implicated as a principal cause. Inhibition of norepinephrine uptake results in adrenergic α1 receptor agonistic effects which can produce a profound vasoconstriction. Vasoconstriction involving the uterine, placental and fetal vasculature in turn leads to reductions in fetal vasculature perfusion with resultant deficiencies in conceptal tissue oxygenation and tissue damage. It is thus of interest that, in experimental animals, cocaine appears to cause the same type of hind limb abnormalities that are producible by vascular clamping, α1-adrenergic agonists, epinephrine, uterine handling following laparotomy and by hyperbaric oxygen. Fantel et al. [103] suggested that intermittent (episodic) exposures to cocaine could result in reperfusion hyperoxic effects on rodent hind limbs – analogous to the extensively investigated reperfusion effects producible in adult cardiac, cephalic and other tissues in which excess reactive oxygen species (ROS) are generated and cause tissue damage. Other investigators also have suggested that ROS-related free radicals are implicated in the conceptotoxic effects of cocaine [104, 105]. The status of these ideas has been the subject of a recent extensive review by Fantel [106]. It was concluded that much further study will be required before the exact role of ROS in cocaine-elicited birth defects can be precisely defined.

It is clear that cocaine can elicit toxic effects by a variety of other mechanisms, and it seems probable that at least some of these mechanisms would be implicated as contributory factors in the conceptotoxic effects producible by cocaine. Related to its local anesthetic activity, cocaine can prevent the generation and conduction of nerve impulses via actions on the cell membrane. The block in conduction is effected via decreasing or preventing the large transient increases in the permeability of excitable membranes to Na^+ that normally is produced by a slight depolarization of the membrane. This action is due to direct interaction with voltage-gated Na^+ channels. In addition, cocaine can also block K^+ channels, albeit higher concentrations are required. Whether any of these actions are significantly involved in the conceptotoxic effects of cocaine is not known at present, although hypothetical scenarios for involvement are not out of the question. Cocaine is also capable of blocking neuronal dopamine uptake and dopamine transport systems and appears to alter the metabolism of a variety of neurotransmitter substances. These and other effects of cocaine are described in pharmacology textbooks, but the extent to which any of these effects are mechanistically involved in cocaine teratogenicity remains for future investigations. Because cocaine and ethanol are so frequently abused concomitantly, it is of interest that enzymatic cocaine-ethanol transesterification catalyzed by tissue carboxylesterase(s) results in the generation of cocaethylene, a metabolite that may be implicated in the mechanistic process [107]. This issue assumes increased importance in view of the opinions of several (e.g. [108] and cited references) that cocaine alone is an extremely weak neuroteratogen and may be important primarily in terms of combinatorial effects with other agents such as ethanol, tobacco smoking and so on.

6.14   Miscellaneous agents

Four chemicals not discussed above are currently listed as established human teratogens, at least on some lists regarded as authoritative [1–5]. These four substances (penicillamine, lithium, toluene and methylene blue) do not fit neatly into any of the above discussed categories. Their status as established human teratogens is, in general, more questionable; their importance in the field is not as great as judged from the numbers of citations addressing their teratogenic activities, most are not generally regarded as highly effective teratogens at doses and exposure levels approximating those normally expected for human populations, and information pertaining to mechanisms whereby they produce teratogenic effects is relatively scarce. For these reasons, agents in this category will be discussed only briefly.

6.14.1   Penicillamine

This substance (D-β,β-dimethylcysteine), a metabolite of penicillin, has seen fairly extensive use in the treatment of heavy metal poisoning, especially for arsenic, lead, copper and mercury and some cadmium poisoning cases. It is a metal chelating agent that also has been used to chelate copper in the treatment of Wilson's disease (hepatolenticular degeneration). It also effectively chelates zinc, which may feasibly be related to its teratogenic effects. It crosses membranes readily and is orally effective. It is also capable of forming a relatively water-soluble cysteine-penicillamine mixed disulfide which is the basis for its use in the treatment of cystinuria. Uses in the treatments of rheumatoid arthritis, primary biliary cirrhosis and scleroderma appear related to its immunomodulating properties. In experimental animals (rats), as well as apparently also in humans, prenatal exposure to penicillamine can result in an unusual kind of abnormality referred to a cutis laxa. This is characterized by a wrinkled and folded skin that gives the general appearance of senescence and shows similarities to the Ehlers-Danlos syndrome. Lax skin, joint hyperflexibility, vein fragility, varicosities and impaired wound healing are each characteristic (but not always primary) abnormalities and are indicative of a generalized connective tissue defect. The effects in humans are reportedly largely reversible, but only five cases have been reported and three of the infants did not survive. It has been suggested that the mechanism for the elicitation of the defect is via chelation of copper to deplete copper stores in the body, resulting in the derangement of normal collagen biosynthesis [109]. It is established that copper stores are depleted and that collagen synthesis is abnormal, but the interrelationships between these two phenomena appear not to have been well defined, and the precise manner in which they may be mechanistically involved in the teratogenic effects observed is also not understood at present. In experimental animals, penicillamine interferes with condensation of both collagen and elastin cross-links by compressing free lysine-derived aldehydes [109], and these effects also may feasibly be involved. Clearly, much remains to be learned concerning mechanistic aspects.

6.14.2   Lithium salts

Concern for teratogenic effects of lithium salts at the exposure levels and dosage regimens normally encountered in therapy (primarily for treatment of manic-depressive illness – bipolar disorder) appears to be steadily decreasing. Unfortunately, the decreased concern does not appear to be due to the results of recent investigations demonstrating a lack of effective teratogenicity. Also, the known toxic effects of higher dosages and exposures to lithium salts, lack of long-term follow-up studies of persistence of functional deficits and the possible interactive effects with other agents should counteract complacency. Currently recommended adjuncts or alternatives to lithium therapy in bipolar disorder are valproic acid and carbamazepine, two agents that are also regarded as established human teratogens. The use of natriuretics and/or low sodium diets in combination with lithium therapy can significantly contribute to maternal and neonatal lithium intoxication.

Lithium is known to have several effects on thyroid function, the most important of which appear to be decreased secretion of thyroxine and triiodothyronine [110]. As such, lithium salts may be regarded as antithyroid agents, and teratogenic effects would be expected to include those discussed for other antithyroidals discussed in Section 6.6 above. It is thus noteworthy that fetal/neonatal goiter is frequently mentioned as a concomitant of exposure to lithium during pregnancy – particularly during the latter part of gestation [1–5]. As with other antithyroidals, substantial concern for persistent effects on mentation and behavior must therefore also be reserved for lithium salts.

On the other hand, diminished concerns for the cardiovascular abnormalities that have been historically attributable to prenatal lithium exposure during early gestation appear to be somewhat justified. The risk of Ebstein''s anomaly (malformed tricuspid valve, often with a septal defect) may be increased – estimated as not above 1 per 5000 versus 1 per 20,000 as basal risk – but is detectable *in utero* and is often surgically correctable. Several other kinds of defects have been "associated" with prenatal lithium exposures, but cause-effect relationships have not been established. Mechanistic aspects of lithium-elicited teratogenic effects have not yet received sufficient investigative attention to warrant substantive comments and can therefore only be described as speculative at present.

6.14.3 Toluene

This chemical is one of the most recent additions to lists of established human teratogens [2]. Microcephaly, CNS dysfunction, growth retardation, blunted fingertips and craniofacial and limb abnormalities appear to be the defects most frequently associated with *in utero* toluene exposures, although several others also have been reported. Often, the craniofacial abnormalities resemble those of fetal alcohol syndrome. Exposures can be "recreational", exemplified by toluene sniffing, workplace-related, exemplified by exposures to "organosilicon" varnishes, laboratory environments or product handling. In adults, the very high levels of toluene encountered by glue sniffers can result in cerebellar damage as well as changes in CNS integrative functions. The CNS appears to be a prime target for toluene toxicity. Although the teratogenic potency appears to be low, exposure levels encountered in the above-described situations can be very high and are thus not extremely uncommon. More detailed descriptions of the teratogenic effects associated with toluene exposure have appeared in the relatively recent literature [111–113].

This author is unaware of reported investigations that have focused on mechanistic aspects of the teratogenic effects of toluene. Elicited developmental defects may be due to the general solvent properties inherent in such organic chemicals and/or may also be due to more specific effects elicited by toluene metabolites, although most toluene metabolites appear to have a low order of toxicity. The primary route of metabolism is oxidation at the methyl group followed by a series of oxidations leading to the generation of benzoic acid. Benzoic acid undergoes conjugation with glycine to yield hippuric acid, which is readily excretable in the urine. Generation of toxic reactive intermediary metabolites appears not to have been reported, and toluene has tested negatively as a mutagen in the Ames test. It also appears to be only very weakly or negatively genotoxic in other systems. Wood [114] has recently reviewed toluene toxicity. At present, it seems safe to assert that any descriptions of the mechanism(s) whereby toluene elicits teratogenic effects must remain speculative. Much future research will be needed to provide substantiated, definitive statements.

6.14.4   Methylene blue

This redox dye is also a very recent addition to lists of established human teratogens [2]. It acts as a weak cyanide antidote, presumably by virtue of its capacity to accelerate the conversion in vivo of hemoglobin to methemoglobin, which has a far higher affinity than hemoglobin for cyanide and thus diverts the effects of cyanide from the mitochondrial electron transport systems to binding with methemoglobin. Interestingly, this chemical can also act as a reducing agent in vitro to facilitate the reduction of methemoglobin and its action as a cyanide antidote is thus not completely understood. In humans, the teratogenic effects reported have followed amniocentesis-associated intra-amniotic injections of methylene blue. Three separate groups [115–117] reporting studies in The Netherlands, Australia, Italy and Great Britain reported intestinal (jejunal, most frequently) atresia in the offspring of women who had received intra-amniotic injections of methylene blue during the second trimester of their pregnancies. In twin pregnancies, intra-amniotic injections of a dye have been used to mark one twin and ensure that amniotic fluid is sampled from each sac. In virtually every verifiable case, the twin that was dye-marked was also the twin that exhibited intestinal atresia. The data reported appear to be quite convincing for a cause-effect relationship, although the extent to which intra-amniotic injections of other dyes may cause a similar effect is not entirely clear.

The mechanism(s) by which methylene blue could produce intestinal atresia is not known, but it has been suggested that it could be due to release of norepinephrine, which in turn could effect intestinal vasoconstriction with a possible spasm of the mesenteric artery. The clinical features of the defect do suggest a vascular genesis. Injections into the amniotic fluid during the third trimester have been associated with some hemolysis and hyperbilirubinemia – possibly due to conversion of hemoglobin to methemoglobin. First-trimester amniotic injections appear not to have been causally implicated in birth defects in humans. The advent of more sophisticated techniques for amniocentesis may obviate the dangers associated with intra-amniotic dye injections and, unfortunately, may also discourage further investigations of the mechanistic aspects of this interesting phenomenon.

7   Future research

It is clear that during a period of only 4 years since the previous review [1], considerable advances in our understanding of mechanisms whereby chemical agents elicit developmental defects are evident. It is also clear, however, that for many of the agents discussed, an understanding of teratogenic mechanisms is very primitive and that much research will be needed prior to acquisition of a suitable understanding. Exciting progress has been made in the understanding of or potential to understand teratogenic mechanisms involving thalidomide, and progress in understanding mechanisms for nearly all of the other discussed established human teratogens is also evident. In terms of primary, initiating biochemical and molecular mechanisms, we now appear to have a reasonable understanding for the folic acid antagonists, tetracyclines, antithyroid agents and ACEIs. A fair amount of mechanistic information is also now available for alkylating agents, base analogs, organic mercurials, androgens, retinoids, estrogens, coumarin derivatives, cocaine and perhaps lead and penicillamine. Even for those agents for which the statement must be made that mechanisms are not or only very poorly understood (alcohols, thalidomide, anticonvulsants, polyhalogenated aromatic hydrocarbons, tobacco and tobacco products, lithium, toluene and methylene blue), progress toward elucidation of mechanisms has been notable in several cases. However, it is clear, especially in terms of the elucidation of pathogenic mechanisms, that our understanding remains very poor and that considerable future research will be necessary to achieve a satisfactory understanding of both primary and pathogenic mechanisms.

8   Summary and conclusions

In this review, an attempt has been made to summarize our current understanding of the mechanisms whereby certain chemicals cause birth defects. The chemicals selected for consideration were those that have been designated as established or recognized human teratogens. It is clear that our current understanding of mechanisms whereby these agents cause teratogenic effects (birth defects) can vary dramatically from one agent to the next. Extremes include the folic acid antagonists, which are now well established as agents that produce birth defects by virtue of potent inhibition of dihydrofolate reductase as a primary biochemical mechanism. An example at the other extreme is ethanol, for which very few definitive statements can be made with regard to teratogenic mechanisms, and the probability exists that a large number of interacting, contributory mechanisms can be invoked. For nearly all chemical teratogens, the critical links in the chains of events between the initial, primary biochemical and molecular mechanistic event (e.g. dihydrofolate reductase inhibition) and the manifestations of specific abnormalities (pathogenic mechanisms) remain to be delineated. This will provide an enormous challenge for investigators for years to come.

Acknowledgments

The author wishes to acknowledge the many students and colleagues who have participated in the original research reviewed. Support from the National Institutes of Environmental Health Sciences (ES-04041, ES-07032 and ES-05861) is acknowledged.

References

1 M.R. Juchau: Progr. Drug Res. *41*, 9–50 (1993).
2 T.H. Shepard: Catalog of Teratogenic Agents, 8th ed., The Johns Hopkins University Press, Baltimore (1995).
3 J.L. Schardein: Chemically Induced Birth Defects, 2nd ed., Marcel Dekker, New York (1993).
4 J.M. Rogers and R.J. Kavlock, in: Casarett and Doull's Toxicology: The Basic Science of Poisons, 5th ed. (C.D. Klaassen, Ed.), McGraw-Hill, New York (1996), pp. 302–332.
5 J. Adams: Reprod. Toxicol. *7*, 171–175 (1993).
6 J.G. Wilson: Environment and Birth Defects, Academic Press, New York (1973).
7 H. Nau and W.J. Scott Jr.: Pharmacokinetics in Teratogenesis, vols. 1 and 2, CRC Press, Boca Raton, Florida (1987).
8 D.O. Clarke: Toxicol. Methods *3*, 223–251 (1993).
9 I. Nulman and G. Koren: Teratology *53*, 304–308 (1996).
10 International Clearinghouse for Birth Defects Monitoring Systems, Abstracts of the 22nd Annual Meetings, Teratology *53*, 273–281 (1996).
11 M. Dicker and E.A. Leighton: Am. J. Pub. Health *84*, 1433–1439 (1994).
12 C.C. Willhite, M. Dawson and U. Reichert: Drug Metab. Rev. *28*, 105–120, (1996).
13 P.G. Wells and L.M. Winn: Molec. Biol. *31*, 1–40 (1996).
14 M.R. Juchau, Q.P. Lee and A.G. Fantel: Drug Metab. Rev. *24*, 195–238 (1992).
15 M.R. Juchau: Drug Metab. Rev. (in press).
16 Paracelsus (Theophrastus ex Hohenheim Eremita): Von der Besucht, Dillingen (1567).
17 D.A. Karnofsky: Ann. Rev. Pharmacol. *5*, 447–472 (1965).
18 F. Teixeira, M.T. Hojyo, R. Arenas, M.E. Vega, R. Cortes, A. Ortiz and L. Dominguez: Lancet *344*, 196–197 (1994).
19 T.D. Stephens: Teratology *41*, 239–246 (1988).
20 R.J. D'Amato, M.S. Loughnan, E. Flynn and J. Folkman: Proc. Soc. Natl. Acad. Sci. USA *91*, 4082–4085 (1994).
21 R. Neubert, N. Hinz, R. Thiel and D. Neubert: Life Sci. *58*, 295–316 (1996).
22 A.C. Nogueira, R. Neubert, A. Felies, U. Jacob-Mueller, E. Frankus and D. Neubert: Life Sci. *58*, 337–348 (1996).
23 R.R. Arlen and P.G. Wells: J. Pharmacol. Exper. Therap. *277*, 1649–1658 (1996).
24 R.R. Arlen and P.G. Wells: Fed. Am. Soc. Exp. Biol. J. *4*, A608 (1990).
25 L. Liu and P.G. Wells: Free Rad. Biol. Med. *19*, 639–648 (1995).
26 T. Parman, C. Guoman, T.M. Bray and P.G. Wells: App. Toxicol. *30* (Suppl. 1, P. 2: The Toxicologist) *246* (No. 1260) (1996).
27 B. Vaisman: Teratology *53*, 283–284 (1996).
28 J. Ashby and H. Tinwell: Nature *375*, 453 (1995).
29 M. Lishner, D. Zemlickis, P. Degendorfer, T. Panzarella, S.B. Sutcliffe and G. Koren: Br. J. Cancer *65*, 114–117 (1992).
30 A.J. Zanov, J. Anderson, D.F. Cella, E. Zuckerman, A.B. Kornblith, J.C. Holland, A.F. Kantor and F.P. Li: Cancer *70*, 688–692 (1992).
31 J.M. Piper, E.F. Mitchell and W.A. Ray: Obstet. Gynecol. *82*, 348–352 (1993).
32 P. Burtin, A. Taddio, O. Ariburnu, T.R. Einarson and G. Koren: Am. J. Obstet. Gynecol. *172*, 525–529 (1995).
33 J. Waalen: J. Nat. Cancer Inst. *83*, 900–902 (1991).

34   H.O. Nicholson: J. Obst. Gynecol. Br. Com. *75*, 307–312 (1968).

35   J.N. Yamazaki and W.J. Schull: J. Amer. Med. Assn. *264*, 605–610 (1990).

36   D. Zemlickis, M. Lishner, R. Erlich and G. Koren. Teratogen. Carcinogen. Mutagen *13*, 139–143 (1993).

37   M. Schmidt and F.M. Salzano: Acta Genet. Med. Gemellol. (Roma) *29*, 295–297 (1980).

38   C. Harris, K.L. Stark and M.R. Juchau: Teratology *37*, 577–590 (1988).

39   R. Hiranruengchok and C. Harris: Teratology *52*, 205–214 (1995).

40   E. Chu, J.L. Grem, P.G. Johnston and C.J. Allegro: Stem Cells *14*, 41–46 (1996).

41   J.M. DeSesso and G.C. Goeringer: Teratology *45*, 271–283 (1992).

42   J.M. DeSesso and G.C. Goeringer: Teratology *43*, 201–215 (1991).

43   M.R. Juchau, Q.P. Lee and A.G. Fantel: Drug Metab. Rev. *24*, 195–238 (1992).

44   B.A. Chabner, in: Cancer Chemotherapy: Principles and Practice, 2nd ed. (B.A. Chabner and D.L. Longo, Eds.), J.P. Lippincott Co., Philadelphia (1996), pp. 234–268.

45   T. Mikita and G.P. Beardsley: Biochemistry *27*, 4698–4705 (1988).

46   R.M. Zucker, K.H. Elstein, D.L. Shuey and J.M. Rogers: Teratology *51*, 37–45 (1995).

47   D.L. Shuey, A.R. Buckalew, T.S. Wilke, J.M. Rogers and B.D. Abbott: Teratology *50*, 379–386 (1994).

48   W. Bollag: FASEB J. *10*, 938–940 (1996).

49   D.R. Soprano and K.J. Soprano: Ann. Rev. Nutr. *15*, 111–132 (1995).

50   A.L. Means and L.J. Gudas: Ann. Rev. Biochem. *64*, 201–233 (1995).

51   G.M. Morriss–Kay and N. Sokolova: FASEB J. *10*, 961–968 (1996).

52   J.M. Creech Kraft and M.R. Juchau: Drug Metab. Dispos. *23*, 1058–1072 (1995).

53   K. Eckhardt and G. Schmitt: Tox. Letts. *70*, 299–308 (1994).

54   G.V. Raymond, B.A. Buehler, R.H. Finnell and L.B. Holmes: Teratology *51*, 55–56 (1995).

55   P.G. Wells and L.M. Winn: Crit. Rev. Biochem. Mol. Biol. *31*, 1–40 (1996).

56   B.R. Danielsson, K. Danielsson and T. Tomson: Teratology *52*, 252–259 (1995).

57   M. Sato, M. Shirota and T. Nagao: Teratology *52*, 143–148 (1995).

58   G.L. Barnes Jr., B.D. Mariani, R.S. Tuan: Teratology *54*, 93–102 (1996).

59   D.K. Hansen, T.F. Grafton, S.L. Dial, T.A. Gehring and P.H. Siitonen: Teratology *52*, 277–285 (1995).

60   R.H. Finnell, G.D. Bennett, J.T. Slattery, B.M. Amore, M. Bajpai and R.H. Levy: Teratology *52*, 324–332 (1995).

61   D.K. Hansen, S.L. Dial, K.K. Terry and T.F. Grafton: Teratology *54*, 45–51 (1996).

62   W.A. Chen, K.H. Andersen and J.R. West: Teratology *50*, 250–255 (1994).

63   L.E. Kotch and K.K. Sulik: Am. J. Med. Genet. *44*, 168–176 (1992).

64   L.E. Kotch, S–Y. Chen and K.K. Sulik: Teratology *52*, 128–136 (1995).

65   M.R. Juchau and H.L. Yang: Fund. Appl. Toxicol. *34*, 166–168 (1996).

66   S.P. Carpenter, J.M. Lasker and J.L. Raucy: Molec. Pharmacol. *49*, 260–268 (1996).

67   L. Deltour, H.L. Ang and G. Duester: FASEB J. *10*, 1050–1057 (1996).

68   H. Chen, H.L. Yang, M.J. Namkung and M.R. Juchau: Teratology *54*, 12–19 (1996).

69   H. Chen, M.J. Namkung and M.R. Juchau: Alcoholism: Clin. Exp. Res. *20*, 942–948 (1996).

70   T.A. Slotkin, F.J. Seidler, R.J. Kavlock and J.V. Bartolome: Teratology *45*, 303–312 (1992).

71   J.M. Creech Kraft, C.C. Willhite and M.R. Juchau: J. Craniofac. Gen. Dev. Biol. *14*, 75–86 (1994).

72   H.F. Chambers and M.A. Sande, in: The Pharmacologic Basis of Therapeutics, 9th

ed. (J.G. Hardman and L.E. Limbird, Eds.) McGraw-Hill, New York (1996), pp. 1103–1121.

73 H.C. Neu and C.L. Bendush: J. Infect. Dis. *134*, S206–S218 (1976).

74 S.Q. Cohlan, G. Bevelander and T. Tiamsic: Am. J. Dis. Child. *105*, 453–461 (1963).

75 R.A. Goyer, in: Casarett and Doull's Toxicology: The Basic Science of Poisons, 5th ed. (C.D. Klaassen, Ed.), McGraw-Hill, New York (1996), pp. 691–736.

76 T.M. Burbacher: Appl. Toxicol. *25*, 168–171 (1995).

77 D. Bellinger: Teratology *50*, 367–374 (1994).

78 E.K. Silbergeld and L. Watson: Fund. Appl. Toxicol. *25*, 167–168 (1995).

79 E.K. Silbergeld: FASEB J. *6*, 3201–3206 (1992).

80 R.E. Peterson, H.M. Thoebald and G.L. Kimmel: Crit. Rev. Toxicol. *23*, 293–335 (1993).

81 O. Hankinson: Toxicol. *35*, 307–340 (1995).

82 Y.L. Guo, G.H. Lambert and C. Hsu: Env. Health Persp. *103*, 117–122 (1995).

83 B.D. Abbott, G.H. Perdew and L.S. Birnbaum: Toxicol. Appl. Pharmacol. *126*, 16–25 (1994).

84 L. Wilkins, H.W. Jones, G.H. Holman and R.S. Stempfel: J. Clin. Endocrinol. Metab. *18*, 559–585 (1958).

85 C. Chang, J. Kokontis and S.T. Liao: Science *240*, 324–326 (1988).

86 R. Mittendorf: Teratology *51*, 435–446 (1995).

87 B.K. Beyer, K.L. Stark, A.G. Fantel and M.R. Juchau: Toxicol. Appl. Pharmacol. *98*, 113–128 (1989).

88 W.L. Shaul, H. Emery and J.G. Hall: Am. J. Dis. Child. *129*, 360–362 (1975).

89 J.G. Hall, R.M. Pauli and K.M. Wilson: Am. J. Med. *68*, 122–140 (1980).

90 A.M. Howe and W.S. Webster: Teratology *46*, 379–390 (1992).

91 P.W. Majerus, G.J. Broze Jr., J.P. Miletich and D.M. Tollefsen, in: The Pharmacologic Basis of Therapeutics, 9th ed. (J.G. Hardman and L.E. Limbird, Eds.), McGraw-Hill, New York (1996), pp. 1341–1359.

92 B. Sommer, M. Bickel, W. Hofstetter and A. Wetterwald: Bone *19*, 371–380 (1996).

93 J.R. Cairns and P.A. Price: J. Bone Miner. Res. *9*, 1989–1997 (1994).

94 M. Barr Jr.: Teratology *50*, 399–409 (1994).

95 G.H. Williams: New Engl. J. Med. *319*, 1517–1525 (1988).

96 S.G. Spence, A.G. Zacchei, L.L. Lee, C.L. Baldwin, R.A. Berna, B.A. Mattson and R.S. Eydelloth: Teratology *53*, 245–252 (1996).

97 J.R. DiFranza and R.A. Lew: J. Fam. Pract. *40*, 385–394 (1995).

98 C.R. Wasserman, G.M. Shaw, C.D. O'Malley, M.M. Tolarova and E.J. Lammer: Teratology *53*, 261–267 (1996).

99 C.M. Tolson, F.J. Seidler, E.C. McCook and T.A. Slotkin: Teratology *52*, 298–305 (1995).

100 M.K. Sanyal, Y. Li and K. Belanger: Reprod. Toxicol. *8*, 411–418 (1994).

101 B.B. Little, G.N. Wilson and G. Jackson: Teratology *54*, 145–150 (1996).

102 L. Slutsker: Obstet. Gynecol. *79*, 778–789 (1992).

103 A.G. Fantel, C.V. Barber and B. Mackler: Teratology *46*, 285–292 (1992).

104 J.B. Fisher, R.B. Poturri, M. Collins, E. Resnick and E.F. Zimmerman: Teratology *49*, 182–191 (1994).

105 E.F. Zimmerman, R.B. Poturri, E. Resnick and J.E. Fisher: Teratology *49*, 192–201 (1994).

106 A.G. Fantel: Teratology *53*, 196–217 (1996).

107 M.R. Brzezinski, T.L. Abraham, C.L. Stone, R.A. Dean and W.F. Bosron: Biochem. Pharmacol. *48*, 1747–1755 (1994).

108 W.A. Chen, R.E. McAlhany Jr., S.E. Maier and J.R. West: Teratology *53*, 145–151 (1996).
109 F.W. Rosa: Teratology *33*, 127–131 (1986).
110 H. Takami: Int. Surg. *79*, 89–90 (1994).
111 G.L. Arnold, R.S. Kirby, S. Langendoerger and L. Wilkins–Haug: Pediatrics *93*, 216–220 (1994).
112 J.M. Donald, K. Hooper and C. Hopenhayn-Rich: Perspectives *94*, 237–244 (1991).
113 H.J. Klimisch, J. Hellwig and A. Hoffman: Arch. Toxicol. *66*, 373–381 (1992).
114 R. Wood, in: Neurobehavioral Toxicity: Analyses and Interpretation (B. Weiss and J. O'Donoghue, Eds.), Raven Press, New York (1994), pp. 367–375.
115 U. Nicolini and G. Monni: Lancet *336*, 1258–1259 (1990).
116 P.A.L. Lancaster, E.L. Pedisich, C.C. Fisher and R.D. Robertson: I J. Perinat. Med. *20* (Suppl. 1), 262 (1992).
117 J.G. van der Pol, H. Wolf, K. Boer, P.E. Treffers, N.J. Leschot, H.A. Hey and A. Vos: Br. J. Obstet. Gynaecol. *99*, 141–143 (1992).

Progress in Drug Research, Vol. 49 (E. Jucker, Ed.)
© 1997 Birkhäuser Verlag, Basel (Switzerland)

Recent advances in potassium channel modulation

By Gillian Edwards* and Arthur H. Weston

School of Biological Sciences, G38 Stopford Building, University of Manchester, Manchester M13 9PT, UK

---

*   Author for correspondence.

1   Introduction

The opening and closing of potassium (K) channels is the basic mechanism which underlies the control of many cellular excitatory processes. Since the intracellular $[K^+]$ of approximately 150 mM is much greater than the extracellular value of 5 mM, the opening of a significant number of K channels results in K^+ efflux. This flow of ionic current dominates the influence of other ionic conductances, and the membrane potential of the cell moves towards the potassium equilibrium potential (E_K; approximately −90 mV). The resulting hyperpolarisation reduces the open probability of voltage-sensitive ion channels which are permeable to Ca^{2+} and to Na^+, resulting in inhibition of cellular functions.

In contrast, the closure of K channels which are open when the cell is in a resting or basal state primes the cell for excitation. This occurs because the normal leak of K^+ via open K channels (and which keeps the resting membrane potential slightly positive of E_K) is reduced, and depolarisation is the result.

2   K-channel classification

Native K channels have been historically classified according to their gating characteristics, their pharmacological properties and their unitary conductance. From these features, they were assigned names such as "delayed-rectifier" (K_V), "large-conductance, calcium-sensitive" (BK_{Ca}) and "ATP-sensitive" (K_{ATP}) (see [1]). More recently, however, the genes which encode both for the innermost components (α-subunits) of many subtypes of K channel [2, 3] and their β-subunits [4, 5] have been identified, and the amino acid sequences and structures of the respective gene products have been elucidated. Expression of these genes in heterologous systems such as the *Xenopus* oocyte or HEK (human embryonic kidney) 293 cells results in the formation of functional K channels, and this has allowed a classification system based on the constituent genomic products to be developed [3, 6]. Using these comparisons between cloned and native channels, most K channels can be assigned into one of two superfamilies, irrespective of their diverse electrophysiological and pharmacological properties. Superfamily 1 comprises A channels (K_A), delayed rectifiers (K_V), and both small- and large-conductance, Ca^{2+}-sensitive K channels (BK_{Ca} and SK_{Ca}, respectively). The majority of these are also voltage-sensitive, and most of their (presumed) constituent gene products are abbreviated with the nomenclature Kv1.1...1.n, Kv2.1...2.n etc.

Thus a homomultimeric channel expressed in a heterologous system from four Kv1.1 gene products is known as "Kv1.1". Channels in superfamily 2 comprise the inward rectifiers (K_{IR}) and include the ATP-sensitive K channel (K_{ATP}). Their constituent gene products are designated Kir1.1...1.n, Kir2.1...2.n, etc.

In most instances, it is not known whether native channels comprise a homo- or hetero-multimeric arrangement of α-subunits or whether these have structural features typical of superfamily 1 or 2. As an initial working hypothesis, therefore, it is usual to infer the structure of the innermost part of a native K channel by comparing its electrophysiological and pharmacological properties with those of homo- or heterotetrameric assemblies of α-subunits expressed in heterologous systems. A limitation of this approach is that some K channel gene products are endogenously expressed in *Xenopus* oocytes, and thus the expression system itself can influence the electrophysiological characteristics of the expressed channel.

3   K channel sub-types

3.1   Delayed-rectifier and A-type channels

3.1.1   Channel structure
The central part of these voltage-sensitive K channels is formed from a tetramer of polypeptide α-subunits, and each comprises six hydrophobic, membrane-spanning domains. These are linked, alternately, by extra- and intracellular hydrophilic regions, and both the amino- and carboxy termini are also located within the cell. The fourth transmembrane region (S4) is highly positively charged and is considered to function as a voltage sensor. The linker (P) between the fifth (S5) and sixth (S6) membrane-spanning domains appears to dip into the membrane and is believed to contribute to the lining of the channel pore (Fig. 1).

As with studies on sodium and calcium channels, the purification of K channel proteins has revealed not only the presence of α-subunits, which are presumed to lie at the core of the channel, but also that of additional β-subunits (Fig. 1). The β-subunits which associate with Kv-type channels appear to be intracellular. To date, at least four distinct genes encoding these subunits have been identified (*Kvβ1*, *Kvβ2*, *Kvβ3* and *Kvβ4*), and at least one of these (*Kvβ1*) is alternatively spliced, forming Kvβ1.1, Kvβ1.2 and Kvβ1.3 subunits [7]. The β-subunits appear to enhance the surface expression and stability of the α-subunits [8–10]. In addition, some β-subunits modify the voltage threshold of activation and slow deactivation of

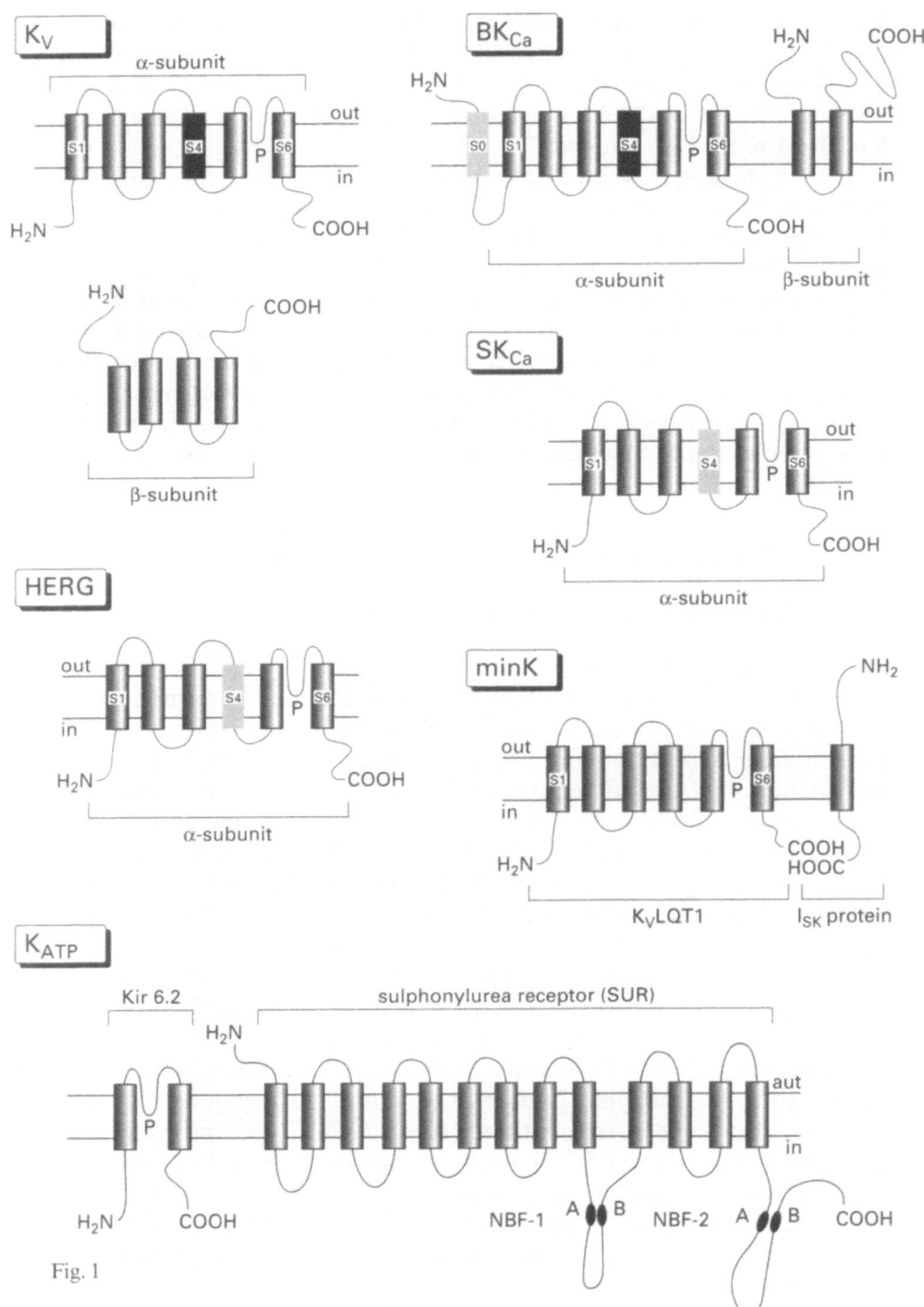

Fig. 1

the channel. They also seem able to impart the property of rapid inactivation on an otherwise non-inactivating or slowly inactivating channel, thus transforming a delayed-rectifier-type channel (such as Kv1.5) into an A-type channel [4, 5, 8].

3.1.2   Pharmacology

To date, no openers of K_V channels have been identified. Recently, however, there has been considerable progress in the recognition and development of K_V inhibitors. Many of these are peptides which have have been isolated from insect or snake toxins and which are selective inhibitors of homomultimeric K_V-like channels. In the immediate future, the primary use of many such drugs is likely to be as tools for deducing the possible distribution and role of individual α-subunits. However, recognition of the role of Kv1.3 (formerly known as the n-type K channel) in the activation of T lymphocytes [11] has led to a search for specific inhibitors of this channel and to the evaluation of their immunosuppressant potential.

In humans, the presence of antigens stimulates a sequence of events which leads to the increased synthesis of cytokines (especially IL-2) and T-lymphocyte proliferation. A critical step in this cascade is believed to be an increase in the intracellular $[Ca^{2+}]$ within the T lymphocyte which is initiated when the antigen interacts with the T-cell receptor (TCR) complex [11]. Until recently, available immunosuppressive agents were only those such as cyclosporin and FK506, which act by suppressing cytokine synthesis at a point in the reaction cascade distal to the increase in $[Ca^{2+}]_i$ (Fig. 2).

Unlike many mammalian cells in which voltage-sensitive Ca channels regulate the influx of Ca^{2+}, the entry of this ion into T lymphocytes is via voltage-insensitive Ca channels, which seem to be somehow activated by the depletion of intracellular Ca stores [12]. Thus, once activated, Ca^{2+} influx through these so-called calcium release-activated channels (CRACs) is governed by prevailing passive forces. Since the Ca^{2+} equilibrium potential (E_{Ca}) is approximately +50 mV, any reduction in the membrane potential of the lymphocyte (from a typical resting value of –60 mV to, say, –30 mV) will reduce the driving force which governs Ca^{2+} influx through any open CRACs [11]. Thus blockade of the Kv1.3 channel leads to mem-

---

Fig. 1
Diagrammatic representation of the postulated basic structures of K channel α- and β-subunits. The linking regions between the membrane-spanning segments (S) are not drawn to scale. P: pore region; NBF: nucleotide-binding fold; A and B: Walker regions. See text for channel abbreviations.

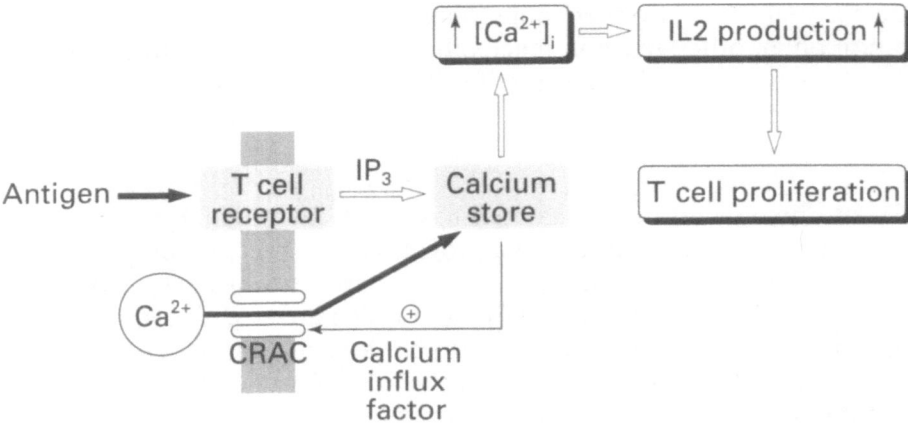

Fig. 2
Antigen-induced activation of a T-cell showing involvement of CRAC. Depolarisation of the cell by inhibition of Kv1.3 reduces calcium influx and store refilling. For further details, see text.

brane depolarisation and to a reduced inward driving force on the extra-cellular Ca^{2+} (Fig. 2).

It has been recognised for some time that charybdotoxin (ChTX; Fig. 3), one of the components of scorpion venom, is a potent inhibitor of Kv1.3 [13]. Using this information, a binding assay was developed using [125I] ChTX and a human lymphoma cell line (Jurkat T cells), and a series of non-peptide molecules was screened for their ability to displace the labelled toxin [14]. From these studies, several molecules were selected for electrophysiological experiments from which WIN 17317-3 (Fig. 3) emerged as the most potent and selective inhibitor of Kv1.3 [14, 15]. Furthermore, this agent inhibited IL-2 production by T lymphocytes [15].

Using information derived particularly from the structures of ChTX and of kaliotoxin (KTX; Fig. 3), the channel vestibule of Kv1.3 has been mapped in detail [16]. This information, together with site-directed muta-genesis of several α-subunit amino acid residues (G380, D386 and H404) within this region enabled the probable mechanism of action of WIN 17317-3 and related molecules such as CP-339,818 to be identified [17]. Based on the correlation between the inactivation time constant of mut-ated channels and their sensitivity to inhibition by CP-339,818, it seems likely that both this agent and (by inference) WIN 17317-3 block Kv1.3 by binding to the inactivated state of the channel [17]. Although WIN 17317-3 and CP-339,818 are potent inhibitors of Kv1.3 and thus of T-cell

```
MgTX   T I I N V KC TS P K Q C L P P C K A Q F G Q S A G A K C M N G K C K C Y P H
NTX    T I I N V KC TS P K Q C S K P C K E L Y G S S A G A K C M N G K C K C Y N N
KTX   GV E I N V KC SG S P Q C L K P C K D - A G M R F G - K C M N R K C H C T P -
ChTX   E F T N V SC TT S K E C WS V C Q R L H N T S R G - K C M N K K C R C Y S -
IbTX   E F T D V DC SV S K E C WS V C K D L F G V D R G - K C M G K K C R C Y Q -
```

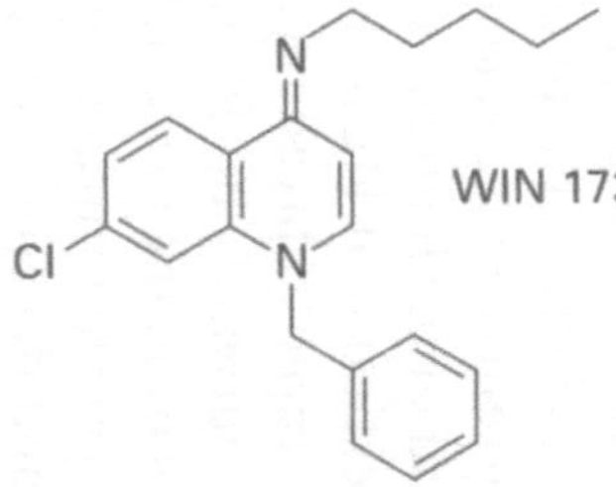

WIN 17317-3

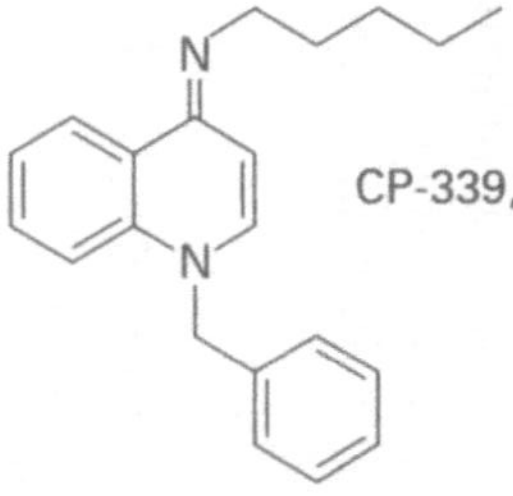

CP-339,818

Fig. 3
Structures of toxin and non-toxin inhibitors of Kv1.3. The amino acid sequence of margatoxin (MgTX) is compared with those of noxiustoxin (NTX), kaliotoxin (KTX), charybdotoxin (ChTX) and the selective BK_{Ca} inhibitor, iberiotoxin (IbTX). Sequence homologies are highlighted. The similarities between the non-toxin Sterling-Winthrop inhibitor, WIN 17317-3, and the Pfizer compound CP-339,818 are evident.

activation, CP-339,818 also reduces current flow through Kv1.4. Since this channel is expressed in the heart, it is unlikely that CP-339,818 or WIN 17317-3 would be free from cardiac side-effects (see [17]).

In parallel with these experiments, Kaczorowski and his co-workers have been searching for peptides which are selective inhibitors of Kv1.3. Although this group showed that ChTX is a potent inhibitor of this channel, it was originally described (and is still widely used) as a blocker of BK_{Ca} [18]. From these studies, margatoxin (MgTX; Fig. 3), extracted from the venom of the scorpion *Centruroides margaritatus* [19, 20], was found to be a potent inhibitor of Kv1.3 (IC_{50} approximately 50 pM) without effect on BK_{Ca} [19]. Although a peptide inhibitor of Kv1.3 would require parenteral administration, preliminary experiments have shown that intravenous infusion of MgTX into minipigs effectively suppresses immune responses [21].

3.2   The human ether-à-go-go-related gene K channel

3.2.1   Channel structure

A mutation which resulted in leg shaking in *Drosophila* allowed the identification of the underlying gene, *ether-à-go-go* (*eag*), and in heterologous systems the products of this gene form a K_V-like channel known as "eag" [22]. The α-subunits encoded by *HERG*, the human ether-à-go-go-related gene, possess six membrane-spanning segments and a voltage-sensor region (Fig. 1). However, the resulting channel is unusual for a delayed rectifier in that it passes little outward current at very depolarised potentials, resulting in a current-voltage relationship which is inwardly rectifying [23, 24]. These and other features such as its inhibition by *D*-sotalol have led to the suggestion that HERG is probably the K channel which underlies the cardiac rapid delayed rectifier current, I_{Kr} [24–26].

The unusual lack of outward current through HERG upon membrane depolarisation results from the extremely rapid inactivation of this channel [24]. However, during membrane repolarisation, channel inactivation is rapidly reversed, and deactivation (closure) occurs. Since the rate of removal of inactivation is faster than the rate of channel closure, a transient K current results, the physiological function of which may be to prevent premature afterbeats [23, 24].

Mutations in *HERG* are now believed to be responsible for one of the inherited types of the long-QT syndrome (the so-called LQT-2 form) [25, 27, 28]. This condition is characterised by delayed ventricular repolarisation during sinus rhythm (hence the long Q-T interval), with intermittent ventricular arrhythmias known as *torsades de pointes* due to the characteristic fluctuating amplitude of the QRS complex in the ECG record. Although the exact basis of the prolonged Q-T interval in patients with LQT-2 syndrome is not known for certain, it is assumed that homotetrameric assemblies of the products of the defective *HERG* gene are not fully functional and that this results in delayed repolarisation and a lengthened Q-T interval. This may also apply to heterotetrameric combinations of the normal and abnormal gene products [25].

3.2.2   *Pharmacology*

I_{Kr} is inhibited by D-sotalol, dofetilide and E4031 (Fig. 4) and these drugs also inhibit HERG (see [29]). Inhibition of I_{Kr} increases cardiac action potential duration, a strategy which reduces the probability of re-entrant arrhythmias. However, excessive prolongation of the Q-T interval can be shown experimentally to predispose to depolarising oscillations on the plateau of the cardiac potential [29], and these are believed to be the basis of *torsades de pointes*. Thus, patients suffering from an inherited LQT syndrome or in those with hypokalaemia (which predisposes them to long Q-T intervals) may be particularly at risk if treated with this group of drugs. The resulting *torsades de pointes* may be fatal.

Agents like D-sotalol, dofetilide and E4031 are open channel blockers of K_r. Since the relative contribution which this channel makes to the net repolarising current diminishes as heart rate increases, these drugs are reverse use-dependent [29]. Thus, under certain conditions, the proarrhythmic potential of agents such as D-sotalol by excessive prolongation of action potential duration at low frequencies may negate the beneficial effect of lengthening the Q-T interval at higher frequencies. Indeed, the increased incidence of sudden death associated with D-sotalol which was noted in the SWORD trials [30] may be due to this property of reverse-use dependence. Currently, the dosage of D-sotalol is restricted to the amount that results in a Q-T interval of 450–500 ms, since values greater than this may result in a higher incidence of adverse effects [25, 31].

It is worth noting that the non-sedating antihistamines terfenadine and astemizole (Fig. 4), both of which may generate cardiac arrhythmias, are potent inhibitors of HERG [32], an action which seems likely to underlie their toxic side-effects.

3.3   The minK K channel

3.3.1   *Channel structure*

In addition to the variant of the inherited long Q-T syndrome associated with HERG (LQT-2; see Section 3.2.1), another form of the disease, LQT-

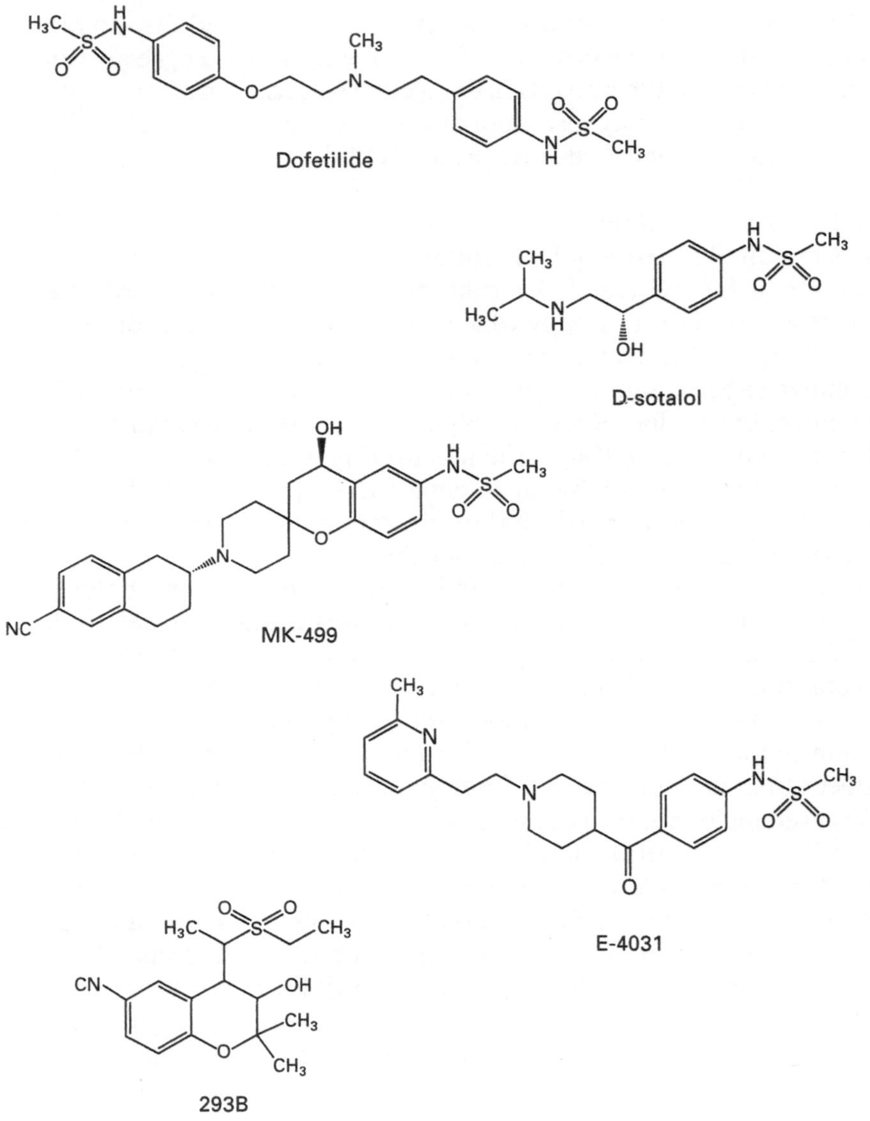

Dofetilide

D-sotalol

MK-499

E-4031

293B

Fig. 4
Structural formulae of the cardiac delayed-rectifier K channel inhibitors mentioned in the text.

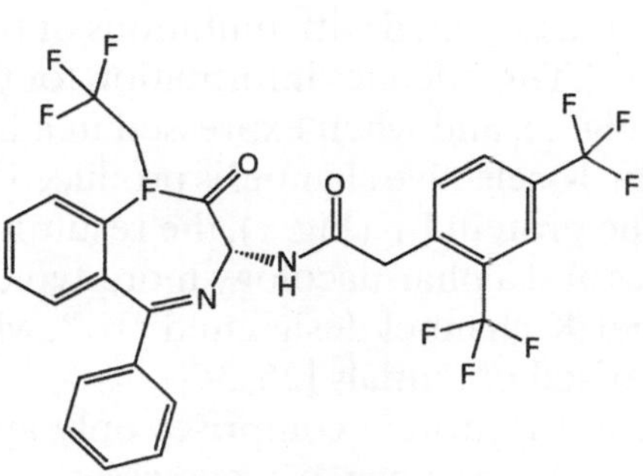

WO-09605839

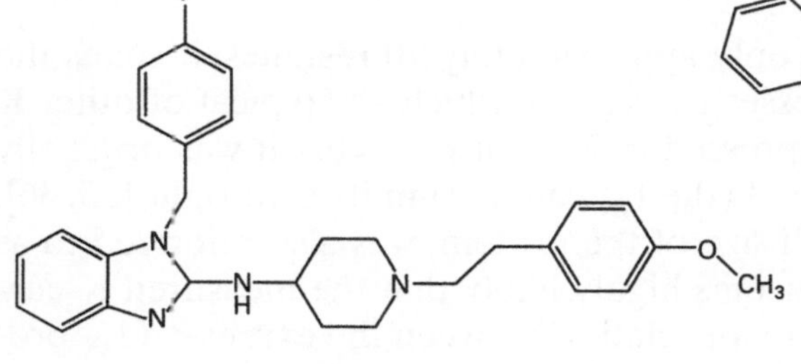

Astemizole

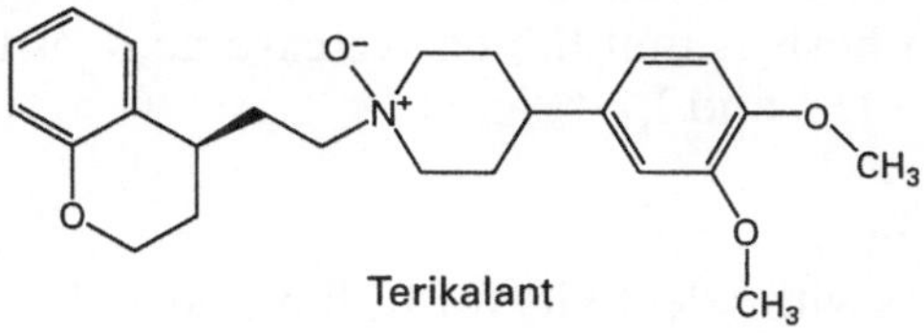

Terikalant

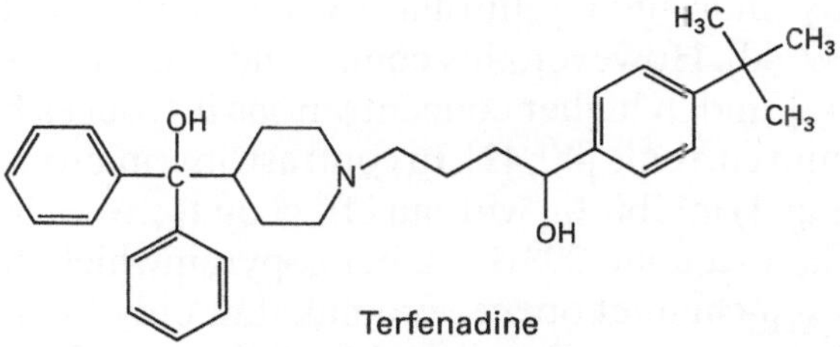

Terfenadine

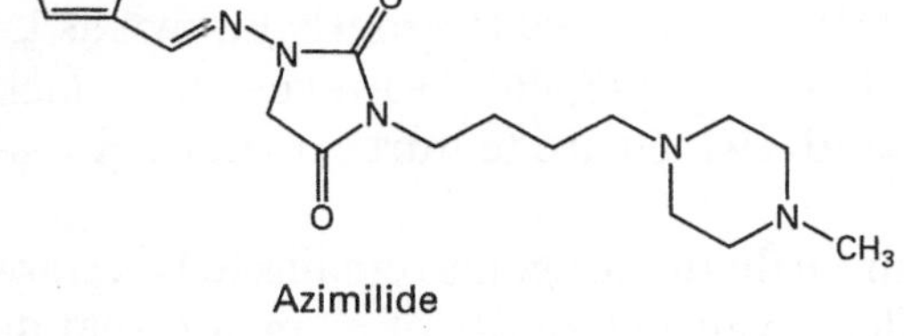

Azimilide

Fig. 4 (continued)

1, is associated with mutations of the K channel gene known as *KvLQT1* [25]. This encodes information for the production of the protein KvLQT1 (Fig. 1), and when expressed in a heterologous system, a rapidly activating K-selective channel is produced [33]. However, when co-expressed with the protein I_{sK} (Fig. 1), the resulting K channel has slow activation kinetics and a pharmacology more typical of the cardiac native delayed-rectifier K channel designated "K_s", which shows little inactivation at depolarised potentials [26, 34].

The I_{sK} protein comprises only approximately 70 residues; it spans the membrane once and possesses no regions which are typical of other K channels (Fig. 1). When expressed in *Xenopus* oocytes, it was originally believed to form a K channel (the I_{sK} channel) in its own right [35, 36], which, because of the small size of the protein, was also referrred to as "minK". However, it now seems highly likely that the measured K-current flow was the result of an association between the expressed I_{sK} protein and a gene product similar to KvLQT1 and endogenous to the oocyte [26, 34, 37]. In the absence of a systematic nomenclature scheme which encompasses a combination of KvLQT1 and I_{sK}, it seems appropriate to use the nomenclature adopted by Busch and Suessbrich [33] in which the resulting cloned channel is termed the "minK channel complex". A reasonable working hypothesis is that the native cardiac K_s is formed from a combination of KvLQT1 and I_{sK} (Fig. 1).

3.3.2   Pharmacology

To date, few modulators with selectivity for K_s have been described. Azimilide (formerly NE-10064; Fig. 4) does inhibit I_{Ks} [38] and is both antiarrhythmic and antifibrillatory in animal models of ventricular arrhythmia [39, 40]. However, this compound also inhibits I_{Kr} with a similar potency [41], and in higher concentrations it reduces both sodium and L-type calcium currents [40, 42]. In contrast, low micromolar concentrations of 293B (Fig. 4) inhibit I_{Ks} without effect on I_{Kr}, even in higher concentrations [43]. The racemate 293B is a benzopyran which differs from the prototypical K_{ATP}-channel opener cromakalim only by the substituent in the 4-position (compare Figs. 4 and 6). Other cardiac K-channel inhibitors which contain a benzopyran moiety (see Fig. 4) include terikalant (which inhibits the cardiac inward rectifier [44]) and MK-499 (formerly known as L-706000 and which blocks HERG and K_r) [45, 46]. However, these lack the substituents in positions 2, 3 and 6 which are features of many K_{ATP}-channel openers (Fig. 6).

The potential of K_s inhibitors as antiarrhythmic agents remains to be established. The slow activation and deactivation kinetics of K_s means that its relative importance in the termination of action potentials increases during tachycardia (see [29]). A relevant feature of this is that the effectiveness of K_s inhibitors would be reduced as heart rate falls, and this might act as a safeguard to prevent the proarrhythmic effect (due to early depolarisation) which is often associated with agents which prolong duration of action potential. Recent chemical developments in this field are the benzodiazepine derivatives described in the patent WO-09605839 (Fig. 5) and which exhibit at least 10-fold greater selectivity for I_{Ks} than for I_{Kr} [47].

3.4   The large-conductance, Ca-sensitive K channel

3.4.1   Channel structure

The structure of the α-subunit of BK_{Ca} has been deduced by studies on the products of the *slo* gene [48, 49]. These place this channel in superfamily 1 with many features similar to those exhibited by delayed-rectifier and A-type K channels [18, 50]. A prominent feature of BK_{Ca} is believed to be the presence of β-subunits. These probably function to increase the calcium sensitivity of BK_{Ca} [51], and they may also be the site of action of drugs like the soyasaponins which modulate the activity of this channel (see [18] and Section 3.4.2). Unlike the cytoplasmically located Kv-type β-subunits, those which associate with *Slo* α-subunits are membrane-bound and appear to comprise two membrane-spanning domains (Fig. 1). Recently, it has been proposed [52] that the α-subunit of BK_{Ca} has an additional membrane-spanning domain at the N-terminus (S0; Fig. 1) which is involved in the interaction of the channel α- and β-subunits.

The channel formed by co-expression of the product of *Slo* and its β-subunit shows only voltage sensitivity in the presence of a low concentration of intracellular Ca^{2+} (<100 nM) [53]). However, above this concentration, calcium increases the open probability of the channel at any given membrane potential (above the voltage activation threshold) in a concentration-dependent manner. It is suggested that calcium promotes the functional association of the α- and β-subunits [53].

3.4.2   Pharmacology

3.4.2.1   Openers

Some naturally occurring K channel openers which appear to be highly selective for BK_{Ca} have been identified. The most potent of these is dehydrosoyasaponin-1 (Fig. 5), a glycosylated triterpene which acts as an allos-

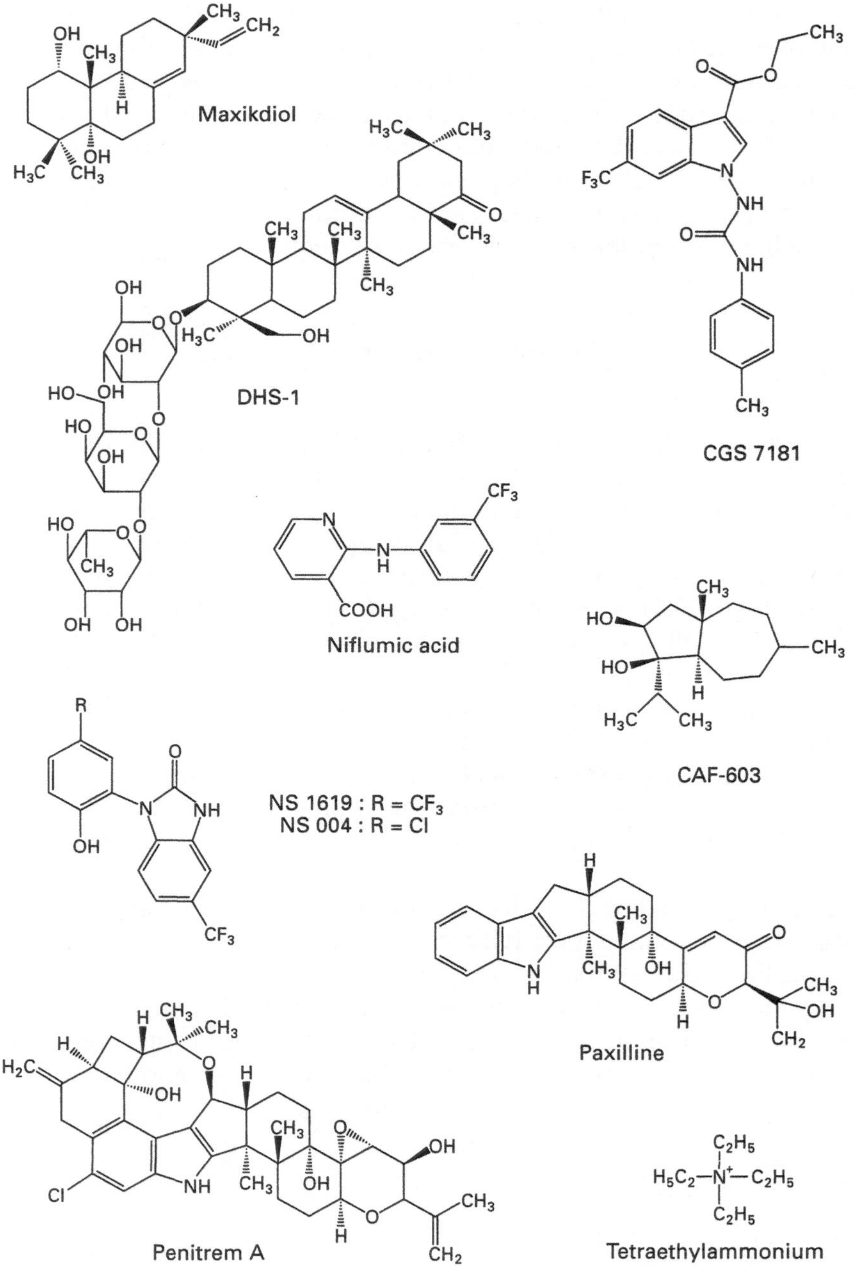

Fig. 5
Structural formulae of BK$_{Ca}$ modulators mentioned in the text.

teric inhibitor of [^{125}I]ChTX binding with a K_i value of approximately 120 nM [54]. Unfortunately, the poor membrane permeability of this compound precludes any therapeutic potential. However, it is a useful tool for electrophysiologists and is of additional interest since it requires the presence of both the α- and β-subunits of BK_{Ca} before the channel will open [55]. Maxikdiol, a diterpene (Fig. 5), is also poorly membrane-permeant, but like dehydrosoyasaponin-1, it is an active opener of BK_{Ca} when applied intracellularly [18, 56]. However, in contrast to dehydrosoyasaponin-1, its action does not require the presence of the channel β-subunit [18]. Little information is available about the carotane sesquiterpene CAF-603 (Fig. 5). It appears to be less potent than maxikdiol or dehydrosoyasaponin-1, but it inhibits ChTX binding, and a concentration of 10 μM, applied to the cytoplasmic side of the channel, does open BK_{Ca} [57, 58].

A series of substituted benzimidazolones which open native BK_{Ca} in a variety of tissues has recently been developed [59, 60]. These agents, typified by NS004 and NS1619 (Fig. 5), act to shift the voltage sensitivity of the BK_{Ca} by a direct interaction with its α-subunit [61]. Both NS004 and NS1619 are membrane-permeable, and their effects are antagonised by various inhibitors, including ChTX, iberiotoxin (IbTX) and penitrem A [59, 62]. They are an interesting development, although careful studies have shown that the benzimidazolones also inhibit a variety of other voltage-sensitive ion channels including K_V and L-type Ca channels [62] and open the cystic fibrosis transmembrane regulator (CFTR) chloride channel [63]. Further modifications of the benzimidazolone nucleus, typified by CGS 7181 (Fig. 4), have recently been described. Under patch-clamp conditions, this agent is a more potent opener of BK_{Ca} than NS1619 in a variety of smooth muscles, but neither its selectivity of action on BK_{Ca} nor its effect in whole-tissue systems has been disclosed [64].

Derivatives of fenamic acid are best known as inhibitors of Ca-sensitive chloride channels. However, these agents, which include niflumic acid (Fig. 5), are also openers of BK_{Ca} (see [65]). Like the benzimidazolones, their site of action is probably the channel α-subunit, although the mechanism involved is not understood [66].

BK_{Ca} openers may prove useful in the treatment of conditions associated with excessive neuronal discharge such as epilepsy and in the irritable bowel and unstable bladder syndromes in which $[Ca^{2+}]_i$ is likely to be greater than in normally-active tissue [50].

3.4.2.2 Inhibitors
With the exception of tetraethylammonium chloride, selective inhibitors of BK_{Ca} are natural plant or animal products. Classically, ChTX and IbTX

(Fig. 3) have been used as inhibitors of BK_{Ca}, and in most tissues inhibition of a K current by these toxins usually indicates that the underlying channel is indeed BK_{Ca}. Early reports that ChTX (isolated from the venom of the scorpion *Leiurus quinquestriatus*) could inhibit delayed rectifier K channels were believed to result from the presence of impurities such as agitoxins [67]. However, using synthetic ChTX it is now clear that this agent is not totally selective for BK_{Ca} and that it can inhibit Kv1.3 with a K_i value of 0.19 nM [68]. IbTX, purified from the venom of the scorpion *Bothus tamulus*, is of a similar size to ChTX, with which it shares approximately 70% sequence homology [69]. Nevertheless, it is a more highly selective inhibitor of BK_{Ca} and is unable to inhibit the binding of ChTX to voltage-sensitive K channels (Kv1.3) in brain or human T lymphocytes [68]. A study on the mode of action of a series of tremorgenic mycotoxins which potentiate neurotransmitter release revealed that these indole alkaloids modify [^{125}I]ChTX binding [70]. Paradoxically, however, both inhibitors (typified by penitrem A; Fig. 5) and enhancers of binding (such as paxilline; Fig. 5) act as potent inhibitors of BK_{Ca} with IC_{50} values in the range 1–10 nM [18, 70]. In whole-cell studies, at least one of the agents, penitrem A (Fig. 5), inhibits current flow through BK_{Ca} induced by the benzimidazolone NS1619 [62].

3.5   The ATP-sensitive K channel

3.5.1   *Channel structure*
The pore-forming region of the ATP-sensitive K channels (K_{ATP}) so far identified places them in superfamily 2, members of which possess α-subunits which comprise only two membrane-spanning domains (M1 and M2). These are linked extracellularly by a membrane-dipping region (P) which forms part of the pore region (Fig. 1). The M1, M2 and P domains share some sequence homology with the S5, S6 and P regions characteristic of superfamily 1, but the S4 voltage-sensor region is missing. Thus, although most members of superfamily 2 are voltage-sensitive in that they are inward rectifiers, very little of this characteristic feature derives directly from the properties of the α-subunits themselves. Instead, it results from the inhibitory effect of intracellular moieties like Mg^{2+} and spermine which are believed to block the pore of the channel at potentials positive to E_K [71, 72].

K_{ATP} opens as the intracellular ATP concentration, $[ATP]_i$, falls (speculatively, under conditions of, say, metabolic stress), whereas under normal conditions, $[ATP]_i$ is probably high enough to ensure that the channel remains closed. Recent evidence suggests that K_{ATP} is formed by the association of Kir6.2 α-subunits with a sulphonylurea receptor (SUR) which can be considered as a β-subunit (Fig. 1). Three of these (SUR1, SUR2 and SUR2B) have been identified to date and found to possess significant amino acid sequence identity [73–75]. Co-expression of Kir6.2 with SUR1 produces channels with properties similar to those of the native K_{ATP} in the pancreatic β-cell, whereas its co-expression with SUR2A produces a K_{ATP} channel more typical of that in skeletal or cardiac muscle [74]. SUR2B is found in several tissues including smooth muscle, and the combination with Kir6.1 or Kir6.2 may represent the native K_{ATP} in this tissue type [75, 76]. It was thought that both ATP and glibenclamide sensitivity is conferred by the presence of the SUR [74, 77] but this has recently been questioned [76].

SUR1 and SUR2 are predicted to have 13 membrane-spanning regions which are divided into two groups (of 9 and 4 transmembrane regions), each of which includes a nucleotide-binding domain (Fig. 1). These structural features place SUR in the family of ATP-binding cassette (ABC) proteins which includes several ABC transporters as well as the CFTR chloride channel [73]. In epithelial cells, K_{ATP} may be formed by the association of a second type of inward-rectifier channel, Kir1.1b, which may be associated with CFTR rather than SUR. Thus it appears that CFTR (which alone forms a chloride channel which is inhibited by glibenclamide) endows glibenclamide sensitivity on Kir1.1b, formerly known as ROMK2 [78]. Interestingly, co-expression of Kir1.1b and SUR1 in HEK293 cells produces a glibenclamide-sensitive K channel, whereas such a channel is not formed after co-expression of these two structures in *Xenopus* oocytes [77, 79]. Presumably this indicates that an additional factor which is provided by the HEK293 cells is required for the coupling or regulation of the Kir1.1b/SUR1 complex.

3.5.2   *Pharmacology*
3.5.2.1 K_{ATP} inhibitors
Most inhibitors of K_{ATP} contain either a sulphonylurea (tolbutamide) or a benzoic acid (meglitinide) moiety or both such structures [80]. The prototypical inhibitor of K_{ATP} is glibenclamide, and although this agent is usually classified as a "sulphonylurea", a benzoic acid residue is also present (Fig. 6). The presence of these two chemical features could indicate that two distinct sites (a benzoic acid *and* a sulphonylurea binding site) are independently associated with inhibition of K_{ATP}.

Photoaffinity labelling of membranes from brain and insulinoma cells has revealed that there are at least two high-affinity sulphonylurea binding

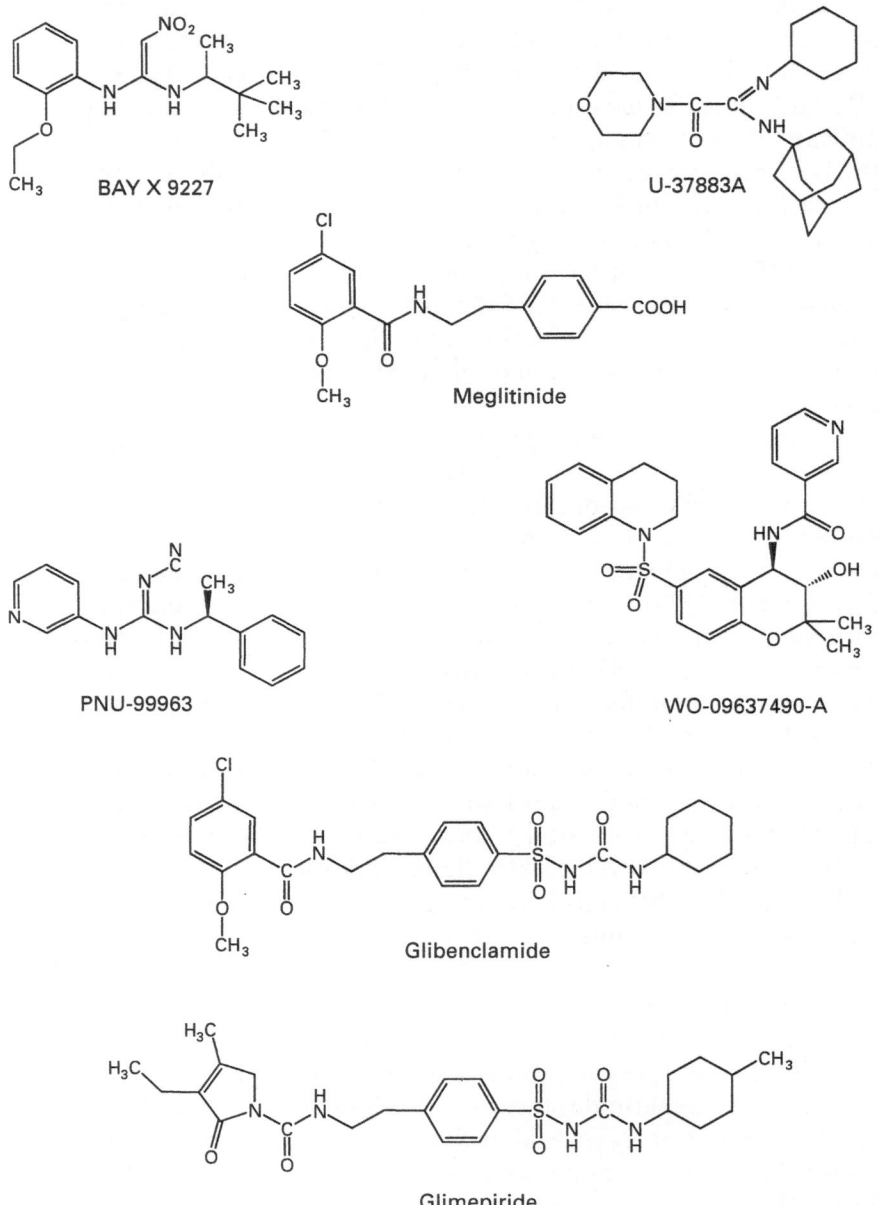

Fig. 6
Structural formulae of established and putative K_{ATP} modulators mentioned in the text. Note the atypical (3R,4S) stereochemistry of BMS 191095 and that the actions of BAY X 9227, BRL 61164 and SB 204269 at K_{ATP} have not been confirmed.

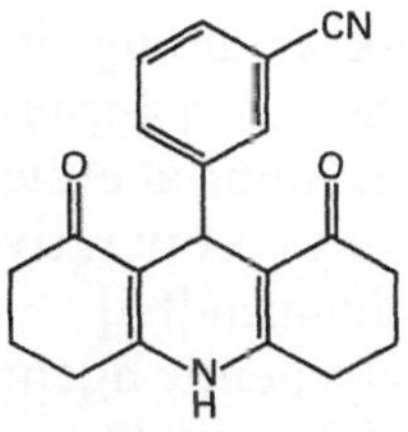

ZM244085

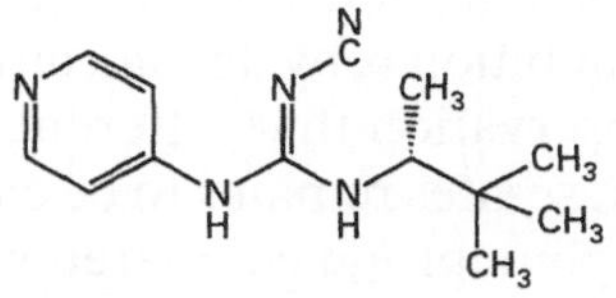

(R)-Pinacidil

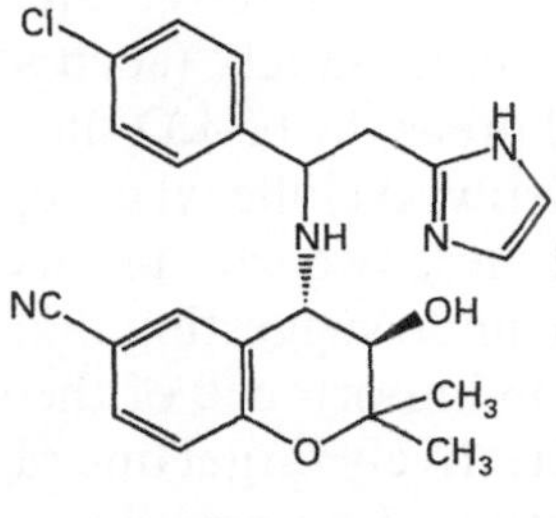

BMS 191095

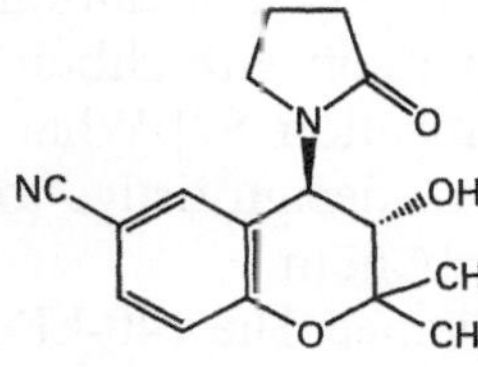

Levcromakalim

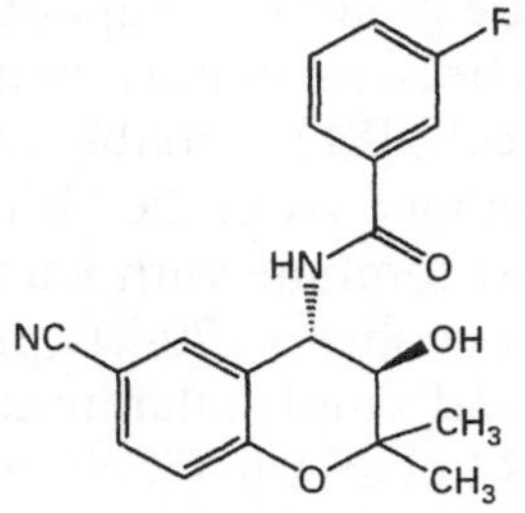

BRL 61164

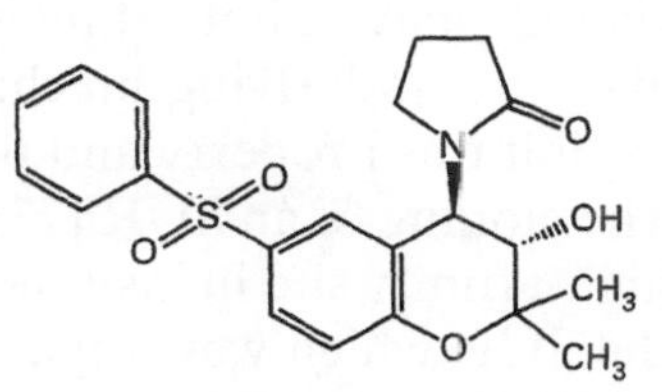

Rilmakalim

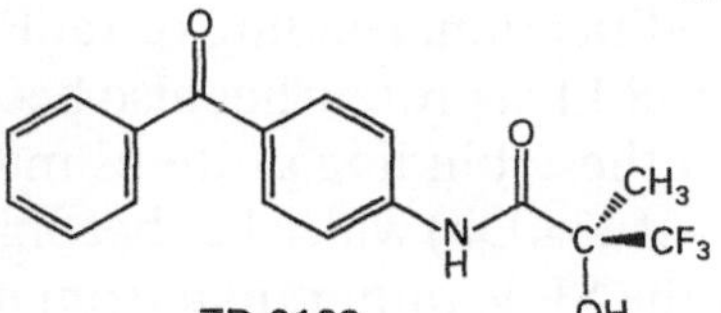

ZD 6169

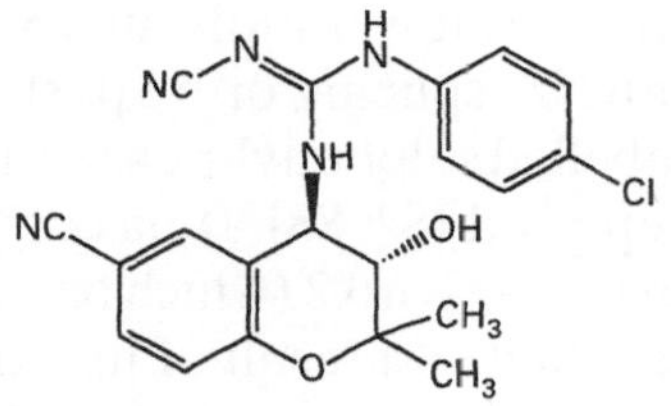

BMS 180448

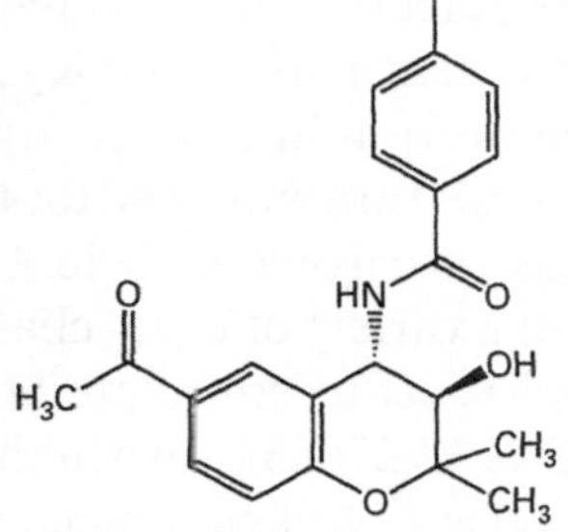

SB 204269

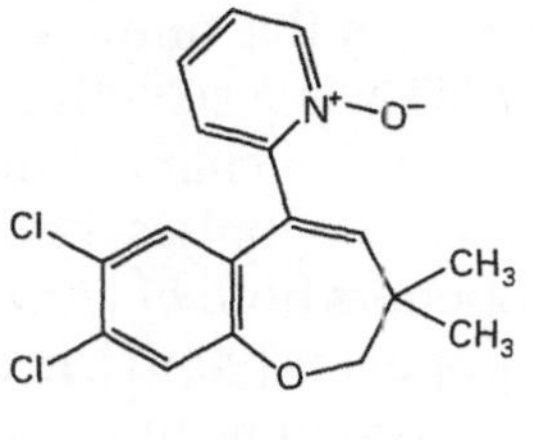

LM-3339

Fig. 6 (continued)

sites [81, 82] (see also [83]). It appears that sulphonylureas with a cyclohexylamino moiety (such as glibenclamide) bind to the 140-kD binding site, whereas the 65-kD site preferentially binds sulphonylureas with a 4-*trans*-methyl cyclohexyl group such as glimepiride (Fig. 6; [84]). Binding at either of these two sites reduces binding at the other in a negatively co-operative manner, suggesting that inhibition is by an allosteric mechanism [85].

The importance of the observation that different hypoglycaemic agents selectively target one of these sites remains to be explored. The prolonged action of a single dose of glimepiride compared with glibenclamide [86] may be a function of its binding site. Alternatively, the higher association and dissociation rates for glimepiride binding in comparison with glibenclamide may be important in reducing receptor desensitisation [87]. Whatever the underlying mechanism, it may be possible to design drugs to exploit this property and provide greater therapeutic benefit.

The cloning of an SUR [73] has been an important advance. The 140-kD, high-affinity site in insulinoma cells [81] probably corresponds to SUR1, the SUR which was originally cloned from the HIT T15 insulinoma cell line [73] and which is thought to combine with Kir6.2 to form the β-cell K_{ATP} (Fig. 1). Although SUR1 encodes a 170-kD protein, the expressed sulphonylurea binding protein had a molecular mass of only 140 kD after transient expression of the SUR1 cDNA in COSm6 cells [73], suggesting that this lower molecular weight form is produced either by differential mRNA splicing or by post-translational modification. Binding of radiolabelled sulphonylureas to a 43-kDa and to a 38-kDa protein has also been reported [82, 88]. It has been proposed that these binding proteins may in fact be Kir6.2 (which has a molecular mass of 43 kDa) which has become labelled as a result of its close contact with the SUR rather than from its direct binding of sulphonylureas [89].

The recent development of K_{ATP} inhibitors which are neither sulphonylureas nor benzoic acid derivatives and which are selective for this channel in smooth muscle suggests that there is much to learn about the K_{ATP} complex in the smooth muscle system. Thus, the morpholino-derivative U-37883A is a selective inhibitor of K_{ATP} in vasculature but is without effect on this channel in either pancreatic β-cells or cardiac muscle. U-37883A antagonises the vascular relaxant effects of a variety of K_{ATP} channel openers both *in vitro* and *in vivo* and inhibits ^{42}K efflux stimulated by K_{ATP} openers [90, 91]. In electrophysiological studies, U-37883A also inhibits K_{ATP} opening in vascular smooth muscle as well as in follicle-enclosed *Xenopus* oocytes in which K_{ATP} is considered to be smooth muscle-like [92, 93]. In contrast, U-37883A is without any effect on the shortening of cardiac action potentials induced by K_{ATP} openers [93] and does not inhibit

$I_{K(ATP)}$ in RINm5F cells [92]. U-37883A also fails to stimulate insulin secretion *in vivo* [94].

Functional and receptor-binding studies with U-37883A suggest that the site at which it modulates K_{ATP} is distinct from that of the sulphonylureas [91, 92, 95]. Thus, radiolabelled U-37883A binds specifically to membranes from follicle-enclosed *Xenopus* oocytes but is not displaced from these by glibenclamide. A low-affinity receptor binding site for U-37883A which is distinct from that of glibenclamide has also been recently described [95]. In contrast, [³H]U-37883A shows no specific binding either to RINm5F membranes [92] or to those from cardiac tissue (Meisheri, personal communication). Furthermore, U-37883A does not compete with [³H]glibenclamide bound to these two tissues. Recently, a brief report on the pinacidil derivative PNU-99963 has appeared (Fig. 6, [96]). This drug exhibits stereoselective inhibition of K_{ATP} in smooth muscle, and further studies with both this agent and with U-37883A should help to clarify the nature of K_{ATP} in smooth muscle.

3.5.2.2 K_{ATP} openers

The prototype K_{ATP}-channel opener is levcromakalim. Many related benzopyrans share similar properties [97], but other structurally-unrelated compounds (Fig. 6) are also active [98]. Until recently, the presence of chiral centres in many of the K_{ATP} openers and particularly those of the benzopyran series (Fig. 6) together with the restriction of channel opening to a single (the 3*S*,4*R*) enantiomer was taken as a clear indication that the site of action for a defined chemical class of opener had precise structural properties. However, the recent disclosure that certain benzopyrans with the 3*R*,4*S* configuration such as BMS191095 (Fig. 6; see page 115) are not only active but also selectively cardioprotective [99] has indicated that a reappraisal of the structure-activity relationships within this group of openers may be required.

Bladder-selective molecules: The involuntary loss of urine or the inability to control the frequency of urination defines the condition of urinary incontinence. Several types of this condition are recognised and urge incontinence, which is associated with involuntary detrusor contractions leading to the rapid desire to urinate even when the bladder is not full, is common. This condition should be ideally suited to correction by an opener of K_{ATP}, since the associated cessation of electrical spike activity should abolish the contractions with little effect on the voluntary voiding of urine. Cromakalim and pinacidil relax bladder smooth muscle *in vitro* without seriously inhibiting the contractile action of acetylcholine [100–102]. However, no bladder selectivity is exhibited by these first-generation K_{ATP} openers [103]. A more recent development, ZD6169 (Fig. 6), shows no bladder selectivity *in vitro*, but it does reduce spontaneous bladder contractions at doses which do not reduce blood pressure [104,105]. This agent is now in phase 2 clinical trials, and the pharmacology of another bladder-active opener of K_{ATP} with a novel structure (ZM244085, Fig. 6) has recently been described [106].

Anti-hyperreactive openers: Recent reports have suggested that certain K_{ATP} openers can prevent the development of the hyperreactive state which is characteristic of certain *in vivo* models of bronchial asthma [107, 108]. As reported [108], a series of benzopyrans, including levcromakalim, reduced the increase in resistance produced by histamine in guinea pig airways made hyperreactive by immune complexes. A distinct potency ratio was described for this effect, with rilmakalim (Fig. 6) being the most potent agent. In a recent patent [109], a series of novel benzopyrans typified by distinctive substituents at the 6-position in the benzopyran nucleus was described. One agent (Fig. 6) was specifically identified, and this may represent the lead compound currently under development by Novartis. Although it has not been disclosed whether these "antihyperreactivity" effects are glibenclamide-sensitive, the doses used, together with the observation that levcromakalim shares this property, strongly suggest that the action does involve the opening of K_{ATP}. LM-3339 is a benzopyran-like K_{ATP} opener (Fig. 6). Preliminary experiments indicate that this agent exhibits airway selectivity [110], and the results of further studies with this agent may prove interesting.

The site at which these *in vivo* effects is exerted is the matter of some debate. Since the development of certain forms of hypersensitivity can be prevented by vagal section, inhibition of the release of mediators involved in the development of the hyperresponsive state is a distinct possibility. In favour of this is the finding that the release of the so-called NANCe transmitter in guinea pig airways can be prevented by levcromakalim [111]. Alternatively, or in addition, a role for platelet-activating factor is a distinct possibility [107, 112]. Whatever their site of action, the successful development of agents [109] which act selectively on hyperresponsive airways without exerting effects on the cardiovascular system can be confidently anticipated.

Cardioselective anti-ischaemic K_{ATP} channel openers: The ability of K_{ATP} openers to protect the ischaemic myocardium has been widely described, and the many data concerning the protective effects of aprikalim, cromakalim and nicorandil have recently been reviewed [113]. One problem with such first-generation drugs is their ability to produce hypotension, and attempts to separate cardioprotective and systemic vascular actions led to the development of agents such as BMS-180448 (Fig. 6) [114]. Recently, however, the agent BMS191095 (Fig. 6) has been described with a claimed 20-fold increase in selectivity for the ischaemic myocardium relative to the vasculature compared with BMS180448 [99]. Of special interest is the disclosure that this agent possesses $3R,4S$ stereochemistry in the benzopyran ring, a feature which would normally confer minimal K_{ATP}-opening activity [97]. In spite of this, the actions of BMS191095 are inhibited by glibenclamide [99], a strong indication that K_{ATP} is indeed the target for this agent.

Benzopyrans as anticonvulsant agents: The potential for the use of K_{ATP} openers in disorders of the CNS is enormous and has recently been comprehensively reviewed [115]. One of the reasons why the development of openers for this important drug target lags behind that of other organ systems is that, until recently, the emergence of novel openers reflected the use of "peripheral" screening systems. Furthermore, existing openers are generally impotent when tested in neuronal systems [115]. However, the pinacidil derivative BAY X 9227 (Fig. 6) is reported to hyperpolarise neurones with picomolar potency [116], and the benzopyran BRL 61164 (Fig. 6) increases the maximal electroshock seizure threshold in mice at a dose which has no effect on rat blood pressure [117]. Although both agents are derived from K_{ATP} openers, the action of BAY X 9227 is not glibenclamide-sensitive [116, 118]. Furthermore, the 3,4 substituents on BRL 61164 are in the trans $3R,4S$ configuration, an arrangement which would not be expected to open K_{ATP} ([97], Fig. 6). However, the $3R,4S$ stereochemistry of BMS191095, together with the glibenclamide sensitivity of this agent (see above), clearly indicates that it cannot be assumed that BRL 61164 does not interact with a centrally located form of K_{ATP}.

More recently, a further series of fluorobenzamides with $3R,4S$ stereochemistry and typified by SB 204269 (Fig. 6) has been described. *In vivo* studies show that this agent is anticonvulsant with negligible hypotensive activity [119]. Using [³H]SB 204269, a unique binding site with no affinity for typical anticonvulsant agents such as diazepam, phenytoin, valproate and phenobarbitone has been identified in the brains of several mammals including that of humans. The binding of SB 204269 to this site is highly enantioselective, with the $3S,4R$ enantiomers SB 204268 exhibiting almost 1000-fold lower affinity [115]. The observation that prototypical K_{ATP}

openers such as levcromakalim, aprikalim and pinacidil have no significant affinity for this site suggests that it does not represent a subtype of K_{ATP}, and the results of further studies with this new series of compounds are awaited with interest.

4   Conclusions

The development of drugs which are capable of modulating K channels constitutes one of the most dynamic areas of modern drug development. This should not be surprising, since the diversity of K channel subtypes and their widespread involvement in altering the excitability of many types of cells offers an unparalleled spectrum of therapeutic targets. These range from arrhythmias and asthma to diabetes, inflammation and urinary tract disorders, and this review represents a personal selection of the most recent advances in the field. However, common to the successful development of all new therapies, selectivity of drug action remains the key, and the ubiquitous presence of K channels means that this is a special challenge. Nevertheless, the latest developments are most exciting, and the results of ongoing clinical trials are awaited with considerable anticipation and optimism.

Acknowledgement

Helpful discussions with Drs. J.M. Evans, G.J. Kaczorowski and K.D. Meisheri are gratefully acknowledged.

References

1   B. Rudy: Neurosci. 25, 729–749 (1988).
2   O. Pongs: Physiol. Rev. 72, S69–S88 (1992).
3   K.G. Chandy and G.A. Gutman, in: Ligand and Voltage-Gated Ion Channels (R.A. North, ed.), CRC Press, London (1995), pp.1–71.
4   L.L. Isom, K.S. De Jongh and W.A. Catterall: Neuron 12, 1183–1194 (1994).
5   O. Pongs: Semin. Neurosci. 7, 137–146 (1995).
6   G.A. Gutman and K.G. Chandy: Semin. Neurosci. 5, 101–106 (1993).
7   S.K. England, V.N. Uebele, J. Kodali, P.B. Bennett and M.M. Tamkun: J. Biol. Chem. 270, 28531–28534 (1995).
8   K. Majumder, M. Debiasi, Z.G. Wang and B.A. Wible: FEBS Lett. 361, 13–16 (1995).
9   M. Fink, F. Duprat, F. Lesage, C. Heurteaux, G. Romey, J. Barhanin and M. Lazdunski: J. Biol. Chem. 271, 26341–26348 (1996).

10 G.Y. Shi, K. Nakahira, S. Hammond, K.J. Rhodes, L.E. Schechter and J.S. Trimmer: Neuron *16*, 843–852 (1996).

11 R.S. Lewis and M.D. Cahalan: Annu. Rev. Immunol. *13*, 623–653 (1995).

12 C. Randriamampita and R.Y. Tsien: Nature *364*, 809–814 (1993).

13 R.J. Leonard, M.L. Garcia, R.S. Slaughter and J.P. Reuben: Proc. Natl. Acad. Sci. USA *89*, 10094–10098 (1992).

14 W.F. Michne, J.W. Guiles, A.M. Treasurywala, L.A., Castonguay, C.A. Weigelt, B. O'Connor, W.A. Volberg, A.M. Grant, C.C. Chadwick, D.S. Krafte and R.I. Hill: J. Med. Chem. *38*, 1877–1883 (1995).

15 R.J. Hill, A.M. Grant, W. Volberg, L. Rapp, C. Faltynek, D. Miller, K. Pagani, E. Baizman, S. Wang, J.W. Guiles and D.S. Krafte: Mol. Pharmacol. *48*, 98–104 (1995).

16 J. Aiyar, J.M. Withka, J.P. Rizzi, D.H. Singleton, G.C. Andrews, W. Lin, J. Boyd, D.C. Hanson, M. Simon, B. Dethlefs, C.L. Lee, J.E. Hall, G.A. Gutman and K.G. Chandy: Neuron *15*, 1169–1181 (1995).

17 A. Nguyen, J.C. Kath, JD.C. Hanson, M.S. Biggers, P.C. Canniff, C.B. Donovan, R.J. Mather, M.J. Bruns, H. Rauer, J. Aiyar, A. Lepple-Wienhues, G. Gutman, S. Grissmer, M.D. Cahalan and K.G. Chandy: Mol. Pharmacol. *50*, 1672–1679 (1996).

18 G.J. Kaczorowski, H.G. Knaus, R.J. Leonard, O.B. McManus and M.L. Garcia: J. Bioenerg. Biomembr. *28*, 255–267 (1996).

19 M. Garcia-Calvo, R.J. Leonard, J. Novick, S.P. Stevens, W. Schmalhofer, G.J. Kaczorowski and M.L. Garcia: J. Biol. Chem. *268*, 18866–18874 (1993).

20 M.A. Bednarek, R.M. Bugianesi, R.J. Leonard and J.P. Felix: Biochem. Biophys. Res. Commun. *198*, 619–625 (1994).

21 G.C. Koo, J.T. Blake, A. Talento, M. Nguyen, S. Lin, A. Sirotina, K. Shah, K. Mulvany, D. Hora, P. Cunningham, D.L. Wunderler, O.B. McManus, R. Slaughter, R. Bugianese, J. Felix, M. Garcia, J. Williamson, G. Kaczorowski, N. Sigal, M. Springer and W. Feeney: J. Immunol. *158*, 5120–5128 (1997).

22 J.W. Warmke and B. Ganetzky: Proc. Natl. Acad. Sci. USA *91*, 3438–3442 (1994).

23 M.C. Trudeau, J.W. Warmke, B. Ganetzky and G.A. Robertson: Science *269*, 92–95 (1995).

24 P.L. Smith, T. Baukrowitz and G. Yellen: Nature *379*, 833–836 (1996).

25 M.W. Russell and M. Dick: Cardiol. *11*, 45–51 (1996).

26 M.C. Sanguinetti, M.E. Curran, A. Zou, J. Shen, P.S. Spector, D.L. Atkinson and M.T. Keating: Nature *384*, 80–83 (1996).

27 M.C. Sanguinetti, M.E. Curran, P.S. Spector and M.T. Keating: Proc. Natl. Acad. Sci. USA *93*, 2208–2212 (1996).

28 C.A. Satler, E.P. Walsh, M.R. Vesely, M.H. Plummer, G.S. Ginsburg and H.J. Howard: Am. J. Med. Gen. *65*, 27–35 (1996).

29 M.C. Sanguinetti and J.J. Salata; in: Potassium Channels and their Modulation: From Synthesis to Clinical Experience (J.M. Evans, T.C. Hamilton, S.D. Longman and G. Stemp, eds.), Taylor & Francis, London (1996), pp.221–256.

30 A.L. Waldo, A.J. Camm, H. deRuyter, P.L. Freidman, D.J. MacNeil, B. Pitt, C.M. Pratt, B.E. Rodda and P.J. Schwartz: Am. J. Cardiol. *75*, 1023–1027 (1995).

31 S.H. Hohnloser and R.L. Woosley: N. Eng. J. Med. *331*, 31–38 (1994).

32 H. Suessbrich, S. Waldegger, F. Lang and A.E. Busch: FEBS Lett. *385*, 77–80 (1996).

33 A.E. Busch and H. Suessbrich: Trends Pharmacol. Sci. *18*, 26–29 (1997).

34 J. Barhanin, F. Lesage, E. Guillemare, M. Fink, M. Lazdunski and G. Romey: Nature *384*, 78–80 (1996).

35 T. Takumi, H. Ohkubo and S. Nakanishi: Science *242*, 1042–1045 (1988).

36   T. Murai, A. Kakizuka, T. Takumi, H. Ohkubo and S. Nakanishi: Biochem. Biophys. Res. Commun. *161*, 176–181 (1989).
37   F. Lesage, B. Attali, J. Lakey, E. Honoré, G. Romey, E. Faurobert, M. Lazdunski and J. Barhanin: Receptors Channels *1*, 143–152 (1993).
38   A.E. Busch, T. Herzer, T, Takumi, P. Krippeit-Drews, S. Waldegger and F. Lang: Eur. J. Pharmacol. *264*, 33–37 (1994).
39   S.C. Black, S.O. Fagbemi, L.G. Chi, G.S. Friedrichs and B.R. Lucchesi: J. Mol. Cell. Cardiol. *25*, 1427–1438 (1993).
40   J.A. Yao and G.N. Tseng: J. Cardiovasc. Electrophysiol. *8*, 184–198 (1997).
41   A.E. Busch, K. Malloy, W.J. Groh, M.D. Varnum, J.P. Adelman and J. Maylie: Biochem. Biophys. Res. Commun. *202*, 265–270 (1994).
42   B. Fermini, N.K. Jurkiewicz, B. Jow, P.J. Guinosso Jr, E.P. Baskin, J.J. Lynch Jr and J.J. Salata: J. Cardiovasc. Pharmacol. *26*, 259–271 (1995).
43   A.E. Busch, H. Suessbrich, S. Waldegger, E. Sailer, R. Greger, H.J. Lang, F. Lang, K.J. Gibson and J.G. Maylie: Pflügers Arch. *432*, 1094–1096 (1996).
44   D. Escande, J.C. Mestre, I. Cavero, J. Brugada and C. Kirchhof: J. Cardiovasc. Pharmacol. *20*, S106– S113 (1992).
45   J.J. Lynch, A.A. Wallace, R.F. Stupienski, E.P. Baskin, C.M. Beare, S.D. Appleby, J.J. Salata, N.K. Jurkiewicz, M.C. Sanguinetti, R.B. Stein and J.R. Gehret: J. Pharmacol. Exp. Ther. *269*, 541–554 (1994).
46   P.S. Spector, M.E. Curran, M.T. Keating and M.C. Sanguinetti: Circ. Res. *78*, 499–503 (1996).
47   D.A. Claremon, N. Liverton and H.G. Selnick: WO–09605839 (1996).
48   A. Butler, S. Tsunoda, D.P. McCobb, A. Wei and L. Salkoff: Science *261*, 221–224 (1993).
49   H.G. Knaus, M. Garcia-Calvo, G.J. Kaczorowski and M.L. Garcia: J. Biol. Chem. *269*, 3921–3924 (1994).
50   G. Edwards and A.H. Weston: Exp. Opin. Invest. Drugs *5*, 1453–1464 (1996).
51   S.I. Dworetzky, C.G. Boissard, J.T. Lumragan, M.C. McKay, D.J. Postmunson, J.T. Trojnacki, C.P. Chang and V.K. Gribkoff: J. Neurosci. *16*, 4543–4550 (1996).
52   M. Wallner, P. Meera and L. Toro: Proc. Natl. Acad. Sci. USA *93*, 14922–14927 (1996).
53   P. Meera, M. Wallner, Z. Jiang and L. Toro: FEBS Letters *382*, 84–88 (1996).
54   O.B. McManus, G.H. Harris, K.M. Giangiacomo, P. Feigenbaum, J.P. Reuben, M.E. Addy, J.F. Burka, G.J. Kaczorowski and M.L. Garcia: Biochemistry *32*, 6128–6133 (1993).
55   O.B. McManus, L.M.H. Helms, L. Pallanck, B. Ganetzky, R. Swanson and R.J. Leonard: Neuron *14*, 645–650 (1995).
56   S.B. Singh, M.A. Goetz, D.L. Zink, A.W. Dombrowski, J.D. Polishook, M.L. Garcia, W. Schmalhofer, O.B. McManus and G.J. Kaczorowski: J. Chem. Soc. Perkin Trans. *1*, 3349–3352 (1994).
57   S.H. Lee, O.D. Hensens, G.L. Helms, J.M. Liesch, D.L. Zink, R.A. Giacobbe, G.F. Bills, S. Stevens-Miles, M.L. Garcia, W.A. Schmalhofer, O.B. McManus and G.J. Kaczorowski: J. Nat. Prod. *58*, 1822–1828 (1995).
58   J.G. Ondeyka, R.G. Ball, M.L. Garcia, A.W. Dombrowski, G. Sabnis, G.J. Kaczorowski, D.L. Zink, G.F. Bills, M.A. Goetz, W.A. Schmalhofer and S.B. Singh: Bioorg. Med. Chem. Lett. *5*, 733–734 (1995).
59   S.P. Olesen, E. Munch, F. Watjen and J. Drejer: Neuroreport *5*, 1001–1004 (1994).
60   S.P. Olesen, E. Munch, P. Moldt. and J. Drejer: Eur. J. Pharmacol. *251*, 53–59 (1994).

61   M.C. McKay, S.I. Dworetzky, N.A. Meanwell, S.-O. Olesen, P.H. Reinhart, I.B. Levitan, J.P. Adelman and V.K. Gribkoff: J. Neurophysiol. 71, 1873–1882 (1994).
62   G. Edwards, A. Niederste-Hollenberg, J. Schneider, Th. Noack and A.H. Weston: Br. J. Pharmacol. 113, 1538–1547 (1994).
63   V.K. Gribkoff, G. Champigny, P. Barbry, S.I. Dworetzky, N.A. Meanwell and M. Lazdunski: J. Biol. Chem. 269, 10983–10986 (1994).
64   S. Hu, C.A. Fink, H.S. Kim and R.W. Lappe: Drug Dev. Res. (in press).
65   A.J. Kirkup, G. Edwards, M.E. Green, M. Miller, S.D. Walker and A.H. Weston: Eur. J. Pharmacol. 317, 165–174 (1996).
66   M. Wallner, P. Meera, M. Ottolia, G.J. Kaczorowski, R: Latorre, M.L. Garcia, E. Stefani and L. Toro: Receptors Channels 3, 185–199 (1995).
67   M.L. Garcia, M. Garcia-Calvo, P. Hidalgo, A. Lee and R. Mackinnon: Biochemistry 33, 6834–6839 (1994).
68   M.L. Garcia, H.G. Knaus, P. Munujos, R.S. Slaughter and G.J. Kaczorowski: Amer. J. Physiol. 38, C1–C10 (1995).
69   A. Galvez, G. Gimenez-Gallego, J.P. Reuben, L. Roy-Contancin, P. Feigenbaum, G.J. Kaczorowski and M.L. Garcia: J. Biol. Chem. 265, 11083–11090 (1990).
70   H.G. Knaus, O.B. McManus, S.H. Lee, W.A. Schmalhofer, M. Garcia-Calvo, L.M.H. Helms, M. Sanchez, K. Giangiacomo, J.P. Reuben, A.B. Smith, G.J. Kaczorowski and M.L. Garcia: Biochemistry 33, 5819–5828 (1994).
71   Y. Kubo, T.J. Baldwin, Y.N. Jan and L.Y. Jan: Nature 362, 127–133 (1993).
72   B. Fakler, U. Brandle, E. Glowatzki, S. Weidemann, H.P. Zenner and J.P. Ruppersberg: Cell 80, 149–154 (1995).
73   L. Aguilar-Bryan, C.G. Nichols, S.W. Wechsler, J.P. Clement, A.E. Boyd, G. Gonzalez, H. Herrerasosa, K. Nguy, J. Bryan and D.A. Nelson: Science 268, 423–426 (1995).
74   N. Inagaki, T. Gonoi, J.P. Clement, C.Z. Wang, L. Aguilar-Bryan, J. Bryan and S. Seino: Neuron 16, 1011–1017 (1996).
75   S. Isomoto, C. Kondo, M. Yamada, S. Matsumoto, O. Higashiguchi, Y. Horio, Y. Matsuzawa and Y. Kurachi: J. Biol. Chem. 271, 24321–24324 (1996).
76   M. Yamada, S. Isomoto, S. Matsumoto, C. Kondo, T. Shindo, Y. Horio and Y. Kurachi: J. Physiol. 499, 715–720 (1997).
77   C. Ämmälä, A. Moorhouse, F. Gribble, R. Ashfield, P. Proks, P.A. Smith, H. Sakura, B. Coles, S.J.H. Ashcroft and F.M. Ashcroft: Nature 379, 545–548 (1996).
78   C.M. McNicholas, W.B. Guggino, E.M. Schwiebert, S.C. Hebert, G. Giebisch and M.E. Egan: Proc. Natl. Acad. Sci. USA 93, 8083–8088 (1996).
79   F.M. Gribble, R. Ashfield, C. Ämmälä and F.M. Ashcroft: J. Physiol. 498, 87–98 (1997).
80   G. Edward and A.H. Weston: Annu. Rev. Pharmacol. Toxicol. 33, 597–637 (1993).
81   W. Kramer, R. Oekonomopulos, J. Punter and H.D. Summ: FEBS Lett. 299, 355–359 (1988).
82   L. Aguilar-Bryan, D.A. Nelson, Q.A. Vu, M.B. Humphrey and A.E. Boyd III: J. Biol. Chem. 265, 8218–8224 (1990).
83   U. Panten, M. Schwanstecher and C. Schwanstecher: Exp. Clin. Endocr. Diabetes 104, 1–9 (1996).
84   W. Kramer, G. Müller, F. Girbig, U. Gutjahr, S. Kowalewski, D. Hartz and H.-D. Summ: Biochim. Biophys. Acta 1191, 278–290 (1994).
85   W. Kramer, G. Muller, F. Girbig, U. Gutjahr, S. Kowalewski, D. Hartz and H.D. Summ: Diabetes Res. Clin. Pract. 28, S67–S80 (1995).

86   K. Geisen: Arzneimittel Forsch. *38*, 1120–1130 (1988).

87   G. Müller, D. Hartz, J. Pünter, R. Ökonomopulos and W. Kramer: Biochim. Biophys. Acta *1191*, 267–277 (1994).

88   M. Schwanstecher, S. Loser, F. Chudziak and U. Panten: J. Biol. Chem. *269*, 17768–17771 (1994).

89   F.M. Ashcroft: Horm. Metab. Res. *28*, 456–463 (1996).

90   K.D. Meisheri, S.J. Humphrey, S.A. Khan, L.A. Cipkusdubray, M.P. Smith and A.W. Jones: J. Pharmacol. Exp. Ther. *266*, 655–665 (1993).

91   C.E. Ohrnberger, S.A. Khan and K.D. Meisheri: J. Pharmacol. Exp. Ther. *267*, 25–30 (1993).

92   E. Guillemare, E. Honore, J. Deweille, M. Fosset, M. Lazdunski and K. Meisheri: Mol. Pharmacol. *46*, 139–145 (1994).

93   N.R. Higdon, X. Xu, S.A. Khan, J. Wang, K.S. Lee and K.D. Meisheri: FASEB J. *9*, A614 (1995).

94   J.H. Ludens, M.A. Clark, M.P. Smith and S.J. Humphrey: FASEB J. *8*, A835 (1994).

95   K. Meisheri, M. Fosset, S. Humphrey and M. Lazdunski: Mol. Pharmacol. *47*, 155–163 (1995).

96   S.A. Khan, N.R. Higdon, J.B. Hester and K.D. Meisheri: FASEB. J. *10*, A6 (1996).

97   J.M. Evans and G. Stemp; in: Potassium Channels and their Modulation: From Synthesis to Clinical Experience (J.M. Evans, T.C. Hamilton, S.D. Longman and G. Stemp, eds). Taylor & Francis, London (1996), pp. 27–55.

98   G. Edwards and A.H. Weston: Trends Pharmacol. Sci. *11*, 417–422 (1990).

99   G.C. Rovnyak, S.Z. Ahmed, C.Z. Ding, S. Dzwonczyk, F.N. Ferrara, W.G. Humphreys, G.J. Grover, D. Santafianos, K.S. Atwal, A.J. Baird, L.G. McLaughlin, D.E. Normandin, P.G. Sleph and S.C. Traeger: J. Med. Chem. *40*, 24–34 (1997).

100 K.-E. Andersson, P.-O. Andersson, M. Fovaeous, H. Hedlund, A. Malmgren and C. Sjögren: Drugs *36*, 41–49 (1988).

101 A. Malmgren, K.E. Andersson, P.O. Andersson, M. Fovaeus and C. Sjögren: J. Urol. *143*, 828–834 (1990).

102 C.D. Foster, K. Fujii, J. Kingdon and A.F. Brading: Br. J. Pharmacol. *97*, 281–291 (1989).

103 G. Edwards, M. Henthorn and A.H. Weston: Naunyn–Schmiedeberg's Arch. Pharmacol. *183*, 2408–2409 (1990).

104 T.L. Grant, C.J. Ohnmacht and B.B. Howe: Trends Pharmacol. Sci. *15*, 402–404 (1994).

105 B.B. Howe, T.J. Halterman, C.L. Yochim, M.L. Do, S.J. Pettinger, R.B. Stow, C.J. Ohnmacht, K. Russell, J.R. Empfield, D.A. Trainor, F.J. Brown and S.T. Kau: J. Pharmacol. Exp. Ther. *274*, 884–890 (1995).

106 J.H. Li, G.D. Yasay, S.T. Kau, C.J. Ohnmacht, D.A. Trainor, A.D. Bonev, T.J. Heppner and M.T. Nelson: Arzneimittel Forsch. *46*, 525–530 (1996).

107 J. Morley: Trends Pharmacol. Sci. *15*, 463–468 (1994).

108 K.-H. Buchheit and A. Hofmann: Naunyn-Schmiedeberg's Arch. Pharmacol. *354*, 355–361 (1996).

109 P.W. Manley: WO-09637490 (1996).

110 J.J. Zeiller, M. Brunet, G. Chavernac, P. Durbin, D. Guerrier, T.N. Luong and M. Noblet: Proc. Am. Chem. Soc. *212*, MEDI 137 (1996).

111 J.F. Burka, J.L. Berry, R.W. Foster, R.C. Small and A.J. Watt: Br. J. Pharmacol. *104*, 263–269 (1991).

112 J.A. Nadel: J. Clin. Invest. *97*, 2689–2690 (1996).

113 G.J. Gross; in: Potassium Channels and their Modulation: From Synthesis to Clini-
     cal Experience (J.M. Evans, T.C. Hamilton, S.D. Longman and G. Stemp, eds). Tay-
     lor & Francis, London (1996), pp. 257–273.

114 K.S. Atwal, G.J. Grover, S.Z. Ahmed, F.N. Ferrara, T.W. Harper, K.S. Kim, P.G. Sleph,
     S. Dzwonczyk, A.D. Russell, S. Moreland, J.R. McCullough and D.E. Normandin: J.
     Med. Chem. *36*, 3971–3974 (1993).

115 H. Herdon, in: Potassium Channels and their Modulation: From Synthesis to Clin-
     ical Experience (J.M. Evans, T.C. Hamilton, S.D. Longman and G. Stemp, eds). Tay-
     lor & Francis, London (1996), pp. 361–382.

116 J.B. Lenfers, V. Muschalek-Letina, E. Niemers, A. Scriabine, J. Chisholm and E. Hun-
     nicutt: EP 0 561 237 A2 (1993).

117 T.P. Blackburn, R.E. Buckingham, W.N. Chan, J.M. Evans, M.S. Hadley, M. Thomp-
     son, N. Upton, T.O. Stean, G. Stemp and A.K. Vong: Bioorg. Med. Chem. Lett. *5*,
     1163–1166 (1995).

118 E.J. Hunnicutt, J.N: Davis and J.C. Chisholm: Eur. J. Pharmacol. *261*, R1–R3 (1994).

119 W.N. Chan, J.M. Evans, M.S. Hadley, H.J. Herdon, J.C. Jerman, H.K.A. Morgan, T.O.
     Stean, M. Thompson, N. Upton and A.K. Vong: J. Med. Chem. *39*, 4537–4539 (1996).

Progress in Drug Research, Vol. 49 (E. Jucker, Ed.)
© 1997 Birkhäuser Verlag, Basel (Switzerland)

Neuronal prostacyclin receptors

By Helen Wise

Department of Pharmacology, The Chinese University of Hong Kong, Shatin, New Territories, Hong Kong

1   Prostacyclin

1.1   Introduction

Prostacyclin is primarily derived from vascular endothelium and has traditionally been regarded as an important regulator of haemostasis due to its potent anti-platelet and vasodilator activity [1]. However, prostacyclin has additional biological activity mediated by receptors located in both the peripheral and central nervous system (CNS), and it is recent developments in the study of these neuronal prostacyclin receptors (IP-receptors) which form the basis of the following review. These are early days still in our understanding of the neuronal function of prostacyclin; I hope therefore that this review will set the scene for what is a rapidly developing and exciting area of research. To date only one IP-receptor has been isolated and cloned [2], and this represents the classical IP-receptor present in platelets. While evidence will be presented for the existence of subtypes of the IP-receptor, to date none of these have been cloned. Therefore to avoid the use of possibly inappropriate nomenclature, I shall refer to the subtypes with respect to their primary location, for example enteric IP-receptors or neuronal IP-receptors.

1.2   Prostacyclin biosynthesis

Prostanoids are formed by the initial conversion of arachidonic acid to a common intermediate, PGH_2, by the enzyme cyclooxygenase (COX) [3]. The subsequent synthesis of the prostanoids prostaglandin D_2 (PGD_2), prostaglandin E_2 (PGE_2), prostaglandin $F_{2\alpha}$ ($PGF_{2\alpha}$), prostacyclin (PGI_2) and thromboxane A_2 (TxA_2) is then dependent on the particular isomerase/reductase complement of various tissues and cells. While many of these prostanoids are non-specific in their ability to interact with prostanoid receptors, each prostanoid shows greatest potency at its own receptor. Accordingly, under the IUPHAR classification of prostanoid receptors, PGD_2, PGE_2, $PGF_{2\alpha}$, PGI_2, and TxA_2 act preferentially at DP-, EP-, FP-, IP- and TP-receptors, respectively [4].

The cyclooxygenase enzyme exists in two forms, the constitutive form (COX-1) and the mitogen-inducible form (COX-2). As we shall see later (Sec. 3.3), it is COX-2 which is of particular interest in relation to the neuronal activity of prostacyclin. Prostacyclin synthase converts PGH_2 to the chemically unstable prostacyclin, which has a half-life of 2 to 3 min, breaking down to 6-oxo-$PGF_{1\alpha}$ [1]. The prostacyclin synthase gene has been assigned to human chromosome 20 [5], and prostacyclin synthase mRNA is widely expressed in human tissues [6], especially in heart, skeletal muscle and lung, which have a high blood flow per mass of tissue. It is therefore surprising to find that prostacyclin synthase mRNA is also highly expressed in ovary and prostate [6]. Inflammatory cytokines such as interleukin (IL)-1, IL-6 and tumor necrosis factor α (TNF$_\alpha$) can enhance the expression of the prostacyclin synthase gene in cultured human and bovine aortic endothelial cells [6], endothelial cells being the most active producers of prostacyclin [1].

1.2   Prostacyclin mimetics

Prostacyclin itself is rarely used when studying IP-receptors because of its short half-life and its ability to stimulate EP- and TP-receptors [7]. Instead, one can use a variety of prostacyclin analogues, some of the more important examples being shown in Figure 1. The most potent and selective of these prostacyclin analogues is cicaprost, primarily because it lacks the potent EP$_1$-agonist activity associated with iloprost, carbacyclin and isocarbacyclin [7]. In addition, cicaprost is also a relatively weak EP$_3$-agonist compared with these other prostacyclin analogues [8, 9]. Surprisingly, cicaprost is a relatively weak agonist of the recently identified IP-receptor in the CNS (see Sec. 3.1); therefore we now need to show some caution in interpreting results from studies using cicaprost and other established IP-agonists.

In addition to these prostacyclin analogues, IP-receptors can be activated by compounds with structures dissimilar to prostacyclin such as EP 157 and EP 185, which are about 50-fold less potent than cicaprost on human washed platelets [10] (Fig. 2). Similar anti-platelet and vasodilator activity is seen with octimibate, which forms the basis of a series of non-prostanoid prostacyclin mimetics developed by Bristol-Myers Squibb (Fig. 2), culminating in BMY 45778 which is merely 10-fold less potent than iloprost in inhibiting human platelet aggregation [11].

2   IP-receptor pharmacology

2.1   The molecular biology of IP-receptors

The deduced amino acid sequences of the cloned IP-receptors infer their membership of the G protein-coupled receptor superfamily. The first IP-receptor to be cloned in 1994 was the mouse IP-receptor [12]; thereafter cDNA for the human IP-receptor [13–15], and rat IP-receptor [16] were rapidly reported. Because the IP-receptor was one of the last of the prostanoid receptor family to be cloned, the screening strategy could make

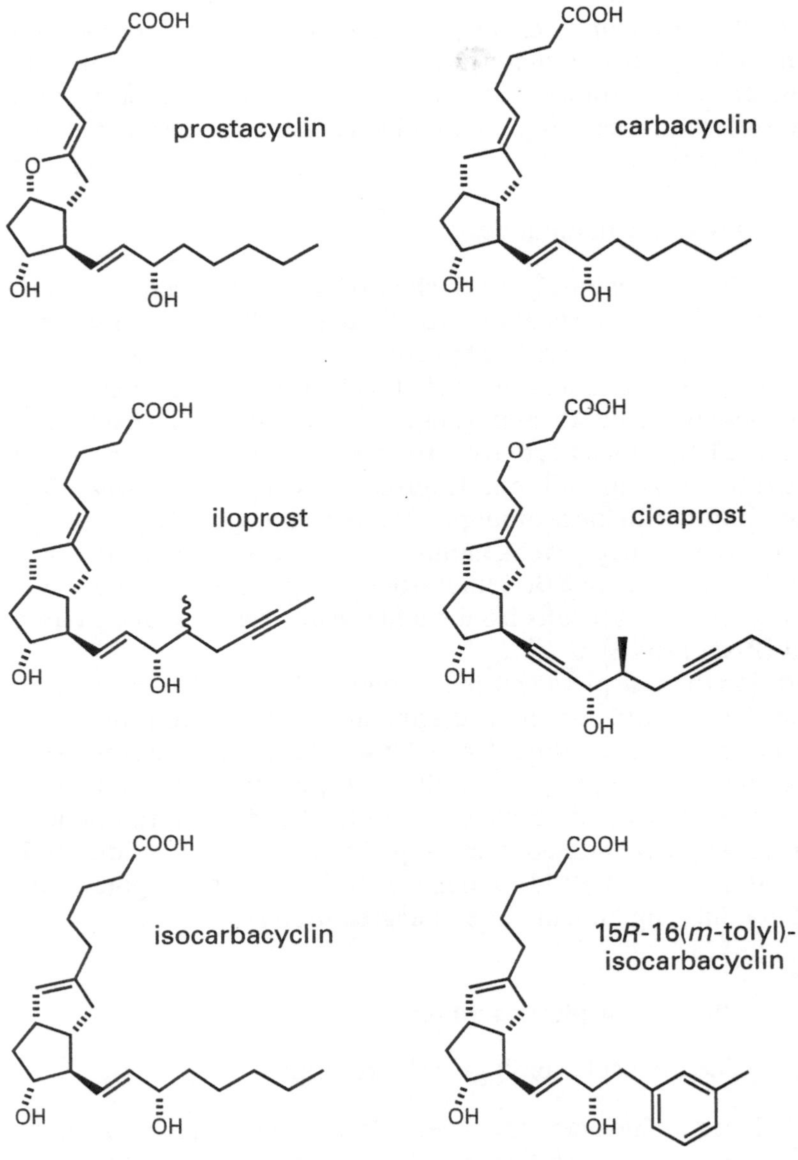

Fig. 1
Prostacyclin analogues.

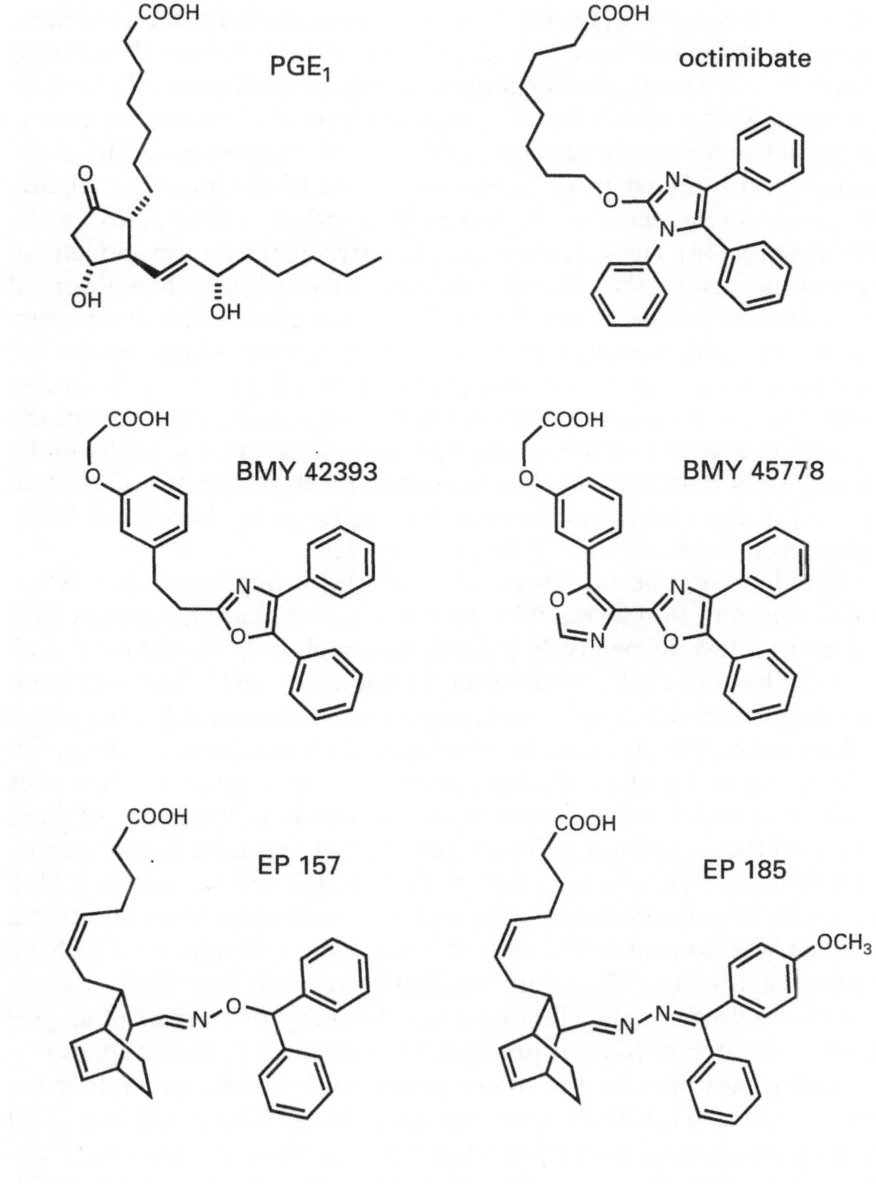

Fig. 2
PGE₁ and non-prostanoid prostacyclin mimetics.

use of the observation that there are highly conserved amino acid sequences in the second and seventh transmembrane-spanning domains of EP- and TP-receptors [17–19]. By using primers corresponding to these conserved sequences, Namba et al. [12] isolated the mouse IP-receptor cDNA by reverse transcription polymerase chain reaction and hybridization screening of a cDNA library prepared from P-815 mouse mastocytoma cells. The human IP-receptor cDNA encodes a polypeptide of 386 amino acids [13–15], whereas the mouse and rat IP-receptors are slightly larger at 417 amino acids for the mouse [12] and 416 amino acids for the rat IP-receptor [16]. The sequence identity between the mouse and human IP-receptors is only 73%, this value being relatively lower than observed in other rhodopsin-type receptors [18]. The human IP-receptor differs from the mouse receptor most notably at the translation initiation site, with the human homologue having an N-terminus which is 30 amino acids shorter than that of the mouse IP-receptor [2]. In general, the clones from the three species are very similar in their primary structure, especially in the second cytoplasmic loop, which may be important for receptor-G protein coupling [2]. The mouse and human IP-receptor genes have been localised on chromosomes 7 and 19, respectively [20].

The cloned mouse and rat IP-receptors display a single class of [^{3}H]iloprost binding site with an equilibrium dissociation binding constant (K_d) of 4.5 and 1.3 nM, respectively [12,16]. Although both Katsuyama et al. [14] and Nakagawa et al. [15] also found a single class of [^{3}H]iloprost binding site (K_d values of 3.3 and 24 nM, respectively), Boie et al. [13] reported that the binding profile could be best fitted with a two-site model yielding Kd values of 1 and 44 nM. Two populations of iloprost binding sites with different affinities have been reported elsewhere, but in one of these studies [21] the same human IP-receptor cDNA was used as that described by Boie et al. [13]. In the other study of Leigh and MacDermot [22], using NCB-20 neuroblastoma cells, [^{3}H]iloprost bound to an additional site which was non-saturable, non-stereospecific and appeared to have no biological function. Therefore we should presently view the two binding sites observed for the cloned human IP-receptor of Boie et al. [13] with some caution until their functional significance becomes clearer.

The binding affinities of the major prostanoid ligands are similar for human, mouse and rat IP-receptors expressed in COS-M6, COS-7 or CHO cells; they compete with [^{3}H]iloprost binding in the following order: cicaprost ≥ iloprost > PGE_1 > carbacyclin >> PGD_2 = PGE_2 = STA_2 or U-46619 (TP-receptor agonists) > $PGF_{2\alpha}$.

Although coupling to G_s and the subsequent production of cyclic AMP is usually considered the principal signalling system used by IP-receptors, these receptors can also couple to a pertussis toxin-insensitive G protein, leading to an increase in inositol phosphates [12, 14, 21]. However, there is a 1000-fold difference in the efficacies of activating the two second-messenger pathways when these cloned IP-receptors are expressed in COS and CHO cell lines [12,14,21]. Namba et al. [12] clearly demonstrated that the IP-receptor couples to multiple G proteins (G_s and G_p), rather than using G_s or its $\beta\gamma$ subunits to generate the inositol phosphate response. This ability of the IP-receptor to couple to more than one G protein may be responsible for the past confusion over the existence of receptor subtypes (see Sec. 2.2).

Given the promiscuous nature of receptor-G protein coupling [23], one could conclude that the IP-receptor activates the turnover of inositol phosphates due to the relatively high expression level of IP-receptors in transfection experiments (typically 2–6 pmol/mg protein). However there is evidence of normal functional coupling of the IP-receptor to G_p; for example, multiple signalling pathways for IP-receptors have been noted in a variety of transformed cell lines, but in this instance there is much closer agreement between the potencies of IP-agonists for stimulating cyclic AMP and IP_3 production [24]. In addition, prostacyclin-mediated depolarization of rat vagus nerve can be mimicked by forskolin or phorbol dibutyrate (see Sec. 4.3.2).

In general though, the biological relevance of this latter G_p-coupled pathway is unclear. It could be responsible for the agonist-dependent protein kinase C (PKC)-mediated phosphorylation of the human IP-receptor, especially as higher concentrations of IP-agonist are also required for this process [21]. This agonist-dependent phosphorylation does not appear to depend on protein kinase A (PKA) activity [21]. Both TxA_2 and phorbol myristate acetate (PMA)-treated platelets show an attenuated cyclic AMP response to iloprost; and desensitization of TP-receptors (which couple to phospholipase C) potentiates the cyclic AMP response to iloprost [25], which suggests that phosphorylation normally desensitizes the IP-receptor. There is a conserved potential PKC phosphorylation site in the carboxy-terminal tails of the mouse, rat and human IP-receptors [2]. Presumably, therefore, the IP-receptor could utilize G_s-coupled pathways for normal cell signalling, but under abnormally high tissue concentrations of prostacyclin could downregulate its responsiveness via activation of the G_p-coupled pathway, leading to agonist-dependent PKC-mediated phosphorylation of the IP-receptor. It is surprising therefore to find that in cultured mouse mast cells (IC2 cells), PKC activation enhances, rather than attenuates, IP-receptor-mediated activation of adenylate cyclase via a calmodulin/MARCKS (myristoylated alanine-rich C kinase substrate) system [26].

In addition to IP-receptor-mediated cell signalling, there exists the potential for non-receptor-mediated processes involving IP-agonists. For example, prostacyclin and prostaglandins in general have a cytoprotective action in the CNS which does not appear to be mediated by cell surface receptors [27] or by cyclic AMP [28]. In non-neuronal tissue, carbacyclin appears unique among IP-agonists such as PGE_1 and other prostaglandins in its ability to regulate the expression of two differentiation-dependent genes in preadipose and adipose cells in a fashion also apparently independent of a cell surface receptor and possibly mediated at the gene level by members of the peroxisome proliferator-activated receptor family (PPAR) [29]. Aubert et al. [29] have already shown that the IP-agonist PGE_1 is unable to mimic the gene-expression response to carbacyclin, and it would therefore clearly be interesting now to extend this study to structurally unrelated IP-agonists such as BMY 45778 and EP 157.

2.2   IP-receptor subtypes

It is perhaps worth pointing out that the existence of IP-receptor subtypes has been claimed many times [10, 30–36], but only a few such claims stand up to scrutiny. The reasons are twofold: (1) there are no IP-antagonists available to confirm pharmacologically the role of an IP-receptor in mediating the response of interest, and consequently (2) all characterization studies rely on the measurement of agonist potency ratios. Unfortunately, the potency of agonists is a highly tissue-dependent and species-dependent phenomenon [37]. Because many of the novel prostacyclin mimetics are partial agonists, one has to take extra care to account for the influence of agonist efficacy in different tissues and in different species before concluding the existence of IP-receptor subtypes. For example, if the same IP-receptor has different coupling efficiencies in different tissues or in different species, then we might incorrectly conclude the existence of IP-receptor subtypes. Indeed, different coupling efficiencies have already been reported for the cloned mouse IP-receptor expressed in CHO cells and the native receptor in P-815 mastocytoma cells [12].
The potency with which prostacyclin inhibits adenosine diphosphate (ADP)-stimulated platelet aggregation in platelet-rich plasma can vary more than 10-fold depending on the species; for example, IC_{50} values in human, rat, rabbit, horse and sheep are 0.8, 5.3, 6.7, 11.5 and 15.2 nM, respectively [38]. Whether this variation in potency of prostacyclin represents different IP-receptors in different species, or represents differences in receptor-effector coupling, still remains to be fully clarified. However, there is now substantial evidence that rodent IP-receptors may differ from

human IP-receptors with respect to agonist specificity, especially considering carbacyclin and PGE_1 compared with iloprost and cicaprost. For example, although iloprost and cicaprost are less potent anti-platelet compounds in rat compared with human platelets, the rat platelet is clearly more sensitive than the human platelet to carbacyclin [30]. Also, in NCB-20 neuroblastoma cells (mouse/hamster hybrid), iloprost and carbacyclin showed similar potencies in competition for [3H]iloprost binding [39, 40] and for stimulation of cyclic AMP production [39], but carbacyclin was at least 10-fold less potent than iloprost for both competition for [3H]iloprost binding and stimulation of adenylate cyclase activity in human platelets [39]. We can also see that PGE_1 and carbacyclin are more potent for competing with [3H]iloprost binding to cloned mouse and rat IP-receptors [12, 16] than to the cloned human IP-receptor [13–15]. Octimibate and related compounds were also able to demonstrate species specificity, being 10- to 50-fold less potent in inhibiting rat and rabbit platelets compared with human platelets [32, 41–43].

When making cross-species comparisons, we also have to be aware of the different characteristics of the assays, which may influence our interpretation of the results. Therefore, while the absolute potency of IP-agonists may differ between species, their order of potency may indicate that the receptors are similar. Using such information, we have previously suggested that IP-receptors are similar on rat neutrophils and human platelets, but differ from IP-receptors on rat platelets and rat enteric neurones ([35] and see Sec. 4.1). Thus we can conclude that, in general, the platelet IP-receptor and the platelet-like IP-receptors, i.e. the cloned IP-receptors and the IP-receptor in neuroblastoma cells, differ between humans and mice/rats.

With hindsight we can now see that the extreme metabolic instability of the endogenous ligand prostacyclin, and the reliance on the use of just one [3H]labelled IP-agonist, i.e. [3H]iloprost, has hampered the assessment of the variety of roles of prostacyclin in the body. As is often the case, pharmacological identification of receptor subtypes is highly dependent on the choice of available agonists and antagonists. In the absence of any IP-receptor antagonists, we have had to rely on the use of a few readily available IP-agonists. As we shall discover later, the synthesis and use of non-prostanoid prostacyclin mimetics has helped identify a potential IP-receptor subtype located on enteric neurones (Sec. 4.1), and the use of [3H]isocarbacyclin in addition to [3H]iloprost has identified a novel IP-receptor subtype in the CNS (Sec. 3.1). In much of the earlier work on characterizing the role of prostanoids, PGE_1 was often used instead of PGE_2 without the authors considering that while both ligands show similar potency at EP-receptors, PGE_1 has much higher affinity than PGE_2 for the prostacyclin receptor [4]. It may be necessary now to re-evaluate these studies in light of our present knowledge on subtypes of the IP-receptor, the increasingly complex organization of the EP-receptor family and the observations that IP-receptors can couple to both G_s and G_p proteins.

3   IP-receptors in the CNS

3.1   Neuronal tissue

Binding sites for [³H]iloprost in the higher centres of rat CNS show a different distribution compared with [³H]PGE_2 binding [44], and presumably therefore serve a different function. For example, as also seen in the sympathetic nervous system (Sec. 4.2), PGE_2 stimulates presynaptic EP_3-receptors to inhibit [³H]noradrenaline ([³H]NA) release in mouse brain cortex, but IP-agonists are without effect [45]. In contrast, there is a much better correlation between the binding sites for [³H]iloprost and [³H]PGE_2 in the nucleus tractus solitarius (NTS), spinal trigeminal nucleus caudalis and dorsal horn as identified by *in vitro* autoradiography of rat brain [44]. Because the binding of [³H]iloprost was not displaced by low concentrations of PGE_2, and because the distribution of [³H]iloprost binding sites in rat CNS differs from that of PGD_2 and $PGF_{2\alpha}$, it seems likely that these [³H]iloprost binding sites represent an IP-receptor located neuronally. It also now seems reasonable to conclude that in the CNS, the primary binding site for [³H]iloprost has the same characteristics as the classical platelet IP-receptor and is located predominantly in the NTS. This conclusion is supported by the more recent data of Takechi et al. [36] and by the extensive *in situ* hybridization studies of Oida et al. [46] of IP-receptor mRNA distribution in mouse tissues.

Let us consider the potential function of this "neuronal" IP-receptor using autoradiographic data. Since the three regions with high density of [³H]iloprost binding sites (see Table 1) possess a common feature in that they receive the primary sensory afferents, Matsumura et al. [44] suggested that the [³H]iloprost binding sites might be located on the presynaptic part of the central terminals of the primary sensory neurones. These authors elegantly demonstrated that [³H]iloprost (and [³H]PGE_2) binding sites were significantly reduced in the NTS 8 days following nodose ganglionectomy, with partial recovery seen afer 49 days. In addition, dorsal rhizotomy produced almost complete loss of [³H]iloprost (and [³H]PGE_2) binding sites in the dorsal horn. In contrast to a lack of effect on [³H]PGE_2 binding

Table 1
Specific binding of [³H]iloprost in rat brain

Region	Mean ± SEM (fmol/mg tissue)
Cerebral cortex	6.9 ± 0.9
Hippocampus	6.5 ± 0.7
Striatum	6.2 ± 0.2
Preoptic area	3.4 ± 0.6
Mediobasal hypothalamus	5.2 ± 0.9
Mammillary complex	4.0 ± 0.8
Thalamus	8.5 ± 0.8
Midbrain	3.8 ± 0.7
Dorsal cochlear nucleus	6.3 ± 0.9
Other pons	2.2 ± 1.0
Nucleus tractus solitarius	111.4 ± 3.5
Area postrema	47.6 ± 5.2
Spinal trigeminal nucleus caudalis	22.4 ± 0.6
Other medulla	1.3 ± 0.3
Cerebellum	2.2 ± 0.4
Dorsal horn (cervical)	29.6 ± 1.3

Reprinted from Neurosci. 65, K. Matsumura, Y. Watanabe, H. Onoe and Y. Watanabe, Prostacyclin receptor in the brain and central terminals of the primary sensory neurons: an autoradiographic study using a stable prostacylin analogue [³H]-iloprost, 493–503, 1995, with kind permission from Elsevier Science Ltd., The Boulevard, Langford Lane, Kidlington OX5 1GB, UK.

sites, ligation of the vagus nerve peripheral to the nodose ganglion (peripheral ligation) yielded an accumulation of [³H]iloprost binding sites proximal to the ligature. And, ligation central to the nodose ganglion (central ligation) also yielded an accumulation of [³H]iloprost binding sites proximal to this ligature. From these results Matsumura et al. [44] suggested that the majority of [³H]iloprost binding sites in the NTS were not located on the postsynaptic neurones of the NTS but were transported by axonic flow to the presynaptic terminals of the primary viscerosensory neurones. Furthermore, the [³H]iloprost binding sites in the dorsal horn are also located presynaptically in the central and peripheral terminals of the unmyelinated or finely myelinated primary sensory fibres. These results are supported by *in situ* hybridization studies showing very high levels of expression of mouse IP-receptor mRNA in the neurones of the dorsal root ganglia (DRG) [46] and studies of IP-agonist-mediated depolarization of rat vagus nerve [47]. All the evidence therefore indicates a role for these "neuronal" IP-receptors in the transmission of sensory signals,

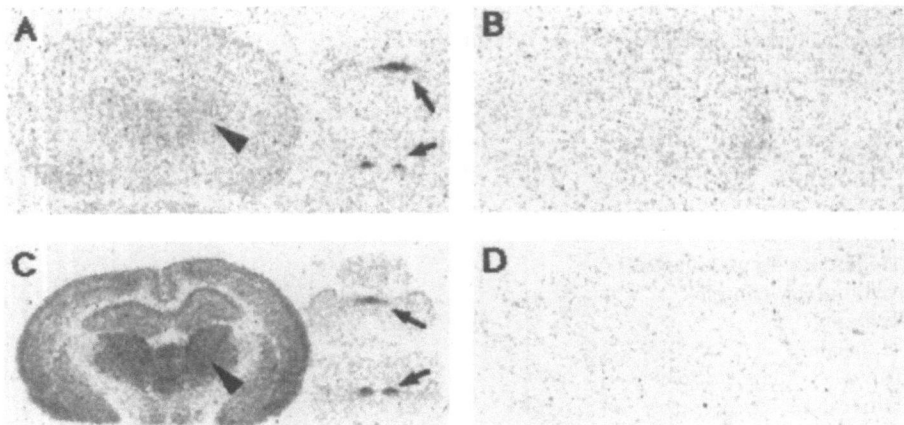

Fig. 3
Differences in autoradiographic features between [³H]iloprost and [³H]isocarbacyclin binding in rat brain sections (from [36] with permission). Cryostat sections were incubated with [³H]iloprost (A, B) or [³H]isocarbacyclin (C, D); non-specific binding (B, D). Arrows indicate the NTS, and arrowheads indicate the thalamus.

and in particular, the transmission or modulation of viscerosensory, nociceptive or thermal signals via unmyelinated or finely myelinated nerve fibres (see Sec. 4.3).

Yasuyoshi Watanabe's group have continued their study of IP-receptors in the CNS, this time using [³H]isocarbacyclin in addition to [³H]iloprost [36]. Although [³H]isocarbacyclin also bound strongly in the NTS and the spinal trigeminal nucleus, it showed considerably higher binding densities than [³H]iloprost in the thalamus, lateral septal nucleus, hippocampus, cerebral cortex, striatum and dorsal cochlear nucleus (see Fig. 3). In addition, the distribution of [³H]isocarbacyclin was quite different from that of [³H]iloprost, [³H]PGD$_2$, [³H]PGF$_{2\alpha}$, [³H]PGE$_1$ and [³H]PGE$_2$. The binding affinity of [³H]isocarbacyclin and its inhibition by other IP-agonists clearly distinguishes this binding site from that recognised by [³H]iloprost (see Table 2). Therefore, Takechi et al. [36] proposed to designate this new subtype, i.e. the [³H]isocarbacyclin binding site, as the IP$_2$-receptor and refer to the classical platelet IP-receptor as the IP$_1$-receptor. For the purpose of this review, I shall however refer to this novel IP-receptor as the neuronal IP-receptor.

Of particular note here is the ability of (15R)-TIC (15R-16-(m-tolyl)-isocarbacyclin) to discriminate between the platelet and the neuronal IP-receptor (see Table 3). Originally the tolyl group was incorporated into

Table 2
Scatchard analysis of [^{3}H]iloprost and [^{3}H]isocarbacyclin binding in rat brain

Brain region	[^{3}H]iloprost		[^{3}H]isocarbacyclin	
	K_d (nM)	B_{max} (fmol/mg)	K_d (nM)	B_{max} (fmol/mg)
NTS	6.8	194	3.9	199
Thalamus	159	163	7.8	230

Data from Takechi et al. [36].

Table 3
Specificity of [^{3}H]iloprost and [^{3}H]isocarbacyclin binding in rat brain

Brain region	Order of potency for competition with [^{3}H]isocarbacyclin binding
NTS	isocarbacyclin = cicaprost = iloprost > carbacyclin > PGE$_1$ > (15R)-TIC > PGE$_2$ > PGD$_2$ = PGF$_{2\alpha}$
Thalamus	isocarbacyclin = (15R)-TIC > carbacyclin > iloprost > PGE$_2$ > PGE$_1$ = cicaprost > PGD$_2$ = PGF$_{2\alpha}$

Data from Takechi et al. [36]. (15R)-TIC is 15R-16-(m-tolyl)-isocarbacyclin.

isocarbacyclin with a view to making a ligand suitable for positron emission tomography [48]. However, (15R)-TIC turned out to be a highly selective ligand for the neuronal IP-receptor, able to compete with [^{3}H]isocarbacyclin binding in rat thalamus and NTS with IC$_{50}$ values of 31 nM and 1.2 μM, respectively [48]. In agreement with these binding experiments, (15R)-TIC was approximately 100-fold less potent than cicaprost and isocarbacyclin in inhibiting human platelet aggregation [48]. Although the (15S) isomer also showed high affinity binding in the thalamus (IC$_{50}$ = 38 nM), it did not discriminate between the platelet and neuronal IP-receptor (IC$_{50}$ = 23 nM in NTS) [48]. The ability of a radioligand binding site to discriminate between isomeric forms of a ligand is one of the pieces of evidence used to suggest that we are indeed looking at a specific receptor site.

To date, activation by low concentrations of cicaprost has always been used as evidence for the role of IP-receptors in mediating a biological response. However, given the relative lack of potency of cicaprost at this neuronal IP-receptor, we will now have to be more cautious in dismissing the role of IP-receptors if cicaprost shows little activity. Another distinction of this neuronal IP-receptor is that it does not appear to couple to changes in cyclic AMP production, phospholipid turnover or calcium concentrations, but the authors make a cautionary note that further experiments are needed to make sure that this is not simply a reflection of low sensitivity assays in cell systems which may have low receptor level expression.

In addition, hemilesion studies of striatal neurones lesioned by kainate or of dopaminergic afferents lesioned by 6-hydroxydopamine revealed that the binding sites for [^{3}H]isocarbacyclin exist on neuronal cells in the striatum, but not on the presynaptic terminals of afferents or on glial cells. Furthermore, electrophysiological studies in the CA1 region of the rat hippocampus revealed that prostacyclin itself, and prostacyclin analogues, have a facilitatory effect on the excitatory transmission through the novel neuronal IP-receptor.

It is interesting now to consider the role of this neuronal IP-receptor in the CNS. Although prostacyclin injected into the third cerebral ventricle (i.c.v.) can cause a surprisingly long-lasting hyperthermic response, it is considerably less potent than PGE_2 and would not appear to be involved in the pathogenesis of fever [49]. Curiously, though, there are behavioural responses in addition to the hyperthermic response to i.c.v. administration of prostacyclin which are species-dependent. For example, prostacyclin (i.c.v.) caused sedation in cats but increased activity in rabbits [49].

The blood-brain barrier permeability of isocarbacyclin and related analogues can be increased by incorporating the prostanoids into lipid microspheres [50, 51]. Thus Japanese pharmaceutical scientists have taken the methyl ester of isocarbacyclin (TEI-9090) [52] and incorporated it into lipid microspheres. The resulting drug (TTC-909) can pass through the blood-brain barrier where it is de-esterified to its active metabolite isocarbacyclin, TEI-7165. When given intravenously 10 min after transient forebrain ischaemia in stroke-prone spontaneously hypertensive rats, TTC-909 dose-dependently protected against pyramidal cell layer death in the hippocampus [50]. Although the attentuation of ischaemic neuronal cell death by TTC-909 may be due to improvement in post-ischaemic events in the local cerebral blood flow and blood-brain barrier permeability, the authors speculate that there may also be a direct effect of TTC-909 on the CNS. Furthermore, when patients with chronic cerebral infarction were treated with this lipid isocarbacyclin preparation, a significant improvement in neurological and mental symptoms was noted after merely 7 days [53]. However, because lipid microspheres containing prostacyclin analogues tend to accumulate at arteriosclerotic lesions in the vascular wall [53], and because isocarbacyclin is nonselective for platelet and neuronal IP-receptors, it is still possible that we are primarily seeing a beneficial cardiovascular effect of IP-agonists, rather than an effect mediated by neuronal IP-receptors.

Prostaglandins do have some protective effect *in vitro* and can protect rat cortical neurones from glutamate-induced toxicity [27], but this cytoprotective effect may not actually be mediated by prostaglandin receptors located in the plasma membrane of cells. Initial studies showed that prostacyclin and its metabolite 6-oxo-PGF$_{1\alpha}$ could protect rat cortical neurones in culture against hypoxia/reoxygenation injury [28]. This cytoprotective action of prostacyclin was not mimicked by cyclic AMP and was surprisingly long-lasting given the short half-life of prostacyclin in these assays. These results need re-evaluating given the possible cyclic AMP-independent neuronal IP-receptor [36], and in light of the ability of carbacyclin to activate PPARs [29]. It would now be interesting to look at the effect of (15*R*)-TIC in various models of neuronal cell death, since this ligand is highly selective for the neuronal IP-receptor.

3.2 Neuronal cell lines

Although relatively little attention has been paid to the role of prostacyclin in the CNS, we already know a great deal about the regulation of IP-receptors and their coupling to adenylate cyclase from studies using neuronal cell lines. Some of the first studies using radiolabelled IP-agonists were performed using neuronal cell lines such as NCB-20 [39] and NG108-15 [54]. The NCB-20 cell line is the result of the fusion of mouse neuroblastoma with foetal hamster brain cells, and usually displays a single class of [^{3}H]iloprost binding sites with a K_d of 5.1–29.9 nM and B_{max} of 183.3–347 fmol/mg protein, equivalent to about 80,000 sites per cell [39,40]. In contrast, Leigh and MacDermot [22] demonstrated the presence of two affinity binding sites for [^{3}H]iloprost in NCB-20 cells; there was a single population of high-affinity receptors (K_d 9.55 nM and B_{max} 431 fmol/mg protein) and an additional second low-affinity, non-saturable, non-stereospecific site of no biological significance. It is likely that this second site is not often seen in other studies due to the need to use relatively high concentrations of radioligand [54]. Iloprost and carbacyclin showed similar EC_{50} values (approximately 90 nM) for stimulation of cyclic AMP production in NCB-20 cells [39]. Although Hall and Strange [39] concluded that there was a broad agreement with data in NCB-20 cells and human platelets, in hindsight we see signs of a species difference in the relative lack of potency of carbacyclin in human cells (see Sec. 2.2). The K_d values for [^{3}H]iloprost binding to membranes of NG108-15 (mouse neuroblastoma × rat glioma hybrid) cells is also approximately 5–15 nM, which is similar to the affinity of [3H]iloprost binding in the NTS rather than in the thalamus [36].

There have been surprisingly few studies attempting to characterize these neuroblastoma IP-receptors using the increasing variety of IP-agonists currently available. Using some of the non-prostanoid prostacyclin mimetics related to octimibate, Wise and Chow [55] showed that the IP-receptor coupled to adenylate cyclase in the human neuroblastoma cell line SK-N-SH was similar to the human platelet IP-receptor. This is perhaps not unexpected, because neuroblastoma cell lines derive from neural crest cells, which ordinarily give rise to spinal ganglionic cells [56], and as we have seen above, the dorsal horn and DRG are well endowed with the classical platelet IP-receptor. However, in light of the discovery of a neuronal IP-receptor with characteristics different from those of the platelet IP-receptor (see Sec. 3.1) and an unknown intracellular signalling pathway, then these neuroblastoma cell lines should now be re-examined to look for (15R)-TIC-displaceable [3H]isocarbacyclin binding to indicate the presence of the neuronal IP-receptor.

NG108-15 cells are the favoured cell line for studying IP-receptor function and regulation. The IP-receptor in NG108-15 cells is present at approximately 100,000 copies per cell, whereas there are some 1.25 million copies of $G_s\alpha$ but only 17,500 copies of adenylate cyclase per cell [57]. Thus the amount of adenylate cyclase present forms the rate-limiting component in the signal transduction pathway following IP-receptor stimulation in these cells. Iloprost causes a concentration-dependent increase in the formation of the complex between $G_s\alpha$ and adenylate cyclase (as measured by specific high-affinity binding of [3H]forskolin) in NG108-15 cells, with an IC_{50} value of 5 nM [58].

Prolonged exposure of NG108-15 cells to iloprost results in subsequent reduction in the capacity for adenylate cyclase activation by iloprost, the adenosine analogue NECA or NaF, whereas the NCB-20 cell only loses its responsiveness to iloprost [54, 59]. The heterologous desensitization seen in NG108-15 cells may, as seen in human platelets, involve the functional loss of $G_s\alpha$ from the cell membrane. The role of IP-receptor internalization in the process of IP-receptor downregulation is still far from clear [60–62], although a major component may be due to the loss of IP-receptors and $G_s\alpha$ [63] and the increased breakdown of existing receptors [64]. In addition to IP-agonist-mediated downregulation of IP-receptors, the cyclic AMP response of NG108-15 cells and human neuroblastoma SH-SY5Y cells to PGE_1 (presumably via activation of IP-receptors) can be increased in opioid-tolerant/dependent cells due to enhanced coupling efficiency between the receptor and G_s [65, 66].

What then are the consequences of IP-receptor-mediated increases in cyclic AMP in NG108-15 cells? Well, iloprost partially inhibits both L- and N-type calcium channel currents, and this effect can be attenuated with PKA inhibitors such as Rp-cyclic AMPS and H89, and by downregulation of Gs [67]. Thus one of the consequences of IP-receptor activation in NG108-15 cells is cyclic AMP-dependent inhibition of calcium channel currents. Whether or not IP-receptors are important in the functioning of glial cells is still unclear. In a review of prostanoid receptors on cultured glial cells, Inagaki and Wada [68] described the presence of EP-, FP- and TP-receptors, but no mention was made of IP-receptors. mRNA for EP_3-, FP- and TP-receptors is present in cultured rat astrocytes and oligodendrocytes, but only EP_3- and TP-receptor mRNA was found in microglia [69]. More recently, Oida et al. [46] found no evidence of IP-receptor mRNA in mouse glial cells *in vivo*. With the IP-receptor being the last of the prostanoid family of receptors to be cloned, we will have to wait a while to gain more information on the expression of IP-receptor mRNA in isolated cultures of glial cells.

3.3   COX activity in the CNS

As there appear to be IP-receptors in the CNS, we should consider the source of the prostacyclin which is necessary to stimulate these receptors. Although we normally think of brain vascular cells as the major source of prostacyclin in the CNS, nonvascular cells such as astrocytes and meningeal cells also potentially produce it [70, 71]. While it had been presumed that production of prostacyclin in neuronal cells was possible because the sympathetic postganglionic neurones could produce it in response to noradrenergic stimulation [72,73], it is only recently that there has been a renewed interest in the role of prostaglandins in the CNS due to the discovery that expression of the *COX-2* gene in the CNS is activity-dependent. COX-2 is expressed throughout the rat forebrain in discrete populations of neurones (being absent in glia and vascular endothelial cells) and is enriched in the cortex and hippocampus [74]. Surprisingly, COX-2 mRNA is constitutively expressed in rat telencephalic neurones even under normal unstimulated conditions [75]. COX-2 expression increases in response to electroconvulsive seizure activity, and in response to high-frequency stimili applied in the hippocampus (blocked by MK-801, an *N*-methyl-D-aspartate (NMDA) receptor antagonist), and is induced by acute stress [74]. In addition, basal expression appears to be regulated by natural synaptic activity and by the adrenocortical axis. Excitotoxin injection into the rat nucleus basalis also causes a marked induction of COX-2 mRNA which is attenuated by MK-801 and by inhibition of glutamate release by lamotrigine [76]. There is also a correlation between the extent of COX-2 mRNA induction in cortical regions at 4 h (attenuated by MK-801) and the severity of tissue damage at 24 h following cerebral ischaemia resulting from permanent middle cerebral artery occlusion in the rat [77]. Furthermore, *COX-2* is a member of a growing family of immediate early genes that are rapidly regulated in brain neurones by synaptic activity but do not appear to encode transcription factors. And as with other immediate early genes, COX-2 mRNA shows a distinct developmental pattern which parallels that of excitatory synapse formation in the rat brain [74].

Unfortunately, *in vivo* studies of COX-2 expression in the CNS tend to offer contradictory evidence concerning the neuronal or glial cell localization of COX-2 mRNA. Lipopolysaccharide (LPS) injection in rats can induce COX-2 mRNA expression in non-parenchymal cells of blood vessels and leptomeninges, and in neuronal cells restricted to telencephalic areas. But it is thought that the constitutive form of neuronal COX-2 presumably does not produce prostaglandins involved in temperature regulation, since non-steroidal anti-inflammatory drugs do not affect normal body temperature. Thus Cao et al. [75] concluded that prostaglandins derived from induced COX-2 in the inner surface of blood vessels and leptomeninges was most likely responsible for fever generation in response to LPS, and later went on to identify endothelial cells as the major source of COX-2 induced in response to IL-1β [78].

When studied in isolation, microglial cultures respond to adenosine $A_{2\alpha}$-receptor agonists with an increase in COX-2 mRNA levels and the synthesis of PGE_2 [79]. However, when studied in mixed primary cultures, prostaglandin endoperoxide synthase protein (i.e. COX) was found predominantly in neurones, not in glial cells, and results suggest that COX is induced mainly in the neurone during the developmental stage with the aid of a certain factor(s) derived from proliferating glial cells, and then is located in both neurones and glial cells in the mature brain [80].

To date there have been few studies concentrating on prostacyclin from neuronal sources, possibly because cultured neuronal cells produce only negligible amounts of prostanoids compared with astrocytes [81]. Eicosanoids, including 6-oxo-$PGF_{1\alpha}$, can be released in micromolar concentrations from brain tissues under hypoxic stress [82, 83], and 6-oxo-$PGF_{1\alpha}$ is detectable in the brain and is increased by pathological conditions such as convulsion [84]. However, the profile of synthesis reported varies markedly among tissues and species [85]. For example, the small blood vessels, choroid plexus and the leptomeninges tend to synthesize more prostacyclin than PGE_2, $PGF_{2\alpha}$ or TxA_2, whereas brain tissue makes mostly PGD_2, PGE_2 or $PGF_{2\alpha}$ depending on the species; thus PGD_2 appears to be the major prostaglandin metabolite in rat brain [82]. It would seem that neuronal IP-receptors are more likely to be activated by prostacyclin released from non-neuronal tissues, but clearly this conclusion requires further clarification.

There are, of course, methodological problems to be encountered when studying prostanoid release from brain tissue, especially with regard to the most appropriate sampling time. For example, in a model of closed head injury in rats, the 6-oxo-$PGF_{1\alpha}$ concentration in cortical slices taken from the injured zone doubles after 15 min and returns to basal levels between 4 and 10 days following injury [86]. In contrast, a much more dramatic increase in PGE_2 does not occur until 18 h post injury, yet this also returns to normal after 4 days [86]. The most marked changes in cerebrospinal fluid (CSF) prostacyclin and TxA_2 occurred during the first 4 h after stroke onset, whereas they were undetectable in CSF samples from non-neurologic patients [87]. Prostacyclin and TxA_2 remained elevated until at least 24 h after stroke onset, and this may indicate damage in the brain vascular compartment and be responsible for the late, vasogenic, component of ischaemic brain oedema [87]. Not only is the correct sampling time required, but the method of sample collection may also influence the interpretation of results. For example, Yergey et al. [88] showed that continuously sampled monkey CSF contains measurable concentrations of PGE_2, $PGF_{2\alpha}$, and 6-oxo-$PGF_{1\alpha}$ (>100 pg/ml), but acutely sampled monkey CSF is similar to human CSF in having immeasurable concentrations of prostaglandins.

Since marked increases in brain eicosanoid synthesis occur during brain hypoxia and convulsive states, Hertting and Seregi [81] concluded that there is a close correlation between neuronal activity and prostanoid formation. Samples of ventricular fluid from patients with head injuries yield some of the highest prostanoid values, especially for prostacyclin [85]. White [85] concluded that prostanoid synthesis is likely to be highest in patients with severe acute injury, to be intermediate when the condition is not life-threatening, to wane as clinical status improves and to be lowest in normal individuals.

Because increased expression of COX-2 would be expected to increase the generation of PGH_2, we clearly need to know more about the distribution of the synthetic enzymes which would convert PGH_2 to prostaglandins, prostacyclin or thromboxane. For example, Fiebich et al. [79] found that activation of adenosine $A_{2\alpha}$-receptors in rat microglial cells led to an increase in COX-2 mRNA levels and the synthesis of PGE_2. However, no measurements of other COX-2 products were made in this study.

As pointed out by Yamagata et al. [74], PGH_2 is highly lipid soluble and could diffuse from neurones to more remote regions of the same neurone, or to adjacent neurones and glial cells. Thus, PGH_2 might diffuse to adjacent oligodendroglia and be converted to PGD_2, or to microvessels and be converted to prostacyclin. When considering the role of the products of COX activity in the CNS, it is worth noting the results from clinical investigations of patients with Alzheimer's disease. There appears to be a beneficial effect for patients taking NSAIDs on the progression of the disease, which may indicate an important pathological role for COX-2 and prostaglandins in neurodegenerative diseases [89].

4   IP-receptors in the peripheral nervous system

4.1   The enteric nervous system

The better-recognized side effects associated with the use of prostacyclin in humans are facial flushing and headaches [1]. In addition, O'Grady [90] noted that colicky central abdominal discomfort, although less frequently experienced, was reproducible in one subject. Thus the following reports on the activity of prostacyclin in the gastrointestinal tract may not be entirely unexpected.

Prostacyclin and $PGF_{2\alpha}$ are predominantly synthesized in the lamina propria of the gastrointestinal tract and are considered as important signal substances in neuroimmune interactions in the intestine (see [91] for references). The lamina propria elements are in close proximity to the submucosal plexus, suggesting that prostaglandins may affect colonic ion transport via actions on colonic submucosal neurones and axon terminals in the mucosa. When prostacyclin is applied directly to submucosal neurones in guinea pig colon (either by pressure microejection or by tissue perfusion), it evokes depolarization of the membrane potential with an enhanced spike discharge [91]. This depolarizing response to prostacyclin was tetrodotoxin-insensitive, indicating a direct postsynaptic effect of prostacyclin on the impaled neurones. Occasionally, fast excitatory postsynaptic potentials (fEPSPs) occurred in an irregular burst, suggesting that part of the response to prostacyclin was due to activation of other neurones which project onto the impaled neurone. The physiological relevance of these observations remains uncertain, given that while the vast majority of neurones responded to prostacyclin, relatively few type-3 neurones were depolarized by prostacyclin. In contrast to these tetrodotoxin-insensitive depolarization responses, electrical field stimulation evoked a tetrodotoxin- and atropine-sensitive increase in short-circuit current which was significantly enhanced in the presence of prostacyclin.

Early reports indicated that prostacyclin could stimulate neuronal structures, such as cholinergic nerves in guinea pig ileum, leading to contraction of the longitudinal muscle [92]. However, further examination by Jones and Lawrence [93] showed that atropine could not abolish the contractile action of cicaprost, whereas morphine and tetrodotoxin could. Studies of prostaglandin activity in guinea pig ileum have been hampered by the coexistence of contractile and relaxant responses to non-selective prostaglandin receptor agonists [8]. However, careful examination of this complicated tissue preparation has revealed that the ileum is more sensitive to the neuronal contractile action of cicaprost (pIC_{25} = 8.89) than to the direct smooth muscle inhibitory action of this IP-agonist (pIC_{25} = 7.66) [8].

Further studies by Lawrence et al. [8] showed that the ganglion-blocking drug hexamethonium had no significant effect on the contractile action of cicaprost, indicating a post-ganglionic target for cicaprost in the guinea pig ileum. Furthermore, the contractile action of cicaprost was partially inhibited by the NK_1-receptor antagonist CP-96,345. It was concluded therefore that cicaprost acted on enteric neurones in guinea pig ileum to release both acetylcholine (ACh) and a tachykinin which activates NK_1-receptors on longitudinal smooth muscle. The involvement of a tachykinin in mediating the response to IP-receptor activation may give us a clue to the potential interaction between IP-receptors and tachykinins in dorsal root ganglia cells (see Sec. 4.3.1).

In the rat colon, IP-agonists also have a neuronal site of action and can inhibit spontaneous contractile activity by activation of enteric neurones and the release of non-adrenergic non-cholinergic (NANC) neurotransmitters [94]. Thus the Na^+ channel blockers saxitoxin and tetrodotoxin virtually abolished the inhibitory action of cicaprost, whereas phentolamine, propranolol and atropine were without effect. After an extensive study to identify the NANC neurotransmitters involved, it was concluded that IP-receptor activation leads to the release of nitric oxide and a second unknown neurotransmitter which is not adenosine, adenosine triphosphate (ATP), pituitary adenylate cyclase-activating peptide (PACAP) or vasoactive intestinal peptide (VIP) [94, 95]. The high potency of cicaprost in this assay (IC_{50} = 3.8 nM) would initially suggest that we are looking at a platelet, rather than a neuronal IP-receptor, because as shown in Section 3.1, cicaprost has relatively low affinity for the neuronal IP-receptor.

However, we now have evidence that the IP-receptor located on rat enteric neurones is not the same as the classical IP-receptor [35]. Having previ-

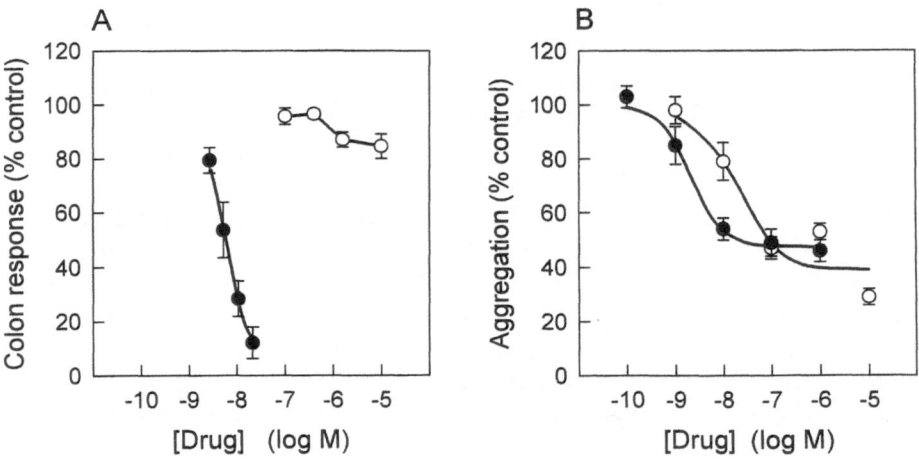

Fig. 4
Concentration-response curves for inhibition by cicaprost (●) and BMY 45778 (○) of rat colon
motility (A) and FMLP-stimulated rat neutrophil aggregation (B). Reprinted from Eur. J. Pharmacol. 278, H. Wise, Y. Qian and R.L. Jones, A study of prostacyclin mimetics distinguishes neuronal from neutrophil IP receptors, 265–269, 1995, with kind permission from Elsevier Science-
NL, Sara Burgerhartstraat 25, 1055 KV Amsterdam, The Netherlands.

ously shown that the non-prostanoid prostacyclin mimetics related to
octimibate (BMY 42393 and BMY 45778) were potent inhibitors of *N*-
formyl-methionyl-leucyl-phenylalanine (FMLP)-stimulated rat neutrophil
aggregation [96], we were surprised to find that along with EP 157, BMY
42393 and BMY 45778 showed very little ability to inhibit the spontaneous contractile activity of rat colon (Fig. 4). These non-prostanoid prostacyclin mimetics are partial agonists for stimulation of adenylate cyclase
in a variety of cells [11,96,97]. Assuming that the inhibitory effect of cicaprost is mediated by cyclic AMP, one might conclude that the partial agonist property of these compounds is responsible for their lack of effect in
rat colon. Such a conclusion would be supported if the non-prostanoid
prostacyclin mimetics could inhibit cicaprost-mediated inhibition of rat
colon with high affinity. However, although BMY 45778 inhibits FMLP-
stimulated rat neutrophil aggregation with an IC_{50} value of 20 nM [96],
BMY 45778 has considerably lower affinity in rat colon, with an apparent K_d of 4 μM [35]. Thus BMY 45778 appears to be able to distinguish
between IP-receptors located on different tissues within the same species, i.e. rat neutrophils and enteric neurones, and this provides good evidence for the existence of an IP-receptor subtype located on enteric neurones.

4.2   The sympathetic nervous system

Sympathetic postganglionic neurones can produce prostacyclin in response to noradrenergic stimulation [73]. In 1993, Jones [98] suggested that in guinea pig vas deferens, the IP-receptor is prejunctional and leads to increased release of neurotransmitter. In contrast, McKay and Poyser [99] showed that although cicaprost could potentiate the first phase of contraction (ATP-dependent) of electrical field-stimulated guinea pig vas deferens, it had no effect on the second (NA-dependent) phase of contraction. Furthermore, cicaprost could potentiate contractions by exogenous ATP, but in contrast to PGE_2 and sulprostone, did not potentiate exogenous NA. It was concluded therefore that the IP-receptors in guinea pig vas deferens were postjunctional rather than prejunctional/neuronal. More recent studies by Tam et al. [100] contradict this work and clearly indicate a prejunctional, and thus neuronal, role for IP-receptors in guinea pig vas deferens.

Although PGE_2 and prostacyclin have many overlapping properties, they clearly differ with regard to modulation of the release of NA from sympathetic nerve endings. In rat vena cava [101] and human saphenous vein or pulmonary artery [102], PGE_2 acting on presynaptic EP_3-receptors inhibits the release of $[^3H]NA$, whereas iloprost has little effect. Additional evidence that EP_3-receptors, but not IP-receptors, are located presynaptically on postganglionic sympathetic nerve fibres comes from studies of electrically induced increase in diastolic blood pressure in pithed rats [103].

4.3   Sensory neurones

4.3.1   Dorsal root ganglia cells

From the data of Matsumura et al. [44] (see Table 1 and Sec. 3.1), we know that the majority of $[^3H]$iloprost binding sites are located on the presynaptic terminals of the primary sensory neurones in the NTS. Furthermore, the $[^3H]$iloprost binding sites in the dorsal horn are also located presynaptically in the central and peripheral terminals of the unmyelinated or finely myelinated primary sensory fibres. These results are supported by *in situ* hybridization studies showing very high levels of expression of mouse IP-receptor mRNA in the neurones of the DRG [46]. Approximately 40% of neurones in mouse DRG expressed IP-receptor mRNA, and about 70% of the substance P (SP)-containing cells co-expressed IP-receptor mRNA. All the evidence therefore indicates a role for these "neuronal" IP-receptors in the transmission of sensory signals and, in particular, the transmission or modulation of viscerosensory, nociceptive or thermal signals via unmyelinated or finely myelinated nerve fibres. These "neuronal" IP-receptors are therefore the classical platelet IP-receptors located neuronally, and are not the same as the CNS neuronal IP-receptor of Takechi et al. [36].

The nociceptive effect of prostacyclin has often been overlooked in favour of PGE_2 and other more readily available prostanoids. For example, intrathecal injection PGE_2 and PGD_2, but not $PGF_{2\alpha}$, produced hyperalgesia in mice [104], but this study failed to examine the effect of prostacyclin despite there being plenty of evidence to suggest an important physiological role for prostacyclin in mediating and regulating nociception. For example, prostacyclin, like PGE_2, can induce hyperalgesia, which is a hypersensitivity response to noxious stimuli as typically measured by a decrease in the nociceptive threshold in the rat paw-withdrawal test [105, 106]. Intraperitoneal injection of zymosan in mice induces a transient writhing response (nociceptive response) accompained by increased levels of 6-oxo-$PGF_{1\alpha}$ in the peritoneal cavity [107, 108]. Much larger increases in prostacyclin than in PGE_2 were reported, and when injected intraperitoneally, prostacyclin (2 µg per mouse) induced a writhing response [107]. Prostacyclin is also much more potent than PGE_2 in potentiating bradykinin-induced pain, as measured by a reflex hypertensive response in anaesthetized dogs [109]. Intraplantar injection of morphine can antagonize both PGE_2 and prostacyclin-mediated hyperalgesia in the rat [110] with morphine clearly having a peripheral rather than a central site of action [111]. COX-2 mRNA has been identified in DRG cells, and its expression in rat spinal cord is markedly increased in the inflammatory model of adjuvant-induced paw swelling [76]. Although it is well known that levels of PGE_2 increase in the spinal cord following adjuvant injection into a rat paw, this study clearly showed that prostacyclin and not PGE_2 is the major inflammatory prostanoid under these conditions [76]. In 1992, Jones and Lawrence [93] suggested that the enteric neuronal stimulant action of cicaprost could indicate a potential role of IP-receptors in enhancing pain in inflammatory conditions. We are now only just beginning to appreciate this statement and to recognize the predominant role of prostacyclin in mediating inflammatory pain.

In addition to prostacyclin, a variety of IP-agonists such as cicaprost and carbacyclin have been shown to produce an increased sensitivity to noxious stimuli: cicaprost potentiates bradykinin-induced excitation of sensory receptors in the isolated rat hind limb preparation [112], and carbacyclin augments bradykinin-, capsaicin- and KCl-induced release of SP and calcitonin gene-related peptide (CGRP) from rat sensory neurones [113].

It is therefore surprising to find that intrathecal injection of cicaprost was much less potent than PGE_2 in inducing allodynia (a state of discomfort and pain evoked by innocuous tactile stimuli) in mice [114].

Ferreira et al. [105] showed that the hyperalgesic effect of prostacyclin was quick in onset but short-lasting, whereas hyperalgesia caused by PGE_2 develops more slowly but is prolonged. These differences in time course of activity also form the basis of the hypothesis that bradykinin-induced hyperalgesia is mediated by the production of PGE_2, whereas noradrenaline-induced hyperalgesia is mediated by the production of prostacyclin [115]. Other differences exist between prostacyclin and PGE_2; thus while both prostanoids can stimulate chemosensitive units, only prostacyclin excites articular mechanonociceptors in the isolated rat hind limb preparation *in vitro* [112].

There are two classes of hyperalgesic response to prostacyclin, first, a rapid direct response and, second, a long-lasting effect possibly caused by stimulation of a sensory nerve sensitization mechanism as used by PGE_2 [105]. Intradermal injection of prostacyclin (1–100 ng) into the rat paw produced a dose-dependent decrease in paw withdrawal thresholds, whereas subcutaneous injection of 10 μg prostacyclin far from the site of testing had no significant effect on nociceptive threshold; results which indicate that prostacyclin produces hyperalgesia by a direct action on primary afferent nociceptors [116]. Both the central and peripheral nerve terminals of sensory neurones have been extensively studied by using DRG cells in culture [117]. Carbacyclin not only has a direct effect in DRG cells, being able to directly stimulate SP and CGRP release, but also has a secondary effect of potentiating bradykinin-, capsaicin- and KCl-induced release of SP [113].

Using slices of rat NTS and patch-clamp methodology, Matsumura et al. [118] concluded that PGE_2 excites NTS neurones by activating cation conductance, with low selectivity to monovalent cations. The long latency of onset and a sustained response after washout suggested that PGE_2 action may be mediated by intracellular messengers. In voltage-clamped *Xenopus* oocytes, both PGE_1 and PGE_2 elicited an outward hyperpolarizing current, caused by an increase in K^+ conductance and appearing to involve cyclic AMP [119]. IP-receptors may couple directly to ion channels, with iloprost-mediated hyperpolarization of canine and rabbit carotid artery being partially inhibited by the K_{ATP} channel blocker glybenclamide [120, 121]. Therefore, one possible mechanism for the hyperalgesic effect of prostacyclin is its ability to inhibit the slow after-hyperpolarization by a cyclic AMP-dependent K^+ conductance mechanism, thus allowing the cell to fire repeatedly [117].

The hyperalgesic responses to both prostacyclin and PGE_2 can clearly be mimicked and prolonged by agents which increase cyclic AMP or Ca^{2+} concentrations at the nociceptive terminals [106, 122, 123]. Such results would be expected given the ability of the IP-receptor to couple to both G_s and G_p proteins (see Sec. 2.1). The role of the adenylate cyclase system in mediating the nociceptive effect of carbacyclin has been well studied in DRG cells in culture. Thus, carbacyclin significantly increased cyclic AMP concentrations in DRG cells at concentrations which also augmented the bradykinin- or capsaicin-evoked release of sensory neuropeptides, and this augmentation response was mimicked by cyclic AMP mimetics such as forskolin, cholera toxin or 8-bromo-cyclic AMP [123].

The association between the platelet IP-receptor, but not the neuronal IP-receptor, and adenylate cyclase suggests that nociception is mediated by the classical IP-receptor. However, given that we still need firmer evidence of the intracellular signalling pathways used by the neuronal IP-receptor, we cannot yet rule out a role for this receptor here in the DRG. Given that there at least two EP-receptors coupled positively to adenylate cyclase (EP_2 and EP_4 [4]), then it may be premature to assume that there is only one IP-receptor so coupled. In addition, since we are also unaware of the intracellular signalling pathway used by the enteric neuronal IP-receptor, and given the high potency of cicaprost in these nociception studies (i.e. as also seen in the enteric nervous system), we clearly need more extensive characterization studies of IP-receptors in the DRG, using a wider range of IP-agonists.

4.3.2 Vagal c-fibres

When given intravenously to anaesthetized dogs, prostacyclin, at doses which produced a substantial fall in systemic arterial blood pressure, also produced marked bradycardia instead of the normal reflex tachycardia response expected in response to hypotensive agents [38]. Prostacyclin must pass through the coronary circulation of the heart to elicit this bradycardia response, and its principal mechanism is thought to be due to activation of a reflexly mediated increase in vagal efferent discharge to the heart, rather than a direct effect on cardiac pacemaker cells, because the bradycardia induced by prostacyclin was abolished by both ganglionic blockade and atropine [124]. Electrophysiological studies have clearly shown that prostacyclin can directly stimulate these vagal cardiac c-fibres [124, 125]; however, additional alternative mechanisms need to be considered. For example, prostacyclin could also influence this vagal reflex by increasing the release of ACh from cardiac parasympathetic nerves or could potentiate the action of ACh by a direct sensitizing action on the cardiac pacemaker cells; both mechanisms would also be blocked by hex-amethonium and atropine.

The vagal afferent receptors which are thought to mediate this reflex brad-ycardia response to prostacyclin are located predominantly in the infer-oposterior wall of the left ventricle. They are termed "chemically sensi-tive receptors" or "chemosensitive endings" and differ from the classical chemosensitive fibres which respond to changes in pO_2, pH, H^+, pCO_2 and so on [124, 125]. Prostanoids seem to stimulate c-fibres in almost all organs tested, and Hintze [124] suggested that this reflex may be evidence of a general biological control mechanism rather than a cardiac-specific reflex. The overall function of this particular cardiac reflex though may be protective in the case of injured or ischaemic myocardium.

More recent studies using the isolated rat vagus nerve clearly confirm IP-receptor-mediated depolarizations of sensory afferents [47]. Prostacyclin and carbacyclin showed much higher affinity than PGE_2 for depolariz-ing the vagus nerve (pEC_{50} values were 8.4, 7.9 and 6.2, respectively). Although prostacyclin-induced depolarizations were slow in onset when compared with ligand-gated ion channels, the maximal response (393 μV) was quite comparable. This prostacyclin-mediated depolarization of rat vagus could be mimicked by forskolin or phorbol dibutyrate, which may relate to the ability of the IP-receptor to couple to both G_s and G_p pro-teins (see Sec. 2.1).

Staszewska-Barczak [125] has suggested that prostanoids, at concentra-tions too low to stimulate vagal afferent nerve endings in the heart, might sensitize them to other chemical stimuli. For example, prostacyclin sig-nificantly potentiated the reflex pressor effects of bradykinin when applied in low doses directly to the surface of the left ventricle in dogs. The dura-tion of this potentiating effect of prostacyclin, unlike that of PGE_2, was extremely brief and disappeared as soon as application of prostacyclin was discontinued. Ferreira et al. [105] noted a similar distinction in the time course of hyperalgesic activity of prostacyclin and PGE_2, which is unlikely to be due entirely to different rates of inactivation of these pros-tanoids. Thus this sensitizing action of prostacyclin on cardiac receptors may relate to the production of hyperalgesia mentioned in Section 4.3.1.

4.4   Miscellaneous

So far in Section 4 it would appear that the actions of neuronal IP-recep-tors are all stimulant, resulting in increased release of neurotransmitters. However, there is an example of a presynaptic IP-receptor which inhib-its neurotransmitter release. Prostacyclin, beraprost and iloprost all relax canine bronchial smooth muscle precontracted with either ACh or KCl [126]. However, at concentrations low enough to have no effect on muscle relaxation, beraprost and prostacyclin reduced the contractile responses to electrical field stimulation, but had no effect on exogenous ACh. Therefore, these IP-agonists appear to inhibit the release of ACh from cholinergic nerve terminals in canine airway.

5   Concluding remarks

To date, only one IP-receptor has been cloned, and this receptor displays all the characteristics of the receptor which mediates the well-known antiplatelet and vasodilator actions of prostacyclin [2]. However, with the availability of an increased variety of chemically distinct prostacyclin mimetics, we are able at last to begin to recognize the existence of species differences and subtypes of the IP-receptor. For example, the platelet IP-receptor in rat and mouse differs in agonist recognition compared with the human IP-receptor, and studies within the same species have identified IP-receptor subtypes in the CNS and in the enteric nervous system of the rat. The discovery of IP-receptor subtypes using conventional pharmacological methods has opened up the field of prostacyclin pharmacology, and forced us to reconsider the precise physiological role of prostacyclin. It is to be hoped that identification of these IP-receptor subtypes using agonist-based pharmacology will soon be followed by more definitive pharmacological characterization using IP-receptor antagonists, supported by evidence from molecular cloning studies. While we can speculate on the functional significance of these various CNS and enteric neuronal IP-receptors, the existence of platelet-like IP-receptors located neuronally in sensory pathways offers more immediate rewards with exciting possibilities in increasing our understanding of the mechanisms involved in conditions of inflammatory pain.

Acknowledgments

I should like to thank Professor R.L. Jones (Pharmacology Department, The Chinese University of Hong Kong) for providing Figures 1 and 2 and for his critical reading of this manuscript, and Professor Y. Watanabe (Osaka Bioscience Institute, Japan) for providing Figure 3. This work was supported by the Research Grants Council of Hong Kong.

References

1   S. Moncada: Br. J. Pharmacol. *76*, 3–31 (1982).
2   M. Hirata, F. Ushikubi and S. Narumiya: J. Lipid Mediators Cell Signal. *12*, 393–404 (1995).
3   P. Needleman, J. Turk, B.A. Jakschik, A.R. Morison and J.B. Lefkowith: Annu. Rev. Biochem. *55*, 69–102 (1986).
4   R.A. Coleman, W.L. Smith and S. Narumiya: Pharmacol. Rev. *46*, 205–229 (1994).
5   L. Wang and L. Chen: Biochem. Biophys. Res. Commun. *226*, 631–637 (1996).
6   T. Tanabe and V. Ullrich: J. Lipid Mediators Cell Signal. *12*, 243–255 (1995).
7   Y.J. Dong, R.L. Jones and N.H. Wilson: Br. J. Pharmacol. *87*, 97–107 (1986).
8   R.A. Lawrence, R.L. Jones and N.H. Wilson: Br. J. Pharmacol. *105*, 271–278 (1992).
9   Y. Kawai and T. Ohhashi: Br. J. Pharmacol. *112*, 635–639 (1994).
10 R.L. Jones, N.H. Wilson, C.G. Marr, G. Muir and R.A. Armstrong: J. Lipid Mediators Cell Signal. *6*, 405–410 (1993).
11 N.A. Meanwell, J.L. Romine and S.M. Seiler: Drugs of the Future *19*, 361–385 (1994).
12 T. Namba, H. Oida, Y. Sugimoto, A. Kakizuka, M. Negishi, A. Ichikawa and S. Narumiya: J. Biol. Chem. *269*, 9986–9992 (1994).
13 Y. Boie, T.H. Rushmore, A. Darmon-Goodwin, R. Grygorczyk, D.M. Slipetz, K.M. Metters and M. Abramovitz: J. Biol. Chem. *269*, 12173–12178 (1994).
14 M. Katsuyama, Y. Sugimoto, T. Namba, A. Irie, M. Negishi, S. Narumiya and A. Ichikawa: FEBS Lett. *344*, 74–78 (1994).
15 O. Nakagawa, I. Tanaka, T. Usui, M. Harada, Y. Sasaki, H. Itoh, T. Yoshimasa, T. Namba, S. Narumiya and K. Nakao: Circ. *90*, 1643–1647 (1994).
16 Y. Sasaki, T. Usui, I. Tanaka, O. Nakagawa, T. Sando, T. Takahashi, T. Namba, S. Narumiya and K. Nakao: Biochim. Biophys. Acta *1224*, 601–605 (1994).
17 K.L. Pierce, D.W. Gil, D.F. Woodward and J.W. Regan: Trends Pharmacol. Sci. *16*, 253–256 (1995).
18 M. Negishi, Y. Sugimoto and A. Ichikawa: Biochim. Biophys. Acta *1259*, 109–120 (1995).
19 F. Ushikubi, M. Hirata and S. Narumiya: J. Lipid Mediators Cell Signal. *12*, 343–359 (1995).
20 T. Ishikawa, Y. Tamai, J.M. Rochelle, M. Hirata, T. Namba, Y. Sugimoto, A. Ichikawa, S. Narumiya, M.M. Taketo and M.F. Seldin: Genomics *32*, 285–288 (1996).
21 E.M. Smyth, P.V. Nestor and G.A. Fitzgerald: J. Biol. Chem. *271*, 33698–33704 (1996).
22 P.J. Leigh and J. MacDermot: Br. J. Pharmacol. *85*, 237–247 (1985).
23 T. Kenakin: Pharmacol. Rev. *48*, 413–463 (1996).
24 H. Wise and R.L. Jones: Trends Pharmacol. Sci. *17*, 17–21 (1996).
25 R. Murray, E. Shipp and G.A. Fitzgerald: J. Biol. Chem. *265*, 21670–21675 (1990).
26 T. Sawai, M. Negishi, N. Nishigaki, T. Ohno and A. Ichikawa: J. Biol. Chem. *268*, 1995–2000 (1993).
27 C. Cazevieille, A. Muller, F. Meynier, N. Dutrait and C. Bonne: Neurochem. Int. *24*, 395–398 (1994).
28 C. Cazevieille, A. Muller and C. Bonne: Neurosci. Lett. *160*, 106–108 (1993).
29 J. Aubert, G. Ailhaud and R. Negrel: FEBS Lett. *397*, 117–121 (1996).
30 R.A. Armstrong, R.A. Lawrence, R.L. Jones, N.H. Wilson and A. Collier: Br. J. Pharmacol. *97*, 657–668 (1989).
31 A. Corsini, G.C. Folco, R. Fumagalli, S. Nicosia, M.A. Noe and D. Oliva: Br. J. Pharmacol. *90*, 255–261 (1987).

32   J.E. Merritt, T.J. Hallam, A.M. Brown, I. Boyfield, D.G. Cooper, D.M.B. Hickey, A.A. Jaxa-Chamiec, A.J. Kaumann, M. Keen, E. Kelly, U. Kozlowski and T.J. Rink: Br. J. Pharmacol. *102*, 251–259 (1991).

33   R.L. Hébert, L. Regnier and L.N. Peterson: Am. J. Physiol. *268*, F145–F154 (1995).

34   E. Ragazzi, A. Chinellato, Ü. Lille, M. Lopp, M.G. Doni and G. Fassina: Gen. Pharmacol. *26*, 703–709 (1995).

35   H. Wise, Y. Qian and R.L. Jones: Eur. J. Pharmacol. *278*, 265–269 (1995).

36   H. Takechi, K. Matsumura, Y. Watanabe, K. Kato, R. Noyori and M. Suzuki: J. Biol. Chem. *271*, 5901–5906 (1996).

37   T.P. Kenakin: J. Pharmacological Methods *13*, 281–308 (1985).

38   B.J.R. Whittle, S. Moncada, K. Mullane and J.R. Vane: Prostaglandins *25*, 205–223 (1983).

39   J.M. Hall and P.G. Strange: Bioscience Reports *4*, 941–948 (1984).

40   P.J. Leigh, W.A. Cramp and J. MacDermot: J. Biol. Chem. *259*, 12431–12436 (1984).

41   S. Seiler, C.L. Brassard, A.J. Arnold, N.A. Meanwell, J.S. Fleming and S.L. Keely Jr: J. Pharm. Exp. Ther. *255*, 1021–1026 (1990).

42   S.M. Seiler, C.L. Brassard, M.E. Federici, J.O. Buchanan, G.B. Zavoico, J.S. Fleming and N.A. Meanwell: Thromb. Res. *74*, 115–123 (1994).

43   N.A. Meanwell, J.L. Romine, M.J. Rosenfeld, S.W. Martin, A.K. Trehan, J.J.K. Wright, M.F. Malley, J.Z. Gougoutas, C.L. Brassard, J.O. Buchanan, M.E. Federici, J.S. Fleming, M. Gamberdella, K.S. Hart, G.B. Zavoico and S.M. Seiler: J. Med. Chem. *36*, 3884–3903 (1993).

44   K. Matsumura, Y. Watanabe, H. Onoe and Y. Watanabe: Neurosci. *65*, 493–503 (1995).

45   H.J. Exner and E. Schlicker: Naunyn-Schmiedeberg's Arch. Pharmacol. *351*, 46–52 (1995).

46   H. Oida, T. Namba, Y. Sugimoto, F. Ushikubi, H. Ohishi, A. Ichikawa and S. Narumiya: Br. J. Pharmacol. *116*, 2828–2837 (1995).

47   K.R. Bley, D.G. Blissard, S.M. Amagasu and R.M. Eglen: Prostaglandins Leuk. Essen. Fatty Acids *55*, S1, p159 (1996).

48   M. Suzuki, K. Kato, R. Noyori, Y. Watanabe, K. Takechi, K. Matsumura and B. Långström: Angew. Chem. Int. Ed. Engl. *35*, 334–336 (1996).

49   A.S. Milton: Ann. N Y Acad. Sci. *604*, 392–410 (1990).

50   K. Yamashita, Y. Kataoka, M. Nakashima, Y. Yamashita, H. Tanabe, H. Araki, M. Niwa and K. Taniyama: Jpn. J. Pharmacol. *71*, 351–355 (1996).

51   T. Minagawa, K. Sakanaka, S. Inaba, Y. Sai, I. Tamai, T. Suwa and A. Tsuji: J. Pharm. Pharmacol. *48*, 1016–1022 (1996).

52   M. Tanaka, C. Kojima, M. Muramatsu and H. Tanabe: Arzneimittel-Forschung *45*, 967–970 (1995).

53   K. Hoshi and Y. Mizushima: Prostaglandins *40*, 155–164 (1990).

54   E. Kelly, M. Keen, P. Nobbs and J. MacDermot: Br. J. Pharmacol. *99*, 309–316 (1990).

55   H. Wise and B.S. Chow, in: Recent Advances in Prostaglandin, Thromboxane, and Leukotriene Research (H. Sinzinger, J.R. Vane, B. Samuelsson, R. Paoletti, P.W. Ramwell and P.Y.-K. Wong, eds.), Plenum Press, New York (in press).

56   R.A. Ross, B.A. Spengler and J.L. Biedler: J. Natl. Cancer Inst. *71*, 741–749 (1983).

57   G.D. Kim, E.J. Adie and G. Milligan: Eur. J. Biochem. *219*, 135–143 (1994).

58   G.D. Kim, I.C. Carr and G. Milligan: Biochem. J. *308*, 275–281 (1995).

59   A. Krane, J. MacDermot and M. Keen: Biochem. Pharmacol. *47*, 953–959 (1994).

60   A. Krane and M. Keen: Br. J. Pharmacol. *115*, 137P (1995).

61   A. Krane and M. Keen: Br. J. Pharmacol. *115*, 138P (1995).

62 M. Keen and A. Krane: Br. J. Pharmacol. *117*, 72P (1996).

63 R.J. Williams and E. Kelly: Eur. J. Pharmacol. *268*, 177–186 (1994).

64 D. Pearce and M. Keen: Br. J. Pharmacol. *116*, 19P (1995).

65 H. Ammer and R. Schulz: Mol. Pharmacol. *43*, 556–563 (1993).

66 H. Ammer and R. Schulz: Brain Res. *707*, 235–244 (1996).

67 J. Luty, M. Hepworth, E. Kelly and G. Henderson: Br. J. Pharmacol. *116*, 355P (1995).

68 N. Inagaki and H. Wada: Glia *11*, 102–109 (1995).

69 J. Kitanaka, H. Hashimoto, M. Gotoh, K. Kondo, K. Sakata, Y. Hirasawa, M. Sawada, A. Suzumura, T. Marunouchi, T. Matsuda and A. Baba: Brain Res. *707*, 282–287 (1996).

70 S. Murphy, J. Jeremy, B. Pearce and P. Dandona: Neurosci. Letts. *61*, 61–65 (1985).

71 S.A. Moore, P.H. Figard, A.A. Spector and M.N. Hart: Ann. N Y Acad. Sci. *604*, 471–473 (1990).

72 K.U. Malik and E. Sehic: Ann. N Y Acad. Sci. *640*, 222–236 (1990).

73 R. Gonzales, C.D. Sherbourne, M.E. Goldyne and J.D. Levine: J. Neurochem. *57*, 1145–1150 (1991).

74 K. Yamagata, K.I. Andreasson, W.E. Kaufmann, C.A. Barnes and P.F. Worley: Neuron *11*, 371–386 (1993).

75 C. Cao, K. Matsumura, K. Yamagata and Y. Watanabe: Brain Res. *697*, 187–196 (1995).

76 J. de Belleroche, J. Adams and Y. Collaço-Moraes: Prostaglandins Leuk. Essen. Fatty Acids *55*, S1, p32 (1996).

77 Y. Collaço-Moraes, B. Aspey, M. Harrison and J. de Belleroche: J. Cerebral Blood Flow and Metabolism *16*, 1366-1372 (1996).

78 C. Cao, K. Matsumura, K. Yamagata and Y. Watanabe: Brain Res. *733*, 263–272 (1996).

79 B.L. Fiebich, K. Biber, K. Lieb, D. van Calker, M. Berger, J. Bauer and P.J. Gebicke-Haerter: Glia *18*, 152–160 (1996).

80 M. Kawasaki, Y. Yoshihara, M. Yamaji and Y. Watanabe: Mol. Brain Res. *19*, 39–46 (1993).

81 G. Hertting and A. Seregi: Ann. N Y Acad. Sci. *604*, 84–99 (1990).

82 P.C. Huttemeier, Y. Kamiyama, M. Su, W.D. Watkins and H. Benveniste: Prostaglandins *45*, 177–187 (1993).

83 C.W. Leffler and H. Parfenova: Am. J. Physiol. *41*, H418–H424 (1997).

84 G. Hertting and A. Seregi, in: Arachidonic Acid Metabolism in the Nervous System (A.I. Barkai and N.G. Bazan, eds.), New York Academy of Science, New York (1989), pp. 84–99.

85 R.P. White: Ann. N Y Acad. Sci. *604*, 131–145 (1990).

86 E. Shohami, Y. Shapira, G. Yadid, S. Cotev and G. Feuerstein: Ann. N Y Acad. Sci. *604*, 485–487 (1990).

87 B.M. Djuričić, V.S. Kostic and B.B. Mršulja: Ann. N Y Acad. Sci. *604*, 435–437 (1990).

88 J.A. Yergey, N. Salem Jr, J.W. Karanian, M. Linnoila and M.P. Heyes: Ann. N Y Acad. Sci. *604*, 497–499 (1990).

89 J.C.S. Breitner: Annu. Rev. Med. *47*, 401–411 (1996).

90 J. O'Grady, S. Warrington, M.J. Moti, S. Bunting, R.J. Flower, A.S.E. Fowle, E.A. Higgs and S. Moncada, in: Prostacyclin (J.R. Vane and S. Bergström, eds.), Raven Press, New York (1979), pp. 409–417.

91 T. Frieling, C. Rupprecht, G. Dobreva, D. Häussinger and M. Schemann: Pflugers Archiv. *431*, 212–220 (1996).

92 R.M. Gaion and M. Trento: Br. J. Pharmacol. *80*, 279–286 (1983).

93 R.L. Jones and R.A. Lawrence: Regul. Pept. *S1*, S83 (1992).

94 Y. Qian and R.L. Jones: Br. J. Pharmacol. *115*, 163–171 (1995).

95   R.L. Jones, Y. Qian, F.S.F. Tam, K. Chan, J.K.S. Ho and J.-P. Bourreau: Neuronal stimulant actions of prostacyclin and its novel mimetics, in: Eicosanoids and Other Bioactive Lipids in Cancer, Inflammation and Radiation Injury 3 (K.V. Honn, R.L. Jones, L.J. Marnette, S. Nigam and P.Y.-K. Wong, eds.), Plenum Press, New York (1997), 211–217.

96   H. Wise: Prostaglandins Leuk. Essen. Fatty Acids *54*, 351–360 (1996).

97   R.A. Armstrong, R.L. Jones, J. MacDermot and N.H. Wilson: Br. J. Pharmacol. *87*, 543–551 (1986).

98   R.L. Jones: Br. J. Pharmacol. 108, 16P (1993).

99   A.M. McKay and N.L. Poyser: Br. J. Pharmacol. *116*, 2679–2684 (1995).

100   F.S.F. Tam, K. Chan, J.-P. Bourreau and R.L. Jones: Br. J. Pharmacol. (in press).

101   G. Molderings, B. Malinowska and E. Schlicker: Br. J. Pharmacol. *107*, 352–355 (1992).

102   G.J. Molderings, E. Colling, J. Likungu, J. Jakschik and M. Göthert: Br. J. Pharmacol. *111*, 733–738 (1994).

103   B. Malinowska, G. Godlewski, W. Buczko and E. Schlicker: Eur. J. Pharmacol. *259*, 315–319 (1994).

104   R. Uda, S. Horiguchi, S. Ito, M. Hyodo and O. Hayaishi: Brain Res. *510*, 26–32 (1990).

105   S.H. Ferreira, M. Nakamura and M.S.A. Castro: Prostaglandins *16*, 31–37 (1978).

106   Y.O. Taiwo, L. Bjerknes, E.J. Goetzl and J.D. Levine: Neurosci. *32*, 577–580 (1989).

107   N.S. Doherty, T.H. Beaver, K.Y. Chan, J.E. Coutant and G.L. Westrich: Br. J. Pharmacol. *91*, 39–47 (1987).

108   K. Tanaka, T. Shimotori, S. Makino, M. Eguchi, K. Asaoka, R. Kitamura and C. Yoshida: J. Pharmacobio–Dyn. *15*, 641–647 (1992).

109   M. Katori, Y. Hori, Y. Uchida, K. Tanaka and Y. Harada: Adv. Exp. Med. Biol. *198*, 393–398 (1986).

110   S.H. Ferreira and M. Nakamura: Prostaglandins *18*, 191–200 (1979).

111   S.H. Ferreira and M. Nakamura: Prostaglandins *18*, 201–208 (1979).

112   G.L. Birrell and D.S. McQueen: Brain Res. *611*, 103–107 (1993).

113   C.M. Hingtgen and M.R. Vasko: Brain Res. *655*, 51–60 (1994).

114   T. Minami, I. Nishihara, R. Uda, S. Ito, M. Hyodo and O. Hayaishi: Br. J. Pharmacol. *112*, 735–740 (1994).

115   Y.O. Taiwo and J.D. Levine: Brain Res. *458*, 402–406 (1988).

116   Y.O. Taiwo and J.D. Levine: Brain Res. *492*, 397–399 (1989).

117   A. Dray: News Physiol. Sci. *11*, 288–292 (1996).

118   K. Matsumura, Y. Watanabe, H. Onoe, S. Tanaka, T. Shiraki and S. Kobayashi: Brain Res. *626*, 343–346 (1993).

119   K. Mori, S. Oka, A. Tani, S. Ito and Y. Watanabe: Biochem. Biophys. Res. Commun. *162*, 1535–1540 (1989).

120   G. Siegel, A. Carl, A. Adler and G. Stock: Eicosanoids *2*, 213–222 (1989).

121   W.F. Jackson, A. König, T. Dambacher and R. Busse: Am. J. Physiol. *264*, H238–H243 (1993).

122   S.H. Ferreira and M. Nakamura: Prostaglandins *18*, 179–190 (1979).

123   C.M. Hingtgen, K.J. Waite and M.R. Vasko: J. Neurosci. *15*, 5411–5419 (1995).

124   T.H. Hintze: Fed. Proc. *46*, 73–80 (1987).

125   J. Staszewska-Barczak: Am. J. Cardiol. *52*, 36A–45A (1983).

126   J. Tamaoki, A. Chiyotani, K. Takeyama, F. Yamauchi, E. Tagaya and K. Konno: Prostaglandins *45*, 363–373 (1993).

Progress in Drug Research, Vol. 49 (E. Jucker, Ed.)
© 1997 Birkhäuser Verlag, Basel (Switzerland)

Effects of NSAIDs on the kidney

By M.D. Murray** and D. Craig Brater*

*Clinical Pharmacology Division, Department of Medicine, Indiana University School of Medicine; **Purdue Pharmacy Programs, Purdue University School of Pharmacy, Indianapolis, Indiana 46202, USA

1   Introduction

Nonsteroidal anti-inflammatory drugs (NSAIDs) produce a variety of renal syndromes [1, 2]. Most of these effects are acute and reversible. Permanent damage to the kidney is rare. Included among these renal syndromes are acute ischemic renal insufficiency that can progress to acute tubular necrosis, alterations in sodium and water homeostasis that can produce edema and increased blood pressure, hyporeninemic-hypoaldosteronism resulting in hyperkalemia, interstitial nephritis and papillary necrosis (analgesic nephropathy) that can cause permanent damage to the kidney. This paper describes the role of NSAIDs in the development of acute ischemic renal insufficiency, its epidemiology and factors that increase patient risk.

NSAIDs are among the most commonly prescribed drugs, and in many countries they are also available for over-the-counter (OTC) use. In the United States, estimated prescription NSAID use over the last 5 years has been stable at about 75 million prescriptions per annum. In 1995, ibuprofen accounted for the largest proportion of NSAID use at 29 per cent followed by naproxen (18%), nabumetone (10%), etodolac (7%) and diclofenac (7%) [3]. Though ibuprofen is widely used, its costs represent only 8% of the $ 4.9 billion spent on prescription NSAIDs in 1995 [3]. NSAID use is especially high among elderly persons for treating rheumatologic disorders incident with aging [4, 5].

The nonsalicylate OTC NSAIDs available in the United States are ibuprofen, ketoprofen, and naproxen. Ibuprofen is the most widely used OTC NSAID. The most popular ibuprofen product (Advil) held 13% of the $2.7 billion OTC analgesic market in 1995, followed by 5.4% share for naproxen (Aleve) [6]. These use and cost estimates reveal the widespread availability and use of NSAIDs. Despite their pervasive use and potential to produce a variety of renal syndromes, explicit warnings to consumers of their effects on the kidney are not included within the consumer product literature [7, 8].

Early reports of the adverse effects of NSAIDs focused on their propensity to cause gastrointestinal effects, with little mention of their renal effects. For example, when ibuprofen was introduced in England in 1967 and in the United States in 1974, its renal effects were unknown [9]. With its increased prevalence of use in susceptible persons and increased use of anti-inflammatory dosages, the renal effects soon became manifest [10, 11]. Similar patterns were observed for other NSAIDs such as benoxaprofen, piroxicam and sulindac with increased usage post-marketing.

2   Renal prostanoids

The physiology of the acute, transient renal effects of the NSAIDs is well known. The sites of autacoid synthesis within the kidney predict their effects. As such, understanding the physiology of these local hormones is important for comprehending the effects of their perturbation with the administration of NSAIDs. Figure 1 shows the nephron's many sites of autacoid production. It is important to recognize two compartments of autacoid synthesis [12, 13]. The acute, reversible hemodynamic effects of NSAIDs emanate from their effects on the vascular compartment, including the afferent arteriole, the glomerulus, the efferent arteriole and the vasa recta. Their effects on electrolyte homeostasis and water metabolism derive from the tubular compartment, including the proximal tubule, the loop of Henle, the distal tubule and the collecting duct.

3   Structure and function of the nephron

3.1   Structure

Figure 1 shows the nephron's sites of prostanoid and cytochrome P-450 monooxygenase synthesis [13, 14]. As shown, synthesis of prostaglandins (PGs) and thromboxane is especially concentrated throughout the vascular compartment, whereas cytochrome P-450 monooxygenase is found in the proximal tubule and the medullary thick ascending loop of Henle [15]. The nephron vasculature comprises the afferent arteriole, the glomerulus and its supportive network of mesangium and matrix, the efferent arteriole and the vasa recta.

3.2   Function

PGs maintain renal perfusion in clinical settings associated with reduced actual or effective circulating volume. PGI_2 (prostacyclin) is the principal vascular prostanoid producing renovascular dilatation by direct effects and by modulation of calcium flux [16, 17]. Both PGI_2 and PGE_2 maintain afferent arteriolar tone by attenuating the effects of norepinephrine and angiotensin II; only PGI_2 affects tone at the efferent arteriole [18]. In patients with chronic glomerular disease, urinary excretion of PGI_2 is positively correlated with glomerular filtration rate [17]. Patients with high circulating concentrations of vasoconstrictors such as angiotensin II, norepinephrine or arginine vasopressin have their renal blood flow and glo-

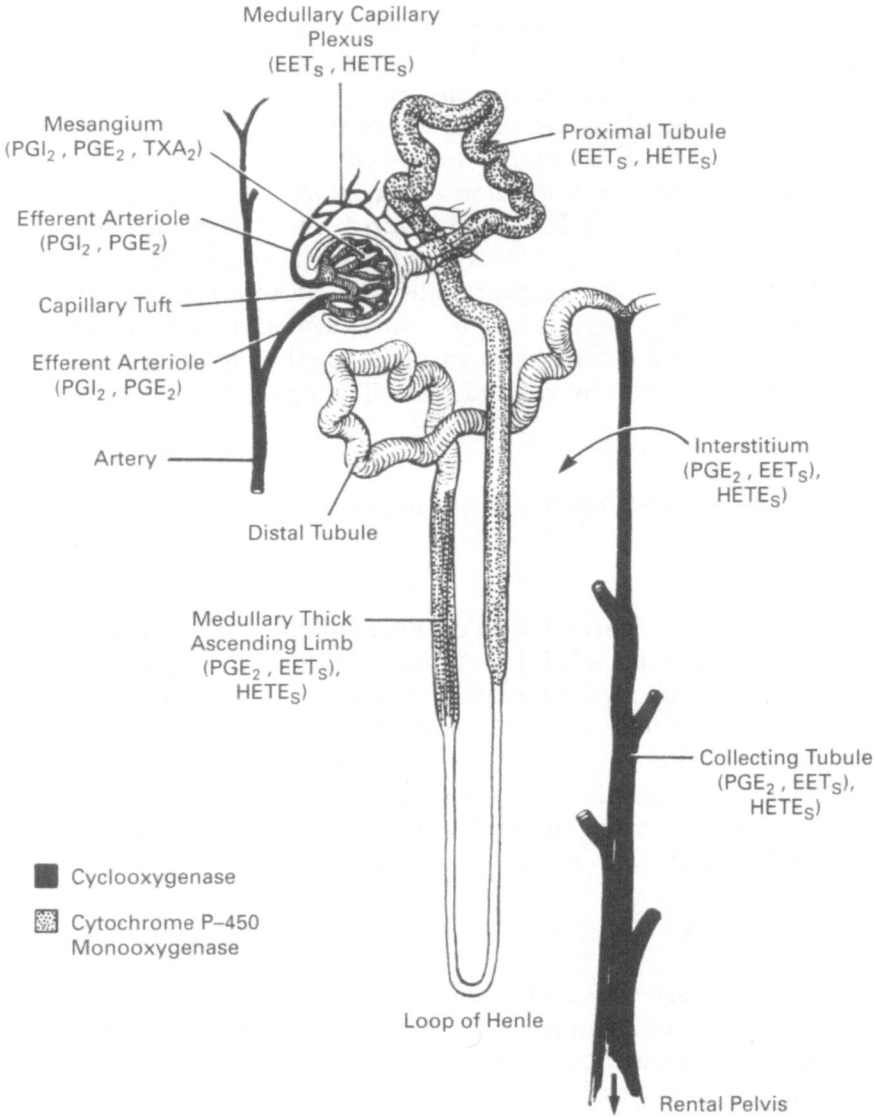

Fig. 1
Distribution of renal autacoids within the nephron vasculature and tubular structures. EETs: epoxyeicosatrienoic acids; HETEs: hydroxyeicosatetraenoic acids; PG: prostaglandin; TX: thromboxane. Reprinted with permission from Annual Reviews, Inc. [2].

merular filtration rendered prostaglandin-dependent. Administration of NSAID reduces this mitigating effect of PGs, thereby decreasing renal blood flow and glomerular filtration in susceptible persons – an effect that can be precipitous [19, 20]. Such patients are susceptible to acute tubular ischemia and necrosis from this hemodynamic effect.

Endothelial-derived substances such as nitric oxide and endothelin-1 also play a role in renal hemodynamics. Nitric oxide produces renal vasodilation and endothelin-1, vasoconstriction [21]. Both nitric oxide and endothelin-1 also interact with prostaglandins in the kidney [22].

4   Cyclooxygenase-1 and -2

It is now apparent that two isoforms of cyclooxygenase synthesize PGs. Cyclooxygenase-1 is a resident or constitutive form that is responsible for normal physiologic functions. Cyclooxygenase-2 is an inducible form that increases with disorders of inflammation [23].

Existing NSAIDs do not distinguish between the isoforms of cyclooxygenase and inhibit both. Therefore, during the course of inhibition of cyclooxygenase-2 to relieve the pain and inflammation of arthritides, cyclooxygenase-1 is also inhibited. When physiologic functions are dependent upon prostaglandins, abrogation of their beneficial effects produces dysfunction. In patients whose renal perfusion is prostaglandin-dependent, NSAID inhibition of both isoforms results in an acute ischemic insult.

It has recently been proposed that the ratio of cyclooxygenase-2 to cyclooxygenase-1 be used as a measure of the relative activities of NSAIDs. NSAIDs with a high cyclooxygenase-2/cyclooxygenase-1 ratio possess more potent inhibition of cyclooxygenase-1. Profiles of cyclooxygenase-2/cyclooxygenase-1 ratios have been proposed [24]. For example, piroxicam's cyclooxygenase-2/cyclooxygenase-1 ratio is 250, ibuprofen's ratio is 15 and diclofenac's ratio is 0.7. The profile of the three NSAIDs implies that piroxicam would more likely produce renal effects than ibuprofen or diclofenac. New NSAIDs are now becoming available with low cyclooxygenase-2/cyclooxygenase-1 ratios. Meloxicam, one of these promising new NSAIDs, has recently been released in South Africa. It remains to be seen whether these NSAIDs will have more favorable risk-to-benefit ratios.

5   Influence of NSAID pharmacokinetics on their renal effects

Generally, the pharmacokinetic characteristics of the NSAIDs include (1) small volumes of distribution, (2) extensive protein binding, (3) low intrinsic clearances, (4) low urinary excretion and (5) variable half-lives [2]. It should be no surprise that the kidney is susceptible to the toxic effects of many drugs; it is the major organ for both concentrating and eliminating xenobiotics. What is surprising is that they have profound effects on renal function despite their extensive metabolism to inactive metabolites with little active drug recovered from the urine.

6   Types of NSAID-associated renal effects

There are four major types of renal impairment from NSAIDs – acute ischemic renal insufficiency; effects on sodium, potassium and water homeostasis with interference of the effects of diuretics and antihypertensive therapy; acute interstitial nephritis; and papillary necrosis. The focus of this chapter will be on acute, transient renal ischemia, the most common adverse renal effect of NSAIDs. Though NSAIDs have produced severe, irreversible syndromes such as papillary necrosis [25] such events are rare and contrast with the multitude of reports of papillary necrosis from phenacetin-containing mixtures [2].

7   Acute renal insufficiency

In susceptible persons, the most common form of NSAID-associated renal impairment is acute ischemic renal insufficiency. It occurs within hours of administration of the first dose of an NSAID and is fully reversible when NSAID administration is discontinued. However, continued administration of an NSAID in this setting can result in sufficient ischemia to cause acute tubular necrosis [26, 27].
Acute hemodynamic effects of NSAIDs are minor in healthy, euvolemic persons who can safely receive these drugs [28–30]. There are, however, a variety of disorders, diseases or drugs that reduce actual or effective circulating volume, thereby setting the stage for an acute ischemic insult to the kidney upon administration of NSAIDs. Diseases that produce a homeostatic increase in the production of catecholamines and activation of the renin-angiotensin system are particularly notorious for putting patients at risk [1]. Clinical settings include dehydration, hemorrhage, congestive heart failure, cirrhosis with ascites and excessive diuresis [1, 2]. Increased concentrations of catecholamine and angiotensin II cause vasoconstriction within the kidney. To counter-regulate this vasoconstriction

and maintain renal blood flow and glomerular filtration, the kidney produces vasodilating PGE_2 and PGI_2 [12,31]. In turn, inhibition of PGs allows unopposed vasoconstriction and an acute ischemic insult.

Administration of thromboxane inhibitors or PGE_1 analogues may have palliative effects. Animal studies suggest that thromboxane synthesis is also involved in the ischemic process [32, 33] and that drugs that inhibit thromboxane synthesis could prevent acute tubular necrosis from occurring. Thromboxane inhibitors have been shown to prevent renal impairment in susceptible humans [34]. Administration of PGE_1 also prevents acute tubular necrosis in rats administered an NSAID [35]. When given to patients with diabetes, PGE_1 administered as misoprostol blunts the reduction in glomerular filtration rate caused by NSAIDs [36].

Renal function deteriorates further when NSAIDs are given to patients with chronic renal insufficiency [19, 20, 37]. In such patients, glomerular filtration is dependent on PGI_2. With NSAID administration, the beneficial effect of PGI_2 is reduced, thereby decreasing renal blood flow and glomerular filtration. We have probed this effect with a variety of NSAIDs. We have performed acute interventional studies of patients with chronic renal insufficiency receiving controlled diets (sodium, potassium and fluid intake) to assess the acute hemodynamic effects of the short-acting NSAIDs flurbiprofen and ibuprofen and the long-acting NSAIDs piroxicam and sulindac. Such studies preselect patients susceptible to the adverse effects of NSAIDs on renal function and, as such, do not provide estimates of their frequency in patients prescribed NSAIDs in the real world of clinical care. We therefore have also performed epidemiologic studies to provide us with estimates of the incidence as well as factors that put patients at risk for the development of NSAID-associated renal impairment. A tandem approach involving acute interventional and epidemiologic methodologies has improved our understanding of the effects of NSAIDs on the kidney.

8 Intervention studies

Acute intervention studies of small groups of susceptible persons have shown reductions in glomerular filtration rate from 9 to 80% from NSAIDs [38, 39]. We have used both clearance and balance techniques in our studies. The reason for using both approaches is that clearance studies are sensitive to the immediate effects of NSAIDs on renal function that may be transient. The effect integrated over the course of a day is best examined using balance techniques. Using these methods, our laboratory has conducted studies of the effects of NSAIDs on renal function in young and elderly persons with and without renal insufficiency.

These studies have all been conducted in a similar manner. NSAID administration is stopped for 1 month prior to the study. Patients are admitted to the carefully controlled conditions of the clinical research center, where they ingest a diet with fixed sodium and potassium intake and up to 3 l of fluid per day. After attaining sodium balance, a clearance study is performed with administration of the first dose of the NSAID. Inulin is used as a marker of glomerular filtration. Following equilibration of the inulin infusion, control collections are obtained to determine the subject's baseline renal function. The first dose of the NSAID is then given followed by serial experimental collections to monitor its effect. Subjects are then discharged from the research center to home where they receive their usual diets and take daily NSAIDs. As outpatients, electrolyte excretion, serum electrolytes and creatinine clearance are carefully monitored for safety. After a month, patients return to the clinical research center for assessment of the chronic effects of the drug. A second clearance study (exactly the same as the first study) is performed with the last dose of the NSAID. The control collection period during this second clearance study represents subjects' renal function with chronic dosing of NSAIDs, and experimental collections represent the effect of a single dose of an NSAID superimposed on the background of chronic dosing. Balance studies consist of 24- to 48-h urine collections and serum samples of sodium, potassium and creatinine.

Our studies of healthy controls and patients with renal insufficiency reveal that the glomerular filtration rate decreases with both the first dose (acute study) and the last dose (chronic study). Decrements in glomerular filtration from the short-acting NSAIDs such as ibuprofen and flurbiprofen are transient and return to baseline, but the effects of longer-acting NSAIDs (piroxicam and sulindac) are sustained [20, 40, 41].

Figures 2 and 3 show the effects of ibuprofen 800 mg three times daily, piroxicam 20 mg daily and sulindac 200 mg twice daily on inulin clearance in 14 elderly persons (73 ± 6 years of age) with preserved renal function (glomerular filtration rate > 70 ml/min) and 15 persons with moderate renal impairment (glomerular filtration rate 30–70 ml/min).

Several important aspects of these time-response profiles are worth noting. First, all three NSAIDs decreased the glomerular filtration rate of patients with and without renal insufficiency. Second, decreases in glomerular filtration were similar for the first and last doses. Third, the effect occurred earlier for ibuprofen and piroxicam as compared with sulindac, presumably owing to the need for sulindac to be metabolized to the active

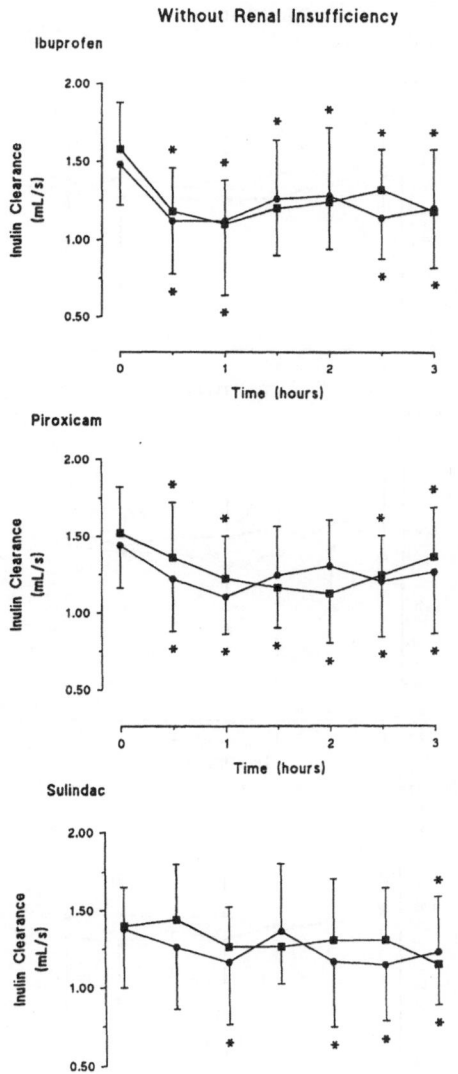

Fig. 2
Inulin clearance after the first dose (blocks) and last dose after 1 month of continuous dosing (circles) in 14 elderly persons without renal insufficiency [(glomerular filtration rate > 1.15 ml/s (70 ml/min)]. Baseline is Time 0.
* = p < 0.05 compared with baseline after correcting for multiple testing. Reprinted with permission from Lippincott Raven Publishers [20].

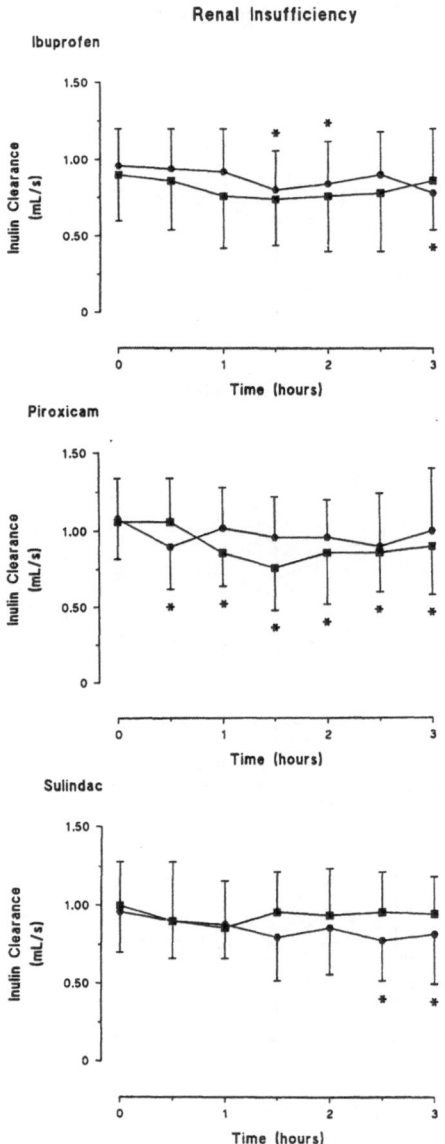

Fig. 3
Inulin clearance after the first dose (blocks) and last dose after 1 month of continuous dosing (circles) in 15 elderly persons with renal insufficiency [(glomerular filtration rate 0.50 to 1.15 ml/s (30–70 ml/min)]. Figure descriptions are the same as in Figure 2.

sulfide form. (Ibuprofen and piroxicam are administered in their active form.) From these results, one would conclude that all of the NSAIDs produce acute and chronic decrements in glomerular filtration. However, the results of the balance studies of glomerular filtration integrated over 2 days revealed that only piroxicam and sulindac produced chronic decreases in glomerular filtration of 0.12 ml/s (7.2 ml/min). The lack of effect from ibuprofen is consistent with the results of our other studies of short-acting NSAIDs [20, 40, 41]. These data indicate that each dose of ibuprofen produced decrements in renal function, but that the effects were transient, so that full recovery to baseline renal function occurred with repeated dosing. In contrast, the longer-acting NSAIDs, sulindac and piroxicam, produced small but statistically significant chronic decrements in glomerular filtration in the elderly patients with renal insufficiency. The results of this study highlight the importance of studying the effects of NSAIDs using both clearance and balance approaches.

Certain patients are extremely susceptible to the renal effects of NSAIDs. Most investigators who have performed acute interventional studies on small numbers of patients have observed a few patients who have dramatic decrements in glomerular filtration. Figure 4 reveals the effect on inulin clearance of an elderly man (73 years old) who was remarkably susceptible to the effects of ibuprofen, piroxicam and sulindac [2]. He had osteoarthritis, hypertension, chronic renal insufficiency and atherosclerosis. He was especially pleased with the pain relief ibuprofen produced. However, his serum creatinine concentration rose from 177 µmol/l to 265 µmol/l (2.0 mg/dl to 3.0 mg/dl) within 3 days, and ibuprofen was stopped. As shown in the figure, his inulin clearance decreased by 65%, 79%, and 64% with sulindac, piroxicam and ibuprofen. This patient's adverse renal response to all three NSAIDs emphasizes the importance of careful monitoring of patients who are susceptible to the acute hemodynamic effects of NSAIDs. Monitoring should occur within days of beginning NSAID administration.

Other investigators who have performed acute interventional studies of small numbers of patients have seen similar effects. Whelton et al. [19] studied the renal effects of ibuprofen, piroxicam and sulindac in 12 women with mild, stable renal insufficiency. In their study, 3 women had their regimen of ibuprofen 800 mg three times daily discontinued within 8 days because of increases in serum creatinine concentration. Of the 3 patients, 2 had exaggerated responses following a dose of 400 mg three times daily. Ciabattoni et al. [37] studied the effects of ibuprofen 1200 mg and sulindac 400 mg per day in 20 patients with chronic renal disease. Following ibuprofen administration, urinary excretion of 6-keto-prostaglandin F1α

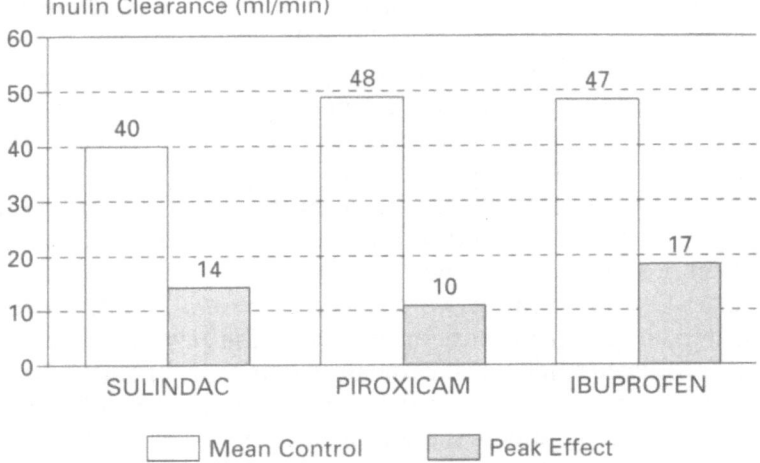

Fig. 4
Effect of single doses of sulindac 200 mg, piroxicam 20 mg and ibuprofen 800 mg on inulin clearance in a patient susceptible to the renal effects of NSAIDs (see text). Each administration of the NSAID was separated by at least 1 month. Mean control represents the patient's baseline measurements, immediately prior to NSAID administration. Peak effect is the nadir response within 3 hours of dosing. Reprinted with permission from Annual Reviews, Inc. [2].

(the stable metabolite of PGI_2) was reduced by 80%, serum creatinine concentration increased by 40%, glomerular filtration was reduced by 28% and renal blood flow was reduced by 35%.

9   Epidemiologic studies

As mentioned previously, the major drawback to acute intervention studies of the effects of NSAIDs on renal function is that they do not provide good estimates of the incidence of these effects in patients likely to be prescribed these drugs and do not provide a complete understanding of the factors that put such patients at risk.
Epidemiologic methodologies permit the study of the frequency of these effects and risk factors. Most rely upon changes in routine laboratory tests such as serum creatinine or blood urea nitrogen concentrations or hospital admitting or discharge diagnoses for renal events. Using a large clinical computing system called the Regenstrief Medical Record System (RMRS), we studied the effects of ibuprofen on renal function in an unselected, adult general medicine clinic population from Indianapolis, Indiana, USA. Within a year of their first ibuprofen prescription, 18% of 1908

patients with available laboratory tests had clinically significant increments of serum creatinine, blood urea nitrogen or both [42]. The distributions of serum creatinine and blood urea nitrogen are displayed in Figure 5. Sixty percent of patients had less than a 30% change in serum creatinine from baseline and 60% of patients had less than a 50% change in blood urea nitrogen (Fig. 5). Factors predictive of renal insufficiency included age, male gender, systolic blood pressure, pre-existing renal insufficiency, coronary artery disease and diuretic use. Two factors were associated with renal insufficiency from ibuprofen, namely age > 65 years and coronary artery disease relative to patients prescribed acetaminophen.

Using linear models, we performed a separate longitudinal analysis of RMRS data for adult general medicine clinic patients prescribed ibuprofen who had multiple serum creatinine measurements. For this analysis there were 17,839 measurements on 1482 patients who had at least two serum creatinine measurements before and after their first prescription for ibuprofen. The linear model that best described the data was one in which there was an abrupt increase in the serum creatinine immediately after the prescription for ibuprofen followed by a decline to baseline. Conceptually, this model fits well with our other studies of short-acting NSAIDs and indicates that following an acute hemodynamic insult, discontinuation of ibuprofen results in a return to baseline values.

Studies using renal diagnoses as the outcome of interest indicate that ibuprofen does not result in hospitalizations or other clinical encounters for important renal disorders. A major problem with such studies is that they are unable to detect lesser, but still clinically important, changes in renal function that might not result in hospitalization [43–45].

Others types of epidemiologic methods have been used to study renal effects of NSAIDs. Sandler et al. [46] studied the risk of chronic renal disease from NSAIDs using a case-control approach. Their primary dependent variable was defined as hospitalization for chronic renal disease and an increase in serum creatinine > 133 µmol/l (1.5 mg/dl). They concluded that NSAIDs increase the risk of chronic renal disease in men > 65 years of age. However, there were too few patients using individual NSAIDs to compute accurate NSAID-specific estimates of risk. Some epidemiologic studies used data from clinical trials that often exclude patients who could be at risk for the renal effects of NSAIDs such as elderly patients, and those with advanced liver disease, heart failure or uncontrolled diabetes [47]. In summary, the results of these epidemiologic studies indicate that NSAID administration rarely leads to hospitalization for renal diagnoses, and consistent with the results of numerous acute intervention studies, young healthy persons tolerate NSAIDs well.

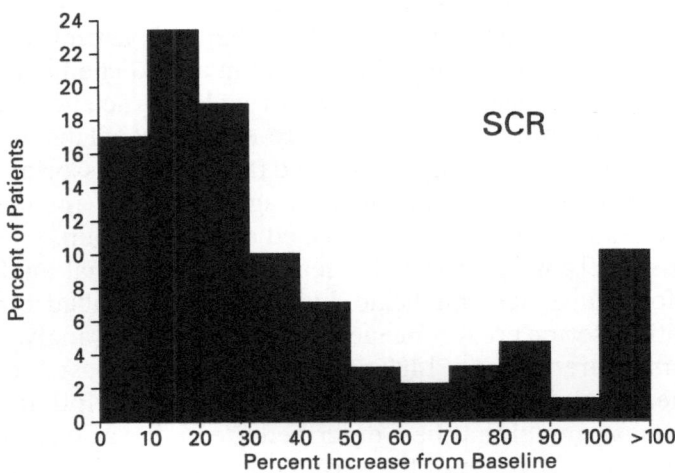

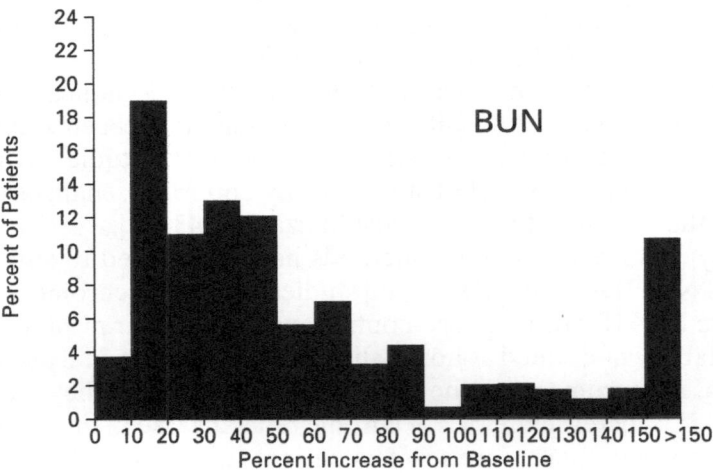

Fig. 5
Percent change from baseline values of serum creatinine (SCR) and blood urea nitrogen (BUN) in outpatients prescribed ibuprofen who had a positive change from baseline. Patients with negative changes from baseline were excluded. Baseline was defined as the value immediately prior to patients' first prescription for ibuprofen and the change from baseline was the percent increase of the first measurement taken after the ibuprofen prescription date.

Elderly persons are an especially vulnerable population. They have the highest prevalence of use (because of arthritis and joint pain), and they also have a greater likelihood of concurrent diseases that make them susceptible to the effects of NSAIDs (such as heart disease). Use of NSAIDs is more than 3.5 times greater in elderly persons than their younger counterparts [48]. Our own surveys of elderly living in the community revealed that NSAIDs were the most frequently used OTC and prescription drugs [4].

Our studies indicate that elderly persons with preserved renal function can safely receive NSAIDs unless they have another risk factor besides old age (such as diabetes or congestive heart failure) for NSAID-associated renal impairment [20]. However, elderly persons with chronic renal insufficiency may have decreases in glomerular filtration from their baseline values when administered NSAIDs. This admonition also applies to young patients with pre-existing renal insufficiency.

To determine the effect of NSAIDs on renal function in elderly persons, Gurwitz et al. [49] performed a prospective study of 114 elderly patients (87 ± 7 years of age). They found that compared with 45 patients who were not prescribed NSAIDs, within a week of starting NSAIDs serum urea nitrogen values increased significantly in 101 NSAID recipients. Serum urea nitrogen was increased > 50% in 13% of the patients compared with baseline. They suggested that risk factors for this effect included concomitant treatment with a loop diuretic and a high NSAID dosage.

10   Summary

NSAID use is pervasive in our society. Existing NSAIDs pose little risk to patients who tolerate them early during their administration. Among persons with normal renal function who have no other risk factors (dehydration) for an acute hemodynamic effect, there is no risk. However, NSAID administration to susceptible persons may cause decrements in renal plasma flow and glomerular filtration rate within hours. This acute hemodynamic effect is the most common renal syndrome caused by NSAIDs. With careful monitoring, this effect is readily detected with routine clinical laboratory tests (serum creatinine and/or blood urea nitrogen concentrations). However, patients who continue administration of NSAIDs in this setting risk acute tubular necrosis and permanent damage to the kidney. Newer NSAIDs that selectively inhibit cyclooxygenase-2: cyclooxygenase-1 ratio may provide a more favorable risk profile for patients who cannot tolerate existing drugs.

References

1   D.M. Clive and J.S. Stoff: New England Journal of Medicine *310*, 563–573 (1984).
2   M.D. Murray and D.C. Brater: Annual Review of Pharmacology and Toxicology *32*, 435–465 (1993).
3   IMS America (1996).
4   J.D. Darnell, M.D. Murray, B.L. Martz and M. Weinberger: Journal of the American Geriatrics Society *34*, 1–4 (1986).
5   L. Girgis and P. Brooks: Drugs & Aging *4*, 101–112 (1994).
6   Anonymous: The Northern New Jersey Record (1995).
7   W.M. Bennett, W.L. Henrich and J.S. Stoff: American Journal of Kidney Diseases *28*, S56–62 (1996).
8   Ad Hoc Committee for the National Kidney Foundation: American Journal of Kidney Diseases *6*, 4–5 (1985).
9   T.G. Kantor: Annals of Internal Medicine *91*, 877–882 (1979).
10 R.T. Schooley, P.F. Wagley and P.S. Lietman: Journal of the American Medical Association *237*, 1716–1717 (1977).
11 R.P. Kimberly, R.E. Bowden, H.R. Keiser and P.H. Plotz: American Journal of Medicine *64*, 804–807 (1978).
12 M.J. Dunn and E.J. Zambraski: Kidney International *18*, 609–622 (1980).
13 E. Änggård and E. Oliw: Kidney International *19*, 771–780 (1981).
14 D. Schlondorff: American Journal of Medicine *81* (Suppl 2B), 1–11 (1986).
15 J.C. McGiff: Annual Review of Pharmacology and Toxicology *31*, 339–69 (1991).
16 J.L. Nadler, M. McKay, V. Campese, J. Vrbanac and R. Horton: Journal of Clinical Investigation *77*, 1278–1284 (1986).
17 C. Patrono, G. Ciabattoni, G. Remuzzi, E. Gotti, S. Bombardieri, O. Di Munn, G. Tartarelli, G. A. Cinotti, B. M. Simonetti and A. Pierucci: Journal of Clinical Investigation *76*, 1011–1018 (1985).
18 B.F. Palmer and W.L. Henrich: Seminars in Nephrology *15*, 214–227 (1995).
19 A. Whelton, R.L. Stout, P.S. Spilman and D.K. Klassen: Annals of Internal Medicine *112*, 568–576 (1990).
20 M.D. Murray, P.K. Black, D.D. Kuzmik, K.M. Haag, A.K. Manatunga, M.A. Mullin, S.D. Hall and D.C. Brater: American Journal of the Medical Sciences *310*, 188–197 (1995).
21 W.L. Henrich: American Journal of the Medical Sciences *302*, 319–328 (1991).
22 J.C. Romero, V. Lahera, M.G. Salom and M.L. Biondi: Journal of the American Society of Nephrology *2*, 1371–1387 (1992).
23 K. Yamamoto, T. Arakawa, N. Ueda and S. Yamamoto: Journal of Biological Chemistry 270, 31315–31350 (1995).
24 J.R. Vane and R.M. Botting: Scandinavian Journal of Rheumatology – Supplement *102*, 9–21 (1996).
25 G.M. Shah, K.K. Muhalwas and R.L. Winer: Arthritis and Rheumatism *24*, 1208–1210 (1981).
26 J. Carmichael and S.W. Shankel: American Journal of Medicine *78*, 992–1000 (1985).
27 X. Chan: The Lancet *2*, 340 (1987).
28 D.C. Brater, S. Anderson, B. Baird and W.B. Campbell: Kidney International *27*, 66–73 (1985).
29 A.P. Passmore, S. Copeland and G.D. Johnston: British Journal of Clinical Pharmacology *27*, 483–490 (1989).

30   A.P. Passmore, S. Copeland and G.D. Johnston: British Journal of Clinical Pharmacology 29, 311–319 (1990).
31   M.J. Dunn: Annual Review of Medicine 35, 411–428 (1984).
32   R.P. Kaufman Jr., H. Anner, L. Kobzik, C.R. Valeri, D. Shepro and H.B. Hechtman: Annals of Surgery 205, 195–198 (1987).
33   J.M. Klausner, I.S. Paterson, L. Kobzik, C. Rodzen, C.R. Valeri, D. Shepro and H.B. Hechtman: Annals of Surgery 209, 219–224 (1989).
34   G. Remuzzi, G.A. Fitzgerald and C. Patrono: Kidney International 41, 11483–11493 (1992).
35   R.P. Kaufman Jr., H. Anner, L. Kobzik, C.R. Valeri, D. Shepro and H.B. Hechtman: Surgery, Gynecology & Obstetrics 165, 404–409 (1987).
36   G.L. Bakris, U. Starke, M. Heifets, D. Polack, M. Smith and S. Leurgans: Journal of the American Society of Nephrology 5, 1684–1688 (1995).
37   G. Ciabattoni, G.A. Cinotti, A. Pierucci, B.M. Simonetti, M. Manzi, F. Pugliese, P. Barsotti, G. Pecci, F. Taggi and C. Patrono: New England Journal of Medicine 310, 279–283 (1984).
38   M.D. Murray and D.C. Brater: Annals of Internal Medicine 112, 559–560 (1990).
39   E. Zambraski and M.J. Dunn, in: J.H. Steward (ed.): Analgesic and NSAID-Induced Kidney Disease, Oxford University Press, Oxford 1993, pp. 145–159.
40   R.D. Toto, S.A. Anderson, D. Brown-Cartwright, J.P. Kokko, D.C. Brater: Kidney International 30, 760–768 (1986).
41   M.D. Murray, P.K. Greene, D.C. Brater, A.K. Manatunga and S.D. Hall: British Journal of Clinical Pharmacology 33, 385–393 (1992).
42   M.D. Murray, D.C. Brater, W.M. Tierney, S.L. Hui and C.J. McDonald: American Journal of Medical Sciences 299, 222–229 (1990).
43   D.A. Fox and H. Jick: Journal of the American Medical Association 251, 1299–1302 (1984).
44   J.H. Johnson, H. Jick, J.R. Hunter and J.F. Dickson: Journal of Rheumatology 12, 549–552 (1985).
45   K. Beard, D.R. Perera and H. Jick: Journal of Clinical Pharmacology 28, 431–435 (1988).
46   D.P. Sandler, F.R. Burr and C.R. Weinberg: Annals of Internal Medicine 115, 165–172 (1991).
47   S.L. Bonney, R.S. Northington, D.A. Hedrich and B.R. Walker: Clinical Pharmacology and Therapeutics 40, 373–377 (1986).
48   C. Baum, D.L. Kennedy and M.B. Forbes: Arthritis and Rheumatism 28, 686–692 (1985).
49   J.H. Gurwitz, J. Avorn, D. Ross-Degnan and L.A. Lipsitz: Journal of the American Medical Association 264, 471–475 (1990).

Progress in Drug Research, Vol. 49 (E. Jucker, Ed.)
© 1997 Birkhäuser Verlag, Basel (Switzerland)

G protein coupled receptors as modules of interacting proteins: A family meeting

By Olivier Valdenaire* and Philippe Vernier**

*Hoffmann-La Roche, PRPV, Grenzacherstrasse 124, CH-4070 Basel, Switzerland, and
**Institut Alfred Fessard, UPR 2212, CNRS, F-91198 Gif-sur-Yvette, France

1 Introduction

The emergence on earth of the first true cell would not have been possible without the presence of molecules ensuring exchanges of information between this membrane-limited, metabolically organized system and its surrounding environment. The function of message recognition and transmission inside the cell is allotted to receptors, most of which are embedded in the plasma membrane and allow hydrophilic compounds to act as extracellular messengers. The evolutionary success of these transmission systems is strikingly evidenced by the tremendous number of membrane receptors which have been described to date in all the organisms from bacteria to mammals. Incidentally, receptors are among the molecules of utmost interest for the pharmacologist, since in most cases a compound must bind a receptor to be biologically active (best stated by Ehrlich's famous aphorism "*Corpora non agunt nisi fixata*" [Ehrlich, 1906]).

During the past 20 years, the illuminating progress of biochemistry and genetics has revealed the molecular structure of these membrane receptors, turning into accessible objects what pharmacology considered previously as operational concepts only. Implications of molecular approaches to receptors are wide and deep, and they are yet far from being fully integrated in pharmacological and therapeutic practice.

One of the most powerful notions advanced by the application of molecular biological methods to membrane receptors was the demonstration that they form protein families encoded by corresponding gene families. Indeed, the very large molecular diversity exhibited by membrane receptors is built up from only a few receptor prototypal structures. The main "superfamilies" made of membrane receptors are those of ligand-gated ion channels, membrane tyrosine kinases, Janus kinase-coupled receptors, guanylate cyclase receptors and, last but not least, G protein-coupled receptors (GPCR). This latter family, on which we will focus here, is by far the largest membrane protein family known. A recent estimation [Clapham et al., 1996] proposed that more than 1000 of such receptors might exist in the human genome out of about 100,000 different genes. In addition, receptor members of the G protein-coupled superfamily are the targets of the majority of drugs of therapeutic use. Studies on GPCR have implications for drug classes ranging from neuroleptics, antihypertensives, antiasthmatics and anorexigens to antimitotics, immunosuppressors and others. No aspects of therapeutics is completely unfamiliar to the biology of GPCR. Accordingly, a tremendous effort has been applied to better understanding GPCR structure-activity relationships.

In this review, we will concentrate first on some recent aspects of the structure-activity relationships of GPCR with a special emphasis on monoamine receptors as a prototypal GPCR. Second, we will examine the interactions of receptors with intracellular proteins. It is an essential issue, since signal transmission is ensured by a module of interacting proteins, and not by the sole "receptor". Third, some implications of the molecular diversity of GPCR for physiology and pharmacology will be addressed. Finally, the problem of receptor classification will be briefly discussed.

2   General mechanisms of signal transmission by GPCR

GPCR-mediated transmission of extracellular signals to the cell is achieved through the use of at least three interacting components: the membrane receptor itself, the G protein and the effector. The so-called receptor consists of a monomeric protein structurally characterized by the presence of seven transmembrane segments. The term "receptor" is questionable if one refers to its pharmacological meaning. Indeed, pioneer investigators at the beginning of this century defined the receptor as an entity able to both recognize relevant extracellular ligands and transmit an effect inside organs or cells [Ehrlich, 1913; Langley, 1905]. Clearly, what we call a receptor in the case of GPCRs is unable to transmit any information in the absence of the G protein and the effector. GPCRs should be conceived more correctly as modules of interacting proteins designed to ensure the transduction, that is the transformation of a signal, the extracellular messenger, into a signal of another nature inside the cells. The seven-transmembrane protein is essentially a binding unit whose conformational changes, stabilized by agonists, are part of the transduction process that will result in an intracellular effect. The complete transduction function requires the presence of three essential components which constitute the transmission module (Fig. 1). In this respect, GPCRs are not significantly different from the other superfamilies of membrane receptors, such as tyrosine kinase receptors or ligand-gated ion channels, which also require the interaction of different proteins or subunits to transduce extracellular signal.

2.1   Receptor activation triggers the G protein cycle

Whereas the ligand-binding receptor is a single protein, the G protein is made up of the three subunits, α, β and γ. The α subunit is able both to bind guanylic nucleotides (5'-diphosphate, or GDP, and 5'-triphosphate,

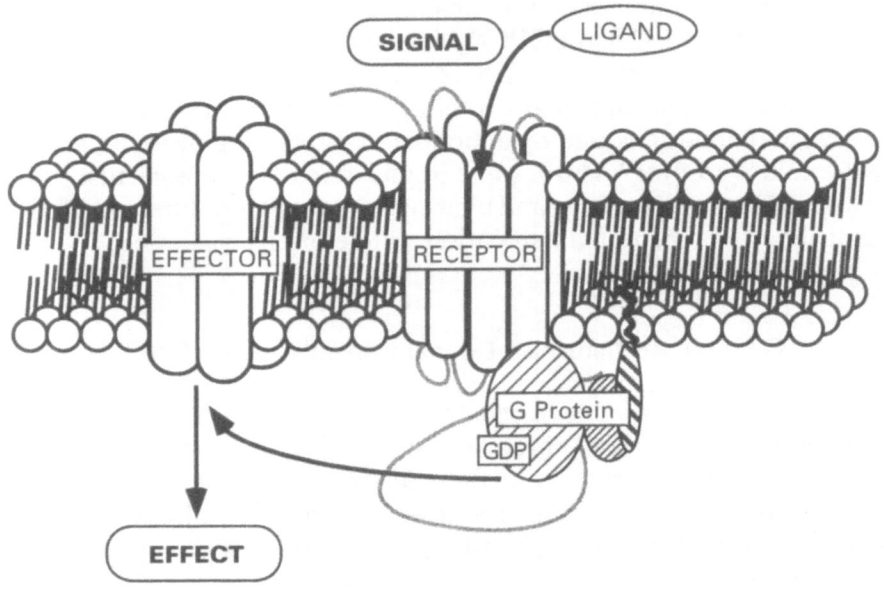

Fig. 1
G protein-coupled receptors are made of three fundamental components: the receptor, the G protein and the effector. Their association constitutes a transmission module which performs the transduction of incoming signals (represented by the binding of various ligands to the receptor) into intracellular effects.

or GTP) and to hydrolyze GTP. The β and γ subunits are tightly connected together so as to form a single functional entity.

At the resting state, the heterotrimeric G protein binds to the receptor through both α and βγ, the α subunit bearing a GDP nucleotide. Stimulation of the receptor, i.e. binding of an agonist, provokes, or more correctly stabilizes, its isomerization in an "activated form". The activated receptor, which has a high affinity for the agonist when bound to the heterotrimeric G protein, promotes in turn a modification of the α subunit conformation, which decreases its affinity for GDP. Due to the higher concentration of GTP in cells, GDP tends to be replaced by GTP. The precise nature of this catalytic function of the receptor is still unclear. However, Birnbaumer proposed that the intimate function of receptor in "activating" the α subunit of the G protein when bound to its βγ partners would be to decrease the magnesium concentration required to promote GDP-GTP exchange on the nucleotide site [Birnbaumer et al., 1990]. An important aspect of this pseudo-catalytic process is the ability of the receptor

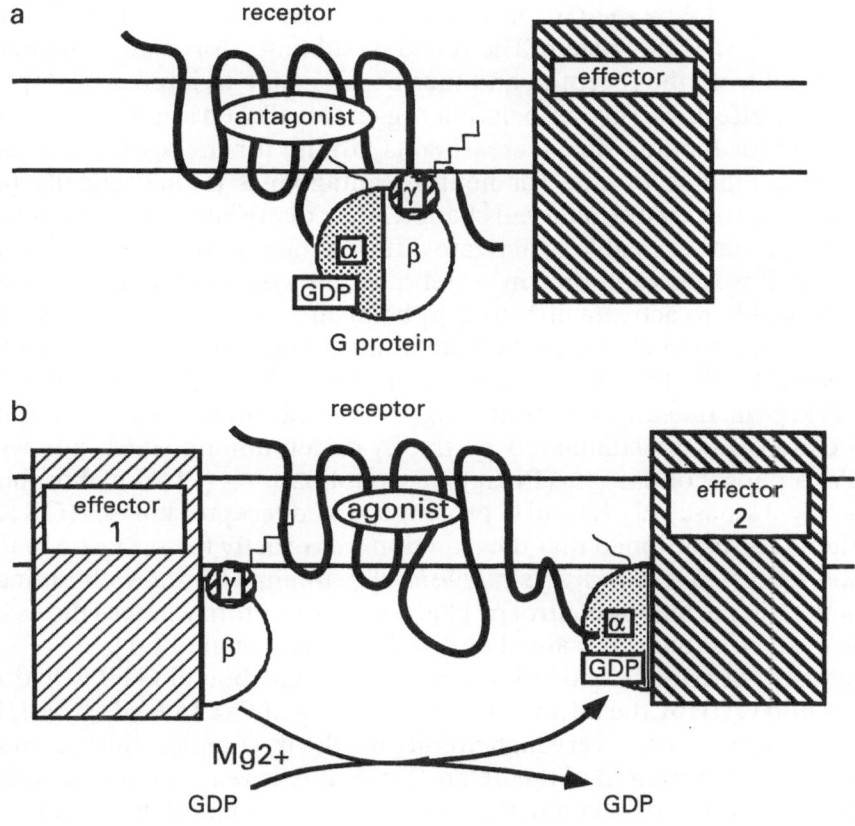

Fig. 2
According to a schematic view derived from the allosteric theory, the receptor "oscillate" between two functional states. The "inactive" state (a), where the receptor is associated to the G protein in its heterotrimeric form, is stabilized by antagonist. The "active" state (b) is stabilized by agonists and favors the dissociation of the receptor-G protein heterotrimer complex triggered by the magnesium-dependant binding of GTP on the a subunit. Then, both α and βγ subunits can, independantly or synergistically, modulate the activity of different effectors.

to activate several G proteins upon stimulation by a single agonist molecule, as has been shown for transducin (the photoreceptor heterotrimeric G protein) activation by rhodopsin [Vuong and Chabre, 1990], and for the α_{2A}-adrenergic receptor [Chabre et al., 1994]. This capacity, which varies from one receptor to another for a given agonist, and from one agonist to another for a given receptor, represents in fact the true efficacy of receptor activation by an agonist (Fig. 2).

Binding of GTP by the Gα protein has a dramatic impact on the whole configuration of the system. The α and βγ subunits dissociate from each other and from the receptor, and thus become able to interact with promiscuous effectors. This dissociation triggers an allosteric modification of the receptor binding site, decreasing its affinity for the agonist. In contrast, the binding of true (or neutral) antagonists is theoretically not affected by this conformational change. After dissociation, the free α and βγ subunits are each able to activate different target effectors. Until very recently, it was thought that, in vertebrates, only the GTP-binding α subunit was able to activate effectors, βγ being at best a negative regulator. Demonstration in 1987 that the muscarinic K^+ channel could be directly activated by the βγ subunit [Logothetis et al., 1987] turned this dogma upside down. Indeed, in the following years, it was shown that many other effectors could be stimulated by the βγ dimer, among which adenylyl cyclase, phospholipase $C_β$ ($PLC_β$), phospholipase A_2 (PLA_2), phosphoinositide-3 kinase (PI_3-K) and G protein-coupled receptor kinases (GRK). It should be mentioned that the situation was exactly the opposite in the baker's yeast *Saccharomyces cerevisiae*, βγ subunits having well-defined functions in the mating control by pheromone receptors, whereas the exact role of the α subunit remained elusive [Dohlman et al., 1991].

The phase of effector activation finishes when Gα-bound GTP is hydrolyzed into GDP by the intrinsic GTPase activity of Gα. Indeed, the GDP-bound α subunit has a very high affinity for the βγ complex, thus promoting a rapid reformation of the heterotrimer and its reassociation with the receptor. After reassociation, the receptor-G protein module is ready for a new activation cycle. The kinetic parameters of GTP hydrolysis, which can differ greatly from one α subunit to another [Carty et al., 1990; Linder et al., 1990], are the major determinants of the time course, direction and efficiency of signal transmission through the plasma membrane. Therefore, α subunits should be considered as molecular "controllers" in the true sense of the word. In this respect the α subunit is functionally analogous to the other GTPases which play important roles in various intermolecular recognition processes from protein translation (elongation factors), signaling via tyrosine-kinase receptor (Ras proteins), intracellular membrane transport (Rab proteins), changes of cell shape (Rho/Rac proteins) and so on.

2.2   The structure of G proteins: Implications for receptor and effector interactions

The fact that receptors, G proteins and most of the corresponding effectors are all encoded by gene families, and therefore share similar structural features, suggests that the mechanisms which govern receptor-G protein-effector interactions are general and common to all the GPCRs.

In mammals, more than 20 G protein α subunits have been identified and divided into four classes on structural grounds [Simon et al., 1991]. Differential splicing events may further increase this diversity, as is the case for the α_o subunit [Hsu et al., 1990; Tsukamoto et al., 1991]. Most of the α subunits are widely expressed, and generally each cell type contains at least 4 or 5 different α subunits. Up to now, 5 and 6 different subunits constitute the mammalian β and γ families [Cali et al., 1992; Simon et al., 1991; Watson et al., 1994] respectively. As a consequence, the combinatorial association of the 3 different subunits could theoretically lead to an enormous diversity of the heterotrimeric G proteins. In fact this diversity is probably not as large as might be expected, due to the incompatibility that exists between some of the subunits. It has been shown, for instance, that a dimer such as $\beta_2\gamma_1$ could not be formed [Pronin and Gautam, 1992]. Nevertheless, an exact description of the subunit composition of the G proteins associated to a given receptor is a difficult task and is known in only a very limited number of cases.

The crystal structures of the free α bound to either GDP or GTPγS and of $\beta\gamma$ subunits have been recently obtained [Coleman et al., 1994; Lambright et al., 1994; Noel et al., 1993; Sondek et al., 1996] as well as the structure of two heterotrimers, $\alpha_{i1}\beta_1\gamma_2$ and $\alpha_t\beta_1\gamma_1$ [Lambright et al., 1996; Wall et al., 1995]. This achievement clarified the interactions between the partners of the GPCR signaling module. The α subunit can be divided into two domains. One is the GTPase domain, which also binds the guanylic nucleotides. It closely resembles, and is probably homologous, to the GTPase domains of other G proteins such as p21^{ras}. The second domain, a helical domain, could act as a regulatory element, comparable to some extent to the GTPase-activating protein (GAP) which is required to accelerate GTP hydrolysis on many low molecular weight GTPases such as Ras. The GTPase domain of the α subunit exhibits all the features of the other known GTPases and in particular the so-called switch regions which change their conformation upon exchange of GDP for GTP. The N-terminus of the α subunit is mandatory for its association with $\beta\gamma$, and edges on one side of the $\beta\gamma$ structure, whereas most of the GTPase volume appears to be asymmetrically located in front of the hole, limited by the WD repeats (repetitions of a highly conserved sequence usually bounded by G-H residues at the N terminus and W-D residues at the C terminus) of the β subunits (see below). Numerous evidence suggests that the receptor itself interacts with the C-terminus of the α subunit. First, the toxin from *Bordetella pertussis*, which covalently modifies a cysteine located at the C-terminus of these proteins, uncouples G_i and G_o proteins from receptors [Avigan et al., 1992]. Second, deletions or mutations of the C-terminus of many α subunits prevent G protein-receptor interactions [Denker et al., 1992; Sullivan et al., 1987]. Third, the specificity of receptor recognition by G proteins may be conferred by short stretches of the α subunit C-terminus as tested in chimeric G proteins [Conklin et al., 1992]. However, other parts of the α subunit are probably also involved in its interactions with the receptor [Lee et al., 1995].

In addition to its interaction with the βγ dimer, the α subunit may be associated to the plasma membrane by lipid modifications. This is the case for α_i, α_o and α_z proteins, which are myristoylated close to their N-terminus. In contrast, a protein such as α_s is transiently palmitoylated upon activation by the β_2-adrenoreceptor, so that the corresponding G protein is no longer able to activate its effector, the adenylyl cyclase [Degtyarev et al., 1993]. This kind of mechanism could contribute to the desensitization or to the regulation of transduction specificity at the receptor level. The βγ complex is associated with the plasma membrane by a prenyl group (whose nature varies from one γ protein to another) bound to the C-terminal cysteine of the γ protein. Crystals of the heterotrimeric complex show that the lipid modifications borne by the α and βγ subunits are located on the same side of the G protein, suggesting that they are both used to insert the trimer in the plasma membrane. This membrane association of the βγ complex is probably central to its function.

The β subunit is made of seven 40 amino acid-long repeats, each of which is flanked by glycine and histidine residues on one side and tryptophan and aspartate residues on the other (the so-called WD 40 repeats). The crystals of βγ proteins revealed that the WD repeats form the blades of a propeller exhibiting a highly symmetric ring structure. Different blades of the propeller are thought to contact different partners. A hydrophobic part of the sixth blade might interact with the receptor, while the α subunit would make extensive contact with the β protein. The γ subunit stretches along the surface of blades 1, 5, 6 and 7. This surface probably determines the specificity of the βγ association. This propeller structure is found in many proteins that share the ability to bind another type of conserved protein domain, the "pleckstrin homology domain" (PH domain) (Fig. 3). PH domains are present in many partners of the βγ subunits, such as GRK [Touhara et al., 1994], protein kinase C_μ [Johannes et al., 1995], *Lfc* proto-oncogene [Whitehead et al., 1995] or dynamin [Liu et al., 1994]. The PH domain comprises seven antiparallel β sheets and one C-terminal α helix centered on a tryptophan residue. Its tridimen-

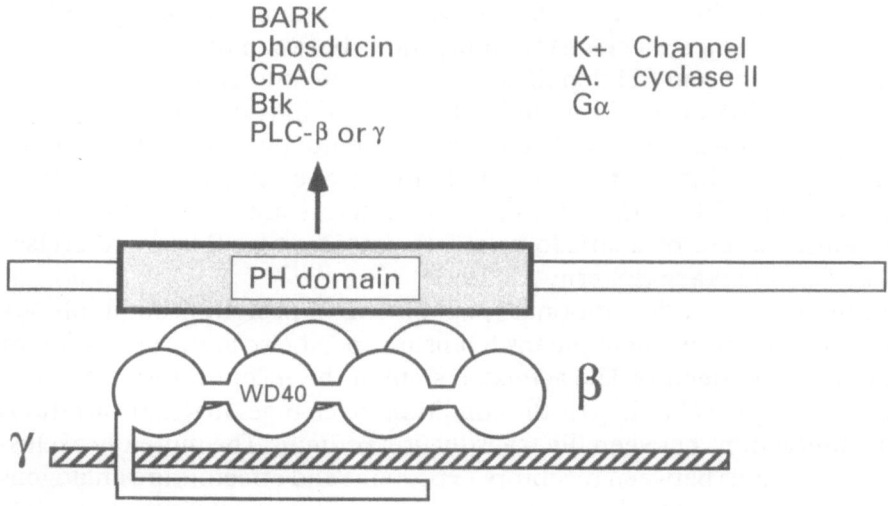

Fig. 3
A schematic representation of the βγ subunits of the G protein and of their association with effectors and regulatory proteins. The WD repeats of the β subunit are shown as bowls. They are the determinants of interactions with the PH domains of many effectors and regulatory proteins indicated by the arrow. The βγ subunits are also able to interact with components which do not bear PH domain such as the a subunit, adenylyl cyclases or potassium channels. The picture has been redrawn from Neer [1995].

sional structure has also been determined in several different proteins, including pleckstrin itself [Yoon et al., 1994].

Interestingly, comparison of the crystallized βγ structures, either free or bound to an α subunit, showed that, in contrast to α, the βγ conformation is almost independent of the G protein activation state. Therefore, βγ subunits should rather be considered as a kind of rigid scaffolding allowing diverse molecular interactions. Such interactions have been shown to take place between the WD repeats of the βγ subunits and the PH domain, which is borne by a large variety of cytosolic proteins.

As suggested by Shaw [1996], the main function of this PH domain would be to promote the membrane relocalization of proteins in response to a given signal. In the case of GPCRs, receptor activation promotes G protein dissociation, which allows the βγ dimer to contact PH domain proteins and to translocate them at the membrane. Thus these proteins become able to interact with other membrane-localized partners as the next step in a signaling pathway. PH domains can be viewed as an alternative to lipid modifications for membrane localization. For instance, the cytosolic β-adrenergic kinases reached the cytoplasmic domains of their target receptor by such a mechanism. Interactions between the WD repeats of the βγ subunits and PH domains may constitute one of the main mechanisms of action of the βγ subunits. The interactions of either the α subunit or the effector to the βγ complex are mutually exclusive, although the corresponding binding sites do not fully overlap [Chen et al., 1995; Sondek et al., 1996]. In addition, some effectors are activated by the G protein in its heterotrimeric form, as is the case for type II adenylyl cyclase or PLC_β [Smrcka and Sternweis, 1993].

In summary, these "conditional" phenomena of protein-protein interactions provide convenient means to ensure specificity in the activation or inhibition of effectors. The activated state of the receptor (generally stabilized by agonist binding) is the condition for changes in the localizations and interactions between the transduction proteins. The mutually exclusive interactions between receptors, G proteins and effectors are analogous to switches in electrical systems. Networks of protein interactions corresponds to what are called signaling pathways. The concept of "protein modules" explains how GPCRs can both activate several different pathways (pleiotropy) and provide the required degree of temporal or spatial specificity to the transmission of messages across the plasma membrane.

3   Structure of the GPCRs

3.1   Seven-transmembrane domains: A common feature

The GPCRs form a large family of integral membrane proteins. Given their sequence similarities and their common function, i.e. interaction with G proteins, they are believed to share the same overall topology. One of their most remarkable features is the presence in their primary structure of seven hydrophobic segments, which likely correspond to transmembrane α-helices, separated by three intracellular and three extracellular loops. The amino termini of these receptors are extracellular, and their carboxy-termini intracellular, as has been shown by enzymatic proteolysis and immunolabeling studies for rhodopsin [Applebury and Hargrave, 1986] and for the β_2-adrenergic receptor [Dohlman et al., 1987; Wang et al., 1989]. The overall topology of GPCRs is assumed to be similar to that of bacteriorhodopsin, which is inserted in the purple membrane of *Halobacterium halobium* [Henderson and Unwin, 1975], whose high-resolution structure was obtained in 1990 [Henderson et al., 1990]. The stereochemical coordinates of bacteriorhodopsin have been used to build up computerized models of several bioamine receptors [Dahl et al., 1991; Hibert et al., 1991; Kuipers et al., 1994]. In these models, the seven α-helices are roughly perpendicular to the membrane. They are tightly packed in a sequential anticlockwise way (when looking from the extracellular part) and face each other across a dihedral cleft. In the case of cationic neurotransmitter receptors, the proteic pocket thus formed in the lipid bilayer is narrow and hydrophobic and constitutes the agonist-binding site. The hydrophobic stretches of bioamine receptor, as well as of other GPCRs and for rhodopsin, are flanked by polar residues which define signal-anchor sequences and are probably sufficient to promote the insertion of the receptor into the membrane of the endoplasmic reticulum [Audigier et al., 1987; Beltzer et al., 1991; von Heijne and Gavel, 1988]. The receptor cytoplasmic loops are positively charged, thus following the "positive inside rule" proposed by von Heijne [von Heijne and Gavel, 1988]. This is especially true for the C-termini of transmembrane domains TM1, TM5 and TM7 and for the N-termini of TM4, TM6 (TM are transmembrane α-helices, numbered 1 to 7 from the N-terminus to the C-terminus of the protein).

Given their length (about 25 residues) and their chemical characteristics [Chothia and Finkelstein, 1990; Engelman et al., 1986], the hydrophobic segments of bioamine receptors are able to spontaneously form transmembrane amphipathic α-helices upon integration in the lipid bilayer. When the sequence of the receptor hydrophobic stretches is represented as a helix (3.6 residues per turn), the side of the helices which faces the inner part of the receptor is constituted of polar residues, while their hydrophobic surface is in direct contact with the lipid environment. The polar side of the helices contains most of the amino acids conserved among the receptors, in agreement with the higher evolutionary variability observed for the membrane-exposed residues of membrane proteins [von Heijne and Manoil, 1990]. These conserved polar residues participate in the overall stabilization of the receptor structure by allowing the formation of crucial interhelix interactions [Hibert et al., 1991]. Thus, the organization of GPCR structure probably follows the two-stage folding mechanism proposed for bacteriorhodopsin [Popot and Engelman, 1990], where the α-helices are the elementary folding components of the protein conformation and are subsequently packed together by interhelix interactions. In most GPCRs a disulfide bridge connecting two conserved Cys residues of the two first extracellular loops also contributes to the overall protein conformation, as suggested by site-directed mutagenesis [Dixon et al., 1987; Dohlman et al., 1990]. In agreement with the presence of strong interhelix interactions, it has been shown that independently expressed frag-

ments of the receptor containing either the first five or the last two transmembrane domains of the β_2-adrenergic receptor could reassemble into
a functional receptor [Kobilka et al., 1988]. The same result was achieved
with the M_2 and M_3 muscarinic receptors [Maggio et al., 1993a]. These
findings support the concept that the receptor structure can roughly be
divided into two parts. One part would include the first five helices strongly
connected together by two short intracellular loops and two extracellular loops themselves linked by a disulfide bond. The other part would comprise the two last transmembrane segments along with the large and variable domain of the third cytoplasmic loop. These two domains would be
able to fold independently and associate to each other, making a functional receptor upon insertion in the lipid bilayer.

The transition from the previous concept to the idea of a potential dim-
erization of GPCR is almost immediate. Indeed, Maggio et al. [1993b]
tested this hypothesis using two chimeras made of the first five helices of
the α_{2C} adrenoceptor associated to the last two helices of the M_3 muscarinic receptor and vice versa. While no binding could be detected after
separate expression of the two chimeric receptors, their co-expression
resulted in high-affinity binding sites for both types of ligands. These observations can only be explained if the two separated domains of one receptor subtype interact with each other in a dimeric structure. In addition, a
recent study demonstrated the existence of β_2-adrenergic receptor dim-
ers, and suggested that agonist stimulation stabilized the dimeric state of
the receptor [Hebert et al., 1996].

The models that have been deduced from bacteriorhodopsin have been
helpful for addressing various questions about GPCRs. Bacteriorhodopsin, however, is not coupled to G proteins, and its primary sequence has
only a low degree of identity with those of GPCRs. Therefore, such models should be considered with caution. The low-resolution structure of
bovine G protein-linked rhodopsin has been obtained [Schertler et al.,
1993]. Although it confirmed the existence and the overall organization
of the seven transmembrane helices, it also suggested significant differences in their topology. These additional data have been used to modify
the previous models [Donnelly et al., 1994].

3.2   The ligand-binding crevice

A large part of the works on bioamine receptors has been devoted to identifying the determinants of drug-binding selectivity. Site-directed mutagenesis has been extensively used to assess the role of candidate residues
selected through the comparison of receptor sequences and three-dimen-

sional modelling. The problem was also approached by the construction of chimeric receptors, to avoid more important conformational disruptions that could result from point mutations and mislead any functional interpretation. These studies, first focused on the β_2-adrenergic receptor and then extended to many other members of the monoamine receptor family, have shown that a limited number of amino acid residues are crucial for binding the receptor's natural ligands. These residues are located in the membrane hydrophobic pocket of the receptor, about one-third of the distance to the extracellular surface. A few key residues were identified in TM3 (one Asp residue), TM5 (Ser residues for the catecholamine receptors) and TM6 (an aromatic residue). The situation is similar for other GPCRs such as peptidergic receptors, where a few residues in the transmembrane helices have been shown to be crucial for binding the agonists. However, in many peptidergic receptors, the extracellular regions are also involved in the binding process, but this situation will not be addressed in this review [rev. in Schwartz et al., 1995].

An aspartic residue located in TM3, conserved in all bioamine receptors but not in other GPCRs, was suspected to be of prime importance because it forms an ion pair between its carboxyl group and the ligand cationic ammonium group. Substitutions of this residue in the β_2-adrenergic receptor resulted in a dramatic decrease in receptor affinity for both agonists and antagonists, but in contrast did not alter agonist efficacy to activate the mutant receptors [Strader et al., 1988, 1991]. Strader et al. could also show that the effect of such mutations was due to a disruption of ligand-receptor interactions, and not to a major structural modification of the receptor. A Ser-mutated β_2 receptor could indeed be fully activated by catechol esters and ketones, which substitute a hydrogen bond to the Asp-ammonium ion pair. The importance of this Asp residue has been demonstrated in the case of other receptors, such as the adrenergic α_2 [Wang et al., 1991], the dopaminergic D_2, the muscarinic M_1 [Fraser et al., 1989], the histaminergic H_1 and H_2 and the serotoninergic 5-HT$_{2A}$ [Wang et al., 1993].

It has been suggested [Hibert et al., 1993] that three conserved aromatic residues, located on TM3 and TM6 and surrounding the Asp residue of TM3, could stabilize the ion pair formed between this residue and the ligand by neutralizing the positive charge of the ligand nitrogen group. These three residues have not been systematically studied. Yet the substitution of the two corresponding aromatic residues on TM6 of the rat muscarinic M_3 receptor severely decreases the affinity of this receptor for acetylcholine [Wess et al., 1990, 1992]. Very recently, Almaula et al. have identified in the 5-HT$_{2A}$ receptor a Ser residue able to form a second inter-

```
199-Y A I A S S I V S F Y V P L V I M V F V-218    β2
     Y A I S S S V I S F Y I P V A I M I V T        D1
     F V V Y S S I V S F Y V P F I V T L L V        D2
     Y V L F S A L G S F Y L P L A I I L V M        α1A
     Y A L F S S L G S F Y I P L A V I L V M        α1B
     Y V I S S C I G S F F A P C L I M I L V        α2A
     Y T I Y S T F G A F Y I P L L L M L V L        5-HT1A
     I T F G T A I A A F Y M P V T I M T I L        M3
     F K V M T A I I N F Y L P T L L M L W F        H1
     Y G L V D G L V T F Y L P L L I M C I T        H2
```

Fig. 4
Alignment of the aminoacid sequences of the fifth transmembrane helix (TM5) of several (human) bioamine receptors. Numerotation with respect to the whole receptor sequence is given for the β_2-adrenergic receptors. Serine residues are underlined.

action (hydrogen bond) with the free amino group of serotonin [Almaula et al., 1996]. This residue is also located in TM3, in the immediate vicinity of the Asp residue. It is of interest to note that another 5-HT$_{2A}$ agonist like lysergic acid diethylamide (LSD] could not establish this second interaction with the receptor.

Modeling of the bioamine receptor binding site has also highlighted the critical role of conserved residues located in the fifth and sixth helices. In the case of catecholamine receptors, two Ser residues (Ser 204 and Ser 207 in Fig. 4) in TM5 are able to form hydrogen bonds with the para and meta hydroxyl groups of the ligand catechol moiety. Mutation of these residues, which lie one helix turn from each other, in the β_2-adrenergic receptor, impairs agonist (but not antagonist) binding, as well as the efficiency of the agonist-mediated activation of the receptor [Strader et al., 1989]. Removal of either of the catechol hydroxyl groups of the ligand resulted in a similar affinity decrease. Serotonin displays a single aromatic hydroxyl group, and a single Ser residue is present in the fifth helix of the 5-HT receptors. Histaminergic and muscarinic receptors do not have a any Ser residue at that same position, which corresponds to the absence of hydroxyl on the aromatic group (in fact to the absence of aromatic group for acetylcholine) in their natural ligands.

Recent observations have, however, raised new questions about the precise role of Ser residues. As shown in the alignment of TM5 sequences (Fig. 4), most of the catecholamine receptors display three Ser residues. The substitution of Ser 203 by Ala in the β_2-adrenergic receptor did not result in the expression of an active protein, making it difficult to draw conclusions. Mutagenesis of the three conserved Ser residues of the D_1 and D_2 receptors affected, although differentially, the binding of dopamine and other agonists to these receptors [Cox et al., 1992; Mansour et al., 1992; Pollock et al., 1992; Tomic et al., 1993; Woodward et al., 1996]. Substitution of the two conserved Ser with Ala (corresponding to Ser 203 and 207 in the β_2-adrenergic receptor) in the α_{2A}-adrenergic receptor affected the binding of catechol agonists [Wang et al., 1991]. From these studies we can conclude that, in spite of their conserved positions, the role of the TM5 Ser residues in ligand binding and in receptor activation can vary from one type of catecholamine receptor to another, or even from one subtype to another, as shown for the α_{1A} and α_{1B}-adrenergic receptors [Cavalli et al., 1996; Hwa and Perez, 1996b].

The Ser residue in TM5 of the 5-HT$_{1A}$ receptor, as well as a neighboring Thr residue, have been shown to play an important role in serotonin binding [Ho et al., 1992]. In addition, residues located in the same region of the fifth helix of the histaminergic receptors (Thr and Asn residues for the H_1 receptor, Asp and Thr residues for the H_2 receptor) have been implicated in the binding of agonists [Gantz et al., 1992; Ohta et al., 1994]. Likewise, the two corresponding Thr residues of the muscarinic receptor M_3 are suspected to form hydrogen bonds through their hydroxyl groups with the ester function of acetylcholine [Wess et al., 1991].

Finally, a Phe residue is conserved in the sixth helix of all the receptors that bind aromatic ligands. Hibert et al. (1993) have suggested that this residue could stabilize the receptor-ligand complex via an interaction with the aromatic nucleus of the ligand. In addition, this residue is replaced in all muscarinic receptors by an Asn, which could form a hydrogen bond with the acetylcholine ester group. Substitution of this Phe residue in the β_2-adrenergic receptor was indeed shown to decrease the affinity of the receptor for agonists [Dixon et al., 1988].

Up to now, most of our knowledge on the structure of the receptor binding site and on the residues implicated in the binding of agonists and antagonists has been obtained from mutagenesis studies. A general scheme for the binding of monoamines to their receptors has been delineated during the last years. According to this scheme, the agonist makes a strong ionic interaction with an Asp residue located in the receptor third helix, and has to contact residues located in the fifth and sixth helices to promote or stabilize the receptor activated state. The residues involved in antagonist binding, on the other hand, are different (except for the conserved Asp of TM3) from those involved in agonist binding. Antagonists are generally supposed to act mainly by preventing access of agonists to residues of TM5 and TM6 involved in receptor activation. If the key determinants of ligand binding are now known, in the case of the bioamine receptors and of some peptidergic receptors, those which may govern class or subtype specificity are far more elusive. Interesting new insights may most likely be expected from techniques such as saturation mutagenesis, coupled or not to chemical modifications, and could compensate for the present lack of crystallographic data. An example of this kind of technique is given by the systematic mapping of the ligand binding crevice undertaken by Javitch et al. in the case of the dopamine D_2 receptor [Javitch et al., 1995a, 1995b].

3.3   Activation of the receptor

The exact mechanisms that drive the conversion of agonist binding into receptor activation are unclear. Site-directed mutagenesis experiments have been carried out on bioamine receptors, and the ability of the resulting mutant receptors to trigger the intracellular signaling pathways has been explored in most cases. Residues required for receptor activation by the agonist have thus been identified. For instance, residues located in the fifth and sixth transmembrane helices (including some of the conserved Ser residues of catecholamine receptors), as well as an Asp residue conserved in the second helix of all GPCRs, were shown to be crucial for the ligand-mediated activation of the receptor. In contrast, the substitution of several other residues was shown to result in a surprising constitutive (i.e. agonist-independent) activation of the receptor, and also in increased affinity of the receptor for agonists. This phenomenon was discovered by changing a short stretch of amino acids in the C-terminal part of the third cytoplasmic loop of the α_{1B} and β_2 adrenergic receptors [Cotecchia et al., 1990]. One of the residues of this region was further shown to be responsible for constitutive stimulation of phospholipase C (via G_q) by the α_{1B} receptor. Indeed, the 19 possible substitutions of this Ala (Ala 293) residue all induced variable levels of constitutive activity [Kjelsberg et al., 1992]. Analogous mutations performed on the β_2 and α_{2A} receptors, which stimulate (G_s) or inhibit (G_i) adenylate cyclase, respectively, yielded comparable results [Ren et al., 1993; Samama et al., 1993].

These observations were extended to other domains of the receptors, and also to other GPCRs. Similar residues located in the C-terminal part of the third intracellular loop were identified for the M_1 muscarinic and for the platelet-activating factor receptors [Hogger et al., 1995; Parent et al., 1996]. Mutagenesis of some residues belonging to the transmembrane helices also proved to result in constitutively activated receptors. This was shown for the muscarinic M_3 and M_5 [Bluml et al., 1994; Spalding et al., 1995], the adrenergic α_{1A} and α_{1B} [Hwa et al., 1996a; Perez et al., 1996] and the angiotensin II AT_{1A} [Groblewski et al., 1997] receptors. Interestingly, the residues responsible for this effect in TM5 and TM6 of α_{1A} and α_{1B} adrenoceptors were already shown to be involved in the agonist specificity of these two receptors subtypes [Hwa et al., 1995]. In the adrenergic α_{1B}, replacement of the Asp residue belonging to the highly conserved DRY motif had similar consequences [Scheer et al., 1996]. A recent study suggested that protonation of this residue could be an important modulator of the receptor activation [Scheer et al., 1997]. Finally, it was suspected that mutations spontaneously activating GPCRs could account for human diseases. Indeed, such mutations have been identified in luteinizing hormone and thyroid-stimulating hormone receptors, and related to familial male precocious puberty and hyperfunctioning thyroid adenomas, respectively [Parma et al., 1993; Shenker et al., 1993].

The agonist-independent activation of some mutant receptors, along with the ability of short peptidergic stretches derived from the intracellular regions of receptors to activate G proteins *in vitro* [Cheung et al., 1991; Okamoto et al., 1991], promoted the emergence of new ideas. It was suggested that, in the absence of agonist, some constraints in the receptor structure may prevent certain cytoplasmic regions to interact with G proteins. The activating mutations would then release these constraints, modifying the receptor structure so as to mimic an active state usually triggered and stabilized by the binding of agonists. The interactions between the three components of the metabotropic signaling module (ligand, receptor, G protein) had previously been modeled by the well-accepted ternary complex model. According to this model, the receptor would be active only when associated with both the ligand and the G protein. The model has been extended by the allosteric ternary complex model [Samama et al., 1993], which introduces an isomerization constant to represent the equilibrium between the inactive and the active states of the receptor (R and R^*). In the absence of an agonist, R predominates; agonists displace the equilibrium towards R^*. Thus, the concept of inverse agonists was also developed, these latter compounds binding preferentially to R, in contrast to "true" antagonists, which bind equally to R and R^*. The allosteric ternary complex model could then also account for the basal levels of activation that had previously been observed for certain GPCRs in the absence of agonists. As a matter of fact, GPCRs display a broad range of basal activity levels. For example, inside the single D_1 class of dopamine receptor, the D_{1B}/D_5 subtype exhibits a significantly higher ability to spontaneously activate adenylyl cyclase than the D_{1A}/D_1 subtype [Cardinaud et al., 1997; Tiberi and Caron, 1994]. The situation could be even more complicated, due to the possible existence of various active states for the receptor, which could be selectively induced by different agonists and could couple to distinct G protein pathways [Perez et al., 1997].

The demonstration that GPCRs display multiple states of functional activation has not had a significant impact on therapeutic strategies so far, as it already has in ligand-gated ion channel pharmacology. It becomes more and more plausible that the poorly understood effects of some drugs could be related to their inverse agonist character. It is, for example, the case of haloperidol, a classical "antagonist" of dopamine D_2 receptors, which turned out to be a potent inverse agonist of the same receptor. Inverse agonists could provide new therapeutic approaches in many instances, and the search for such compounds will be more commonly included in pharmacological screening programs.

3.4   Receptor interaction with G proteins

Many studies, based on the synthesis of chimeric receptors, on site-directed mutagenesis or on the use of synthetic peptides, have attempted to delineate the regions of GPCR structure which interact with G proteins and are directly responsible for their activation. As expected, these regions correspond to the cytoplasmic part of the receptors. In particular, the importance of the N- and C-terminal ends of the third cytoplasmic loop (which would form amphiphilic helices) for the efficiency of coupling was described for many monoamine receptors, including, for instance, the adrenergic α_{1A} [Cotecchia et al., 1990], α_{1B} [Cotecchia et al., 1992], α_{2A} [Eason and Liggett, 1995], β_2 [Kobilka et al., 1988; Strader et al., 1987b] and the muscarinic M_1, M_2 and M_3 [Kubo et al., 1988; Lechleiter et al., 1990; Wess et al., 1990]. In general terms, deletion or mutation of these regions resulted in the uncoupling of the receptor from the G protein [Hausdorff et al., 1990; Shapiro et al., 1993]. Random saturation mutagenesis experiments have indicated the crucial role of stretches of hydrophobic residues belonging to these regions [Burstein et al., 1996; Hill-Eubanks et al., 1996]. A four amino acid motif (VTIL) was identified at the junction between the third cytoplasmic loop and the sixth helix of the M_2 muscarinic receptor that was shown to be essential to G_i and G_o binding [Liu et al., 1996]. Thus, a relative movement of TM6 towards the cytoplasm, as a consequence of agonist-induced receptor isomerization, would expose the VTIL motif at the membrane-cytoplasm interface to enable GTP/GDP exchange on G proteins.

It has been suggested that the N- and C-terminal ends of the third cytoplasmic loop are able to form amphipathic α-helices, reminiscent of the mastoparan structure, a component of wasp venom which is able to directly activate G proteins [Higashijima et al., 1988]. However, the structural determinants of the specificity of the coupling of bioamine receptors with various G proteins are still unclear. Regions of the second intracellular loop and of the C terminal tail of the receptor have also been shown to play a role in coupling with G proteins [Eason and Liggett, 1996; Moro, 1993a; O'Dowd, 1988; Wong et al., 1990]. Receptor chimeras coupled to different G proteins further delineated these determinants. For instance, chimeric receptors (α_{1b} and β_2, M_1 and β_2) have been used to identify several residues at the N terminus of the third cytoplasmic loop which are necessary for the interaction with either G_i or G_s [Cotecchia et al., 1992; Wong et al., 1990].

Some splicing variants of GPCRs, which differ in the sequence and length of the third cytoplasmic loop or the C-terminus, are also natural examples that highlight their functional involvement in G protein activation. In the case of the five variants of the pituitary adenylate cyclase activating polypeptide (PACAP) receptor, the insertion of a 28 amino acid encoding exon suppresses the G protein-mediated activation of phospholipase C and impairs cAMP formation as compared with the other forms of the receptor [Spengler et al., 1993]. The two splicing variants of the D_2 dopaminergic receptor, which differ by an insertion of 29 residues in the middle of the same third intracellular loop, also display different specificity for the G_i proteins. The long isoform of the D_2 receptor seems to preferentially interact with G_{i2} [Guiramand et al., 1995; Montmayeur et al., 1993], although an other group reported exactly the opposite, the long isoform coupling preferentially with G_{i3} and the short one with G_{i2} [Senogles, 1994]. Other cell-specific determinants may account for these discrepancies [Strange, 1996]. Four isoforms of the prostaglandin E3 receptors differs by the length and sequences of their C-terminal tails, as a consequence of alternative splicing. Two of these isoforms are coupled to G_s and activate adenyl cyclase, whereas the third one ($EP3_A$) activates phosphoinositide turnover via a pertussis toxin (PTX)-sensitive G protein and the last one ($EP3_D$) has the same effect via a PTX-insensitive G protein [Namba et al., 1993]. The third cytoplasmic loop and the C-terminal extremity of the bioamine receptors also display many phosphorylable residues which could modify the interaction of the receptor with the G proteins. In the case of the β_2 adrenoreceptor, phosphorylation of the C-terminal end of the third cytoplasmic loop reduces its affinity for Gs and increases its affinity for G_i [Okamoto et al., 1991]. Finally, it should be stressed that these C-terminal regions of the receptors, forming a fourth cytoplasmic loop by their anchorage in the plasma membrane, also contribute significantly to the functional conformation of the receptor and consequently to its intrinsic activity. Many receptor isoforms differing only by their C-terminus exhibit significantly distinct basal activity, such as the prostaglandin E3 receptor [Hasegawa et al., 1996] or the metabotropic glutamate receptor mGluR1 [Prezeau et al., 1996].

The role of GPCR cytoplasmic loops in ensuring some specificity and efficacy in G protein coupling has been confirmed by expressing these regions in cells where they inhibited activation of monoamine receptors [Hawes et al., 1994; Luttrell et al., 1993] or by using corresponding peptides to compete with G protein activation by the cytoplasmic loops of the receptors [Dalman and Neubig, 1991; Kahlert et al., 1990]. A temporary conclusion might be that, although the third cytoplasmic loop and the C-terminus are clearly the key determinants in G protein α subunit recognition and activation, the two other, more conserved cytoplasmic loops also play a role in the receptor's ability to interact with the G protein in its heterotrimeric form. A general feature is that most of the receptors are able to activate several types of different G proteins. Accordingly, strong determinants of a highly specific coupling of receptors with G proteins have not been identified up to now, and it is probable that they simply do not exist.

3.5   Desensitization of the receptor

Desensitization is a general cellular mechanism whose function is to turn off the signaling process triggered by an external stimulus, thus enabling the cell to adapt its behavior to additional or subsequent stimuli. Although a few studies have shown that desensitization could take place at the effector level [Bates et al., 1991], the interruption of the signaling pathway is

---

Fig. 5

A general model of receptor desensitization.

This scheme is based mainly on the data obtained from rhodopsin, the β adrenoreceptors and some related receptors. 1) Phosphorylation of the receptor by second messenger-dependant kinases may occur either in homologous or heterologous desensitization. 2) The sustained presence of the agonist on the receptor triggers the membrane recruitment of GRK by association to the $\beta\gamma$ complex interaction and receptor phosphorylation, the major step for homologous desensitization. RGS proteins (regulators of G protein signaling) also modulate the responses elicited by the GPCR module. 3) Arrestin proteins then bind to the phosphorylated receptor and are thought to be the event required to promote receptor endocytosis, sequestration and recycling.

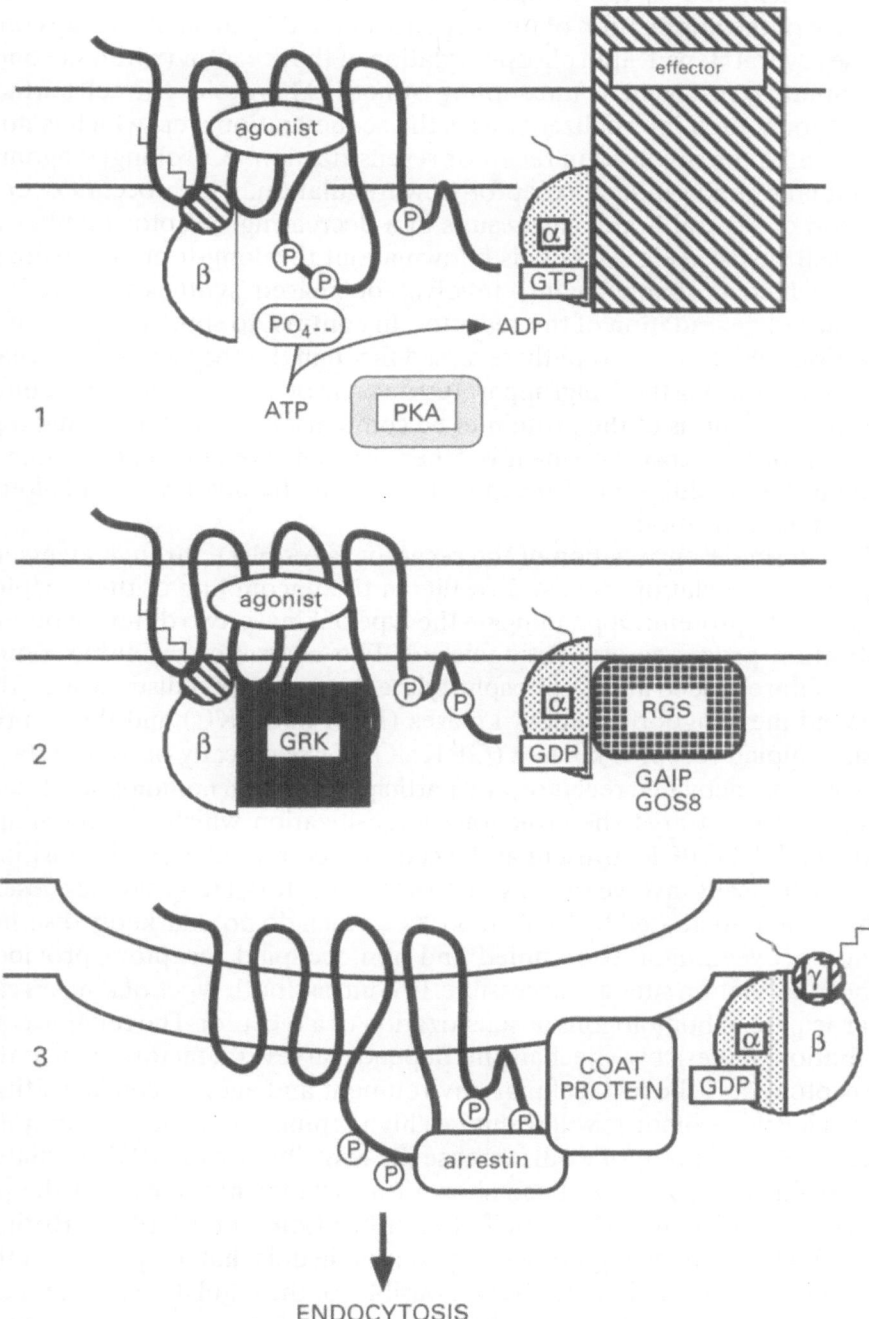

mainly achieved by the receptor itself. In the case of GPCRs, the time course of the attenuation of the response elicited by an agonist may comprise several steps. Rapid phosphorylation of the receptor (within seconds to minutes) results in its uncoupling from the G protein. The cell surface receptor is then internalized; this is the sequestration step, which is now believed to be involved in receptor resensitization. A prolonged agonist stimulation may induce receptor downregulation, which occurs over a period of several hours and results in a decreasing receptor number at the cell surface (Fig. 5). Less is known about this long-term desensitization, which probably mainly involves decreased synthesis as well as increased degradation of the receptor. In contrast to short-term desensitization, which can be rapidly reversed through the recycling of internalized receptors via the Golgi apparatus, reversal of downregulation requires *de novo* synthesis of the protein to be compensated. Transcriptional regulation of the receptor, which is otherwise not thought to play a major role in the modulation of receptor levels, may be involved in this long-term resensitization.

Short-term desensitization of the receptor takes place through an essential phosphorylation step, and results in the uncoupling of the receptor from the G protein. Depending on the type of kinase, two different desensitization processes are distinguished. Two classes of serine/threonine kinases are indeed able to phosphorylate the receptor at distinct sites: the second messenger-dependent kinases (PKA and PKC) and the G protein-coupled receptor kinases (GRK). GRK specifically phosphorylates the agonist-activated receptor, and participates only in homologous desensitization. Contrary to heterologous desensitization, which can potentially affect all the GPCRs present at the cell surface, homologous desensitization specifically involves agonist-activated receptors. Heterologous desensitization is mediated by PKA and PKC, which do not markedly discriminate between agonist-occupied and non-occupied receptors, provided phosphorylation sites are accessible. In contrast, both types of kinases can participate in homologous desensitization of a receptor. The relative contribution of these two mechanisms depends on several factors, such as the receptor itself, the intracellular environment and agonist concentration. High levels of agonists will result in a higher number of agonist-occupied receptors, and therefore will increase the contribution of GRK-mediated desensitization. This has been shown for instance in the case of the β_2-adrenergic receptor [Hausdorff et al., 1989; Lohse et al., 1990a; Roth et al., 1991]. Given the high concentrations of ligands that are present at the synapses, GRKs are likely to be responsible for the regulation of the receptor number which takes place during neurotransmission. This hypothesis is strengthened by the tissue distribution pattern of GRKs, and also by their intracellular (post- and pre-synaptic) localization [Arriza et al., 1992]. Although the contribution of GRKs to homologous desensitization is now better understood, the role of other kinases in this process is not yet clear. In particular, the extent to which activation of one type of GPCR, leading to stimulation of nonspecific kinases such as PKA or PKC, is able to modify the responsiveness of another type of receptor is still a matter of debate. This kind of heterologous desensitization has probably been over-interpreted in the past, and its actual role in receptor regulation remains to be established.

3.5.1   *GRK-activated desensitization*

Recent studies have improved our understanding of GRK-dependent desensitization. GRKs form a family of related proteins, six of which have been identified so far, including rhodopsin kinase (GRK1) and β-adrenergic kinases βARK-1 and βARK-2 (GRK2 and GRK3) [Inglese et al., 1993; Premont et al., 1995]. Many GPCRs, monoamine as well as peptide receptors, are regulated by these kinases, in an essentially nonspecific way. The β_2-adrenergic receptor can, for instance, be desensitized by five of the GRKs, which promote desensitization of rhodopsin [Inglese et al., 1993]. In the absence of agonist-induced stimulation of the cell, GRK1, GRK2 and GRK3 are found in the cytosol. Their necessary translocation to the plasma membrane, triggered by receptor activation, is achieved through different mechanisms. Rhodopsin kinase (GRK1) is farnesylated in its C-terminal region. In the case of the β-adrenergic kinases, targeting to the membrane is mediated via an interaction with the $\beta\gamma$ dimer of G proteins, while isoprenylation mechanisms ensure the association of the γ subunit to the membrane [Pitcher et al., 1992]. The PH of the kinase and the WD domains of the β subunit are probably responsible for the interaction between the two proteins. The three other kinases are thought to be mainly associated with the membrane, independent of the G protein activation state, via either palmitoylation (GRK4, GRK6) [Premont et al., 1996; Stoffel et al., 1994] or a direct interaction between a stretch of basic residues and membrane phospholipids (GRK5) [Premont et al., 1994].

Once translocated to the membrane, GRKs are able to phosphorylate GPCRs at several serine and threonine residues. These residues are generally located at the C terminal tails of the receptors, but can also belong to their third cytoplasmic loops, as for the α_{2A} adrenergic receptor [Liggett et al., 1992]. Palmitoylation and membrane anchoring of the conserved Cys residues of the receptor intracellular ends are probably involved in the mechanisms underlying this specificity of GRKs for activated receptors and GRK specifically phosphorylation activated, i.e. agonist-occupied, receptors. In the case of the β_2-adrenergic receptor, the substitution of this Cys residue resulted in increased basal phosphorylation of the mutant receptor, probably responsible for its inability to activate G_s [Moffett et al., 1993; O'Dowd et al., 1989]. The same mutation in the D_{1A} dopamine receptor resulted in a constitutively desensitized receptor [Jensen et al., 1995]. It was recently proposed [Bouvier et al., 1995] that stimulation of the receptor by an agonist favors depalmitoylation of the receptor, and that the nonpalmitoylated, non-membrane-anchored receptor C-terminus is in a conformation more accessible to phosphorylation. Phosphorylation of the receptor by GRK, although it contributes to receptor desensitization, is not sufficient for its complete inactivation. This full desensitization, as in the case of rhodopsin, requires the binding of additional components, the arrestin proteins. Two arrestins, related to the visual rod and cone arrestins, have been identified so far [Attramadal et al., 1992; Lohse et al., 1990b]. Like GRKs, but by unknown mechanisms, cytoplasmic arrestins are translocated to the plasma membrane, where they preferentially bind to phosphorylated and activated receptors [Lohse et al., 1992], thus resulting in their uncoupling from G proteins. Binding of arrestin to the receptor could be involved in initiation of receptor sequestration [Ferguson et al., 1996]. In this process, arrestin functions as an adapter and favors the association of the receptor with clathrin or other endocytotic vesicle coat proteins and receptor endocytosis.

3.5.2   GPCR sequestration

Short-term resensitization of GPCRs is now believed to be associated with their agonist-induced sequestration. Endosomal internalization was first observed for the β_2-adrenergic receptor, and has since been confirmed for many other members of the GPCR family, including the adrenergic β_1 [Green and Liggett, 1994], endothelin ETA [Chun et al., 1995], luteinizing hormone [Kawate and Menon, 1994] or muscarinic [Goldman et al., 1996; Koenig and Edwardson, 1996] receptors. The low amount of phosphorylated receptors as well as the high phosphatase activity associated with the intracellular sequestration compartment suggested that receptor internalization could be involved in the resensitization process [Sibley et al., 1986]. This concept was grounded on experimental studies where inhibition of receptor sequestration prevented its resensitization [Barak et al., 1994; Yu et al., 1993]. Furthermore, in contrast to what was previously suggested, it seems that only a small part, if any, of the internalized receptors is directed to the lysosomes to be degraded. Indeed, site-directed mutagenesis produced receptors that could still be sequestered but not downregulated and vice versa [Barak et al., 1994; Campbell et al., 1991].

Several stretches of receptor intracellular loops have been found to be crucial for their internalization. A small Ser- and Thr-rich region was identified in the middle of the third cytoplasmic loop of the muscarinic M_1 and M_2 receptors [Lameh et al., 1992; Moro et al., 1993b]. For both M_1 muscarinic and GnRH receptors, the mutation of a Leu residue located in the vicinity of the highly conserved DRY motif (second cytoplasmic domain) impaired sequestration of the receptor [Arora et al., 1995; Moro et al., 1994]. Several receptors (e.g. adrenergic α_{1B}, angiotensin AT_{1A}, neurotensin, GnRH) were also unable to internalize after removal of their cytoplasmic tail [Benya et al., 1993; Hermans et al., 1996; Lattion et al., 1994; Thomas et al., 1995], whereas the same truncation had no effect on M_1 receptor sequestration [Lameh et al., 1992]. It had also a small and cell-type specific influence in the case of the β_2 receptor [Bouvier et al., 1988; Strader et al., 1987a].

The contribution of phosphorylation in sequestration mechanisms has been extensively studied in recent years without providing clear results, except that phosphorylation is not required for internalization. For instance, a β_2 receptor lacking all its PKA/GRK-phosphorylable residues conserved the ability to internalize upon agonist-stimulation in CHO cells [Hausdorff et al., 1989]. On the other hand, overexpression of βARK-1 was shown to facilitate sequestration of the M_2 receptor [Tsuga et al., 1994]. A recent study demonstrated the key role of arrestin in sequestration of the β_2 adrenergic receptor [Ferguson et al., 1996]. Since arrestin preferentially binds to a phosphorylated receptor, GRKs are able to enhance the receptor internalization even if they are not required for this process. For instance, in cells containing high levels of arrestins, receptor sequestration can probably be achieved normally even in the absence of phosphorylation, as is suggested by Ferguson et al. (1996).

Several distinct mechanisms could drive the agonist-induced internalization of the receptor, depending on the type of the receptor but also on its intracellular environment. For instance, sequestered β_2-adrenergic receptors can be harvested both in clathrin-coated vesicles and caveolae [Raposo et al., 1989; von Zastrow and Kobilka, 1992]. Nevertheless, the recently found implication of arrestin proteins in this process [Ferguson et al., 1996], and the demonstration of their ability to promote the endocytosis of the receptor via clathrin-coated vesicles [Zhang et al., 1996], make it possible to describe more precisely one of the internalization pathways of GPCRs. Activation of the receptor by an agonist results in translocation of GRK to the membrane, via the free $\beta\gamma$ dimer in the case of βARK-1 and βARK-2. Receptor phosphorylation increases its affinity for arrestin proteins which, directly or by triggering interactions with other intracellular components, can direct the receptor to the endosomes via clathrin-coated vesicles. In endosomes, receptors are then dephosphorylated and sent back to the plasma membrane. The mechanism underlying this latter transport of the receptor has not been determined, but by analogy with the recycling of other proteins, it may involve sorting of the dephosphorylated receptor from the late endosomes to the trans-Golgi network (TGN) and then from the TGN to the plasma membrane (see below).

3.6   Addressing GPCRs to the plasma membrane

The mechanisms and pathways positions by which GPCRs reach their final positions after synthesis and membrane inclusion in the endoplasmic reticulum remain poorly investigated, essentially because of the lack of good antibodies to allow detailed confocal or electron microscopic cellular studies. However, the techniques of receptor tagging with epitopes recognized by specific antibodies, and the development of sophisticated cell biology techniques, are beginning to provide insights into the intracellular pathways followed by GPCRs. It also appears clearly that regulation of receptor distribution on cell membranes is an important part of the mechanisms by which cells modulate their responsiveness to extracellular signals.

Seven transmembrane receptors are cotranslationally integrated in the membrane of the endoplasmic reticulum (ER). In contrast to some other receptors, like the peptidergic endothelin receptors [Arai et al., 1990; Sakurai et al., 1990], bioamine receptors do not in general display any signal peptides. The reason some receptors bear signal peptides is unknown, but they may facilitate binding of the nascent protein to the signal recognition particle (SRP) and transfer of the first transmembrane segment through the channel formed by the translocation complex [rev. in Schatz and Dobberstein, 1996]. In the absence of signal peptides, integration of receptors into the membrane is promoted just by the alternation of hydrophobic ("signal anchor") and hydrophilic or charged ("top transfer") segments [High and Dobberstein, 1992]. In any case, the final topology of the receptor into the membrane is probably achieved by inserting the first hydrophobic stretch (TM1) alone, and then the six other stretches, two by two, folded into a hairpin structure [Audigier et al., 1987]. How the final oligomerization of the receptor is performed is still unknown. In the case of rhodopsin, a chaperone contributes to the proper folding of mammalian red opsin [Ferreira et al., 1997].

Like any other membrane protein which reaches the lumen of the ER, GPCRs are N- and O-glycosylated [rev. in Abeijon and Hirschberg, 1992]. Prevention of the receptor N-terminus glycosylation in the case of the β_2 adrenoceptor and also of rhodopsin results in decreased receptor density at the cell surface [Liu et al., 1993; Rands et al., 1990]. In general, O-glycosylation is significantly modified, and this difference is often the origin of modified migration patterns in polyacrylamide electrophoresis and Western blot analysis of the receptor proteins. It could also be used to distinguish between "mature" and "immature" receptors in experiments studying the regulation of receptor trafficking [e.g. Fishburn et al., 1995]. Although lipid modification of the C-terminus required for the function of many GPCRs is likely also to occur in the Golgi apparatus, little is known about the mechanisms of this modification.

Finally, when reaching the transgolgi network (TGN), GPCRs are sorted to their final destination, the plasma membrane. Secretory vesicles budding from the TGN will carry the receptors, as well as many other membrane or secreted molecules, to the plasma membrane, where they are integrated or secreted by an exocytotic process. This receptor sorting is of utmost importance, since it governs the spatial organization of the transmission network among cells and since the physiological response of a given cell to the corresponding extracellular messenger will depend on it (see below). It is particularly true for polarized cells such as epithelial cells and neurons, where a "choice" has to been made by the receptor to be localized either to the basolateral or the apical (in the case of the epithelial cells), or the dendritic and the axonal (in the case of neurons), compartments. Unfortunately, mechanisms of receptor sorting in the TGN are completely unknown, although the nature of the protein sequence is likely to play a role [Pelham and Munro, 1993]. It is not known whether the cytoplasmic regions of the GPCR alone could act as a targeting signal or whether the general conformation of the receptors could also contribute to the specificity of membrane transport, as suggested by Munro [1991]. For example, when transfected into polarized epithelial cells, the α_{2A} adrenoceptors are targeted to the basolateral membrane, whereas the adenosine receptor A_{1A} is targeted essentially to the apical pole, exactly where these receptors are localized in cells which naturally express them. Similar results have been obtained for subtypes of serotonin receptors transfected in an epithelial cell line, where the usually presynaptic 5-HT$_{1B}$ receptor is targeted to the apical domain and the generally somatodendritic receptor 5HT$_{1A}$ was observed mainly in the basolateral domain. The regulation of these sorting mechanisms in the TGN could also implicate interactions with heterotrimeric G proteins, as suggested by Huttner and colleagues [Barr et al., 1992; Leyte et al., 1992]. Activation of PTX-sensitive heterotrimeric G proteins or of G_s which are localized in the TGN tends to block the formation of secretory vesicles and the transport of secreted proteins. In contrast, the blockade of G proteins by PTX stimulates vesicle budding. Moreover, different classes of hetrotrimeric G proteins may regulate the polarized localization of membrane proteins in epithelial cells. In MDCK cells, apical addressing is affected by agents interfering with G_s, whereas basolateral transport is altered by PTX [Pimplikar and Simons, 1993].

Although no mechanism has yet been definitely demonstrated, there are now robust evidence that heterotrimeric G proteins may modulate the function of ARF (ADP ribosylation factors). ARF are low molecular weight G proteins which promotes the assembly of coat proteins required for the budding and formation of vesicles from a donor compartment, including the formation of secretory vesicles from the TGN [Boman and Kahn, 1995; Colombo et al., 1995; Galas et al., 1997; Gruenberg and Clague, 1992]. A very attractive hypothesis will be that arrival of GPCRs to the TGN, provided these receptors are in different activation states, could modulate the budding and formation of secretory vesicles "en route" for different compartments of the plasma membrane, by differentially interacting with different sets of heterotrimeric G proteins. In this case, similar mechanisms would exist for both signaling via receptors at the plasma membrane and regulating vesicular transport and sorting inside the cells. "Desensitization" or "downregulation" are just particular cases of more general mechanisms of regulation of receptor localization and activity.

4   The molecular diversity of GPCR-associated transmission modules: A challenge for physiology and pharmacology

The now general observation that GPCRs and their associated proteins exhibit an amazing molecular multiplicity remains puzzling to many pharmacologists and physiologists. What is the physiological counterpart of hundreds of receptors, coupled to dozens of G proteins, themselves potentially able to activate dozens of effectors? It could stand as an insoluble problem for investigators who seek to design experiments to understand the physiological role of these signaling devices. The question of the experimental handling of complex systems, that is, systems made of many different components, cannot be reduced to a few simple elements. A number of observations that have now been made may indicate directions to be followed in the near future.

4.1   GPCRs are potentially coupled to many different signaling systems in cells.

What emerges from structural studies of GPCR and G proteins is that the specificity of interactions between receptors and heterotrimeric G proteins is rather low, a surprising fact at first glance. When *in vitro* assays are considered, the restrictions concerning G protein-receptor interactions are very weak. For example, the β_2-adrenoreceptor activates G_s only two to three times better than G_i in a reconstituted system [Cerione et al., 1985], and the D_2 dopamine receptor does not significantly discriminate among PTX-sensitive G proteins [Senogles et al., 1990]. Numerous experimental evidence has shown that a given receptor does not have a strict specificity with regard to intracellular signaling, and most GPCRs may activate more than one type of heterotrimeric G protein. The only requirement is that G proteins are promiscuous to GPCRs. This property allows investigators to observe, almost invariably, significant activation of intracellular signaling pathways in transfected cells. Obviously, the kind of coupling which is obtained in a highly heterologous context is mainly artificial, and these reconstitution systems may miss some crucial aspects in receptor-G protein interactions. As a representative example, the D_2 dopamine receptor expressed in different cell lines is able to modulate at least six different signaling pathways, including inhibition of adenylyl cyclase, of Na^+/H^+ exchanger and of calcium currents, activation of potassium channels, cell division and phospholipase A_2 [Cali et al., 1992; Chio et al., 1994; Lledo et al., 1994; Piomelli et al., 1991; Vallar et al., 1992]. Receptor transfections remain a useful tool for studying many aspects of receptor biochemistry and structure-activity relationships, but certainly not for predicting the responses that a given drug may elicit in a natural system.

A recent example of the increasing "pleiotropy" of GPCRs has been brought about by showing that $\beta\gamma$ subunits are involved in a broad range of interactions with intracellular effectors and regulatory proteins. Many of them have already been mentioned in this paper. But of general interest is also the demonstration of the modulation by $\beta\gamma$ subunits of the MAP (mitogen-activated protein) kinase pathway, a signaling cascade which is commonly activated by tyrosine-kinase receptors and Ras proteins. Although the complete set of intermediary proteins between $\beta\gamma$ and Ras has not yet been identified, membrane localization of Ras and the different MEK (MAP kinase kinase) proteins is crucial for extracellular signal-regulated kinase (ERK) activation. It involves phosphorylation of the Shc protein on a tyrosine residue and the formation of the Shc-Grb2 complex required for Ras activation. The βγ subunits are likely to provide the substrate for the membrane recruitment of these signaling proteins [Luttrell et al., 1996; van Biesen et al., 1995].

On the other hand, it is equally wrong to state that everything is possible with receptor-G protein interactions. In natural situations, a significant degree of specificity exists both for the association of the α and βγ subunits in the G protein heterotrimer (see 1.2), for interaction of receptors with G protein classes and for the activation of effectors by the various G protein components and subunits. The α_1 adrenoceptors have been reported to interact only with G_q proteins, and receptors such as the muscarinic M_2, α_2 adrenoceptors or dopamine D_2 receptors probably interact only with G_i/G_o proteins. Gudermann et al. [1996] have proposed that preferential association of receptor classes with classes of heterotrimeric G proteins is the rule, though with some exceptions. The TSH receptor has been shown to activate G proteins of each of the known classes [Laugwitz et al., 1996].

Specificity is more apparent for the modulation of effector activity by G proteins. All the subtypes of adenylyl cyclase are activated by $G\alpha_s$, but βγ subunits exert differential effects on the enzyme subtypes. Type II and IV adenylyl cyclase are activated by βγ, which also potentiates the effect of $G\alpha_s$. In contrast, βγ has no effect on type III adenylyl cyclase and inhibits neuronal type I cyclase [rev. in Sunahara et al., 1996]. The case of phospholipase C_β is remarkable by virtue of the fact that both α and βγ subunits activate the enzyme, but by different mechanisms of protein-protein interaction. Different enzyme domains lead to enzymatic activation by either the Gα or Gβγ subunits. It may explain why, in some instances, enzyme activation by GPCR is sensitive to PTX, whereas only toxin-insensitive $G\alpha_q$, $G\alpha_{11}$ or $G\alpha_{16}$ are able to modulate enzyme activity.

Nevertheless, studies which used antibodies or antisense oligonucleotides to specifically disrupt G protein expression have generally revealed a high specificity in the nature of the G protein components implicated in cell responses. G protein interactions with both receptors and effectors are impaired. Schultz used the antisense oligonucleotide technique to show that the effect of a given receptor in a differentiated cell depends on a very specific association of αβγ subunits [Gudermann et al., 1996]. For example, two different isoforms of $G\alpha_o$ are needed to mediate somatostatin and muscarinic receptor effects on calcium channels in GH3 cells. Moreover, the somatostatin receptor was specifically coupled to $\beta_1\gamma_2$, whereas the muscarinic receptor was associated with $\beta_3\gamma_4$ subunits [Kleuss et al., 1991; Kleuss et al., 1992; Kleuss et al., 1993]. In many instances, βγ subunits are required to modulate the activity of ion channels or effector

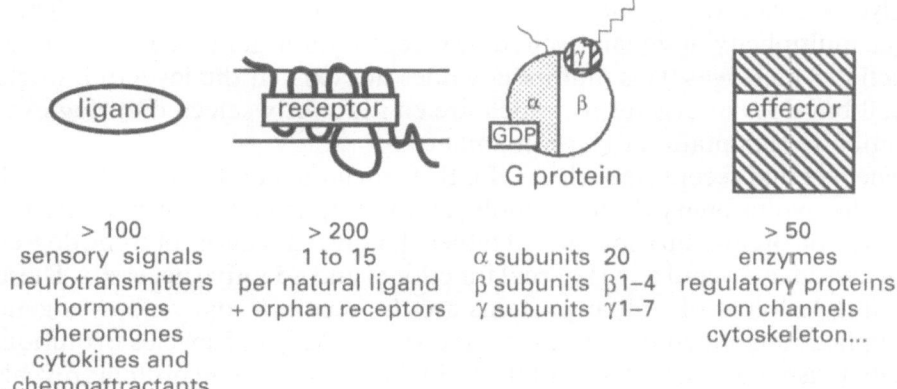

Fig. 6
The components of the transmission modules represented by GPCR exhibit an extremely large degree of molecular diversity and multiplicity. However, not all the combination of interacting molecules is allowed on a structural ground. The required specificity in cell signaling is obtained essentially by the anatomical distribution in the organism and compartmentalization in cells of molecular components, but also by their stochiometry and the timing of their interactions in " signaling pathways".

enzymes, and are likely to play a crucial role in "coincident detection". The precise effect of the βγ complex has not yet been elucidated, but its general contribution to the modulation of the activity of many effector or regulatory proteins is probably related to its rigid structural conformation, a scaffolding for various types of protein-protein interactions.

The fact that the structural requirements for receptor-G protein coupling are less stringent than for G protein ligand recognition has important implications with respect to the evolution of bioamine receptors. In particular, changes in cell-specific expression which may occur during differentiation in different organisms, or after a duplication step in receptor genes, will not result in loss of function, since the receptor will be able to interact with at least one type of G protein at its novel expression site.

4.2   The specificity of transmembrane signaling in organisms
        and cells

The molecular diversity of hormonal or neurotransmission systems is apparent at the very beginning of the chain of events that allows cells to respond to environmental cues in an adaptative manner. In metazoan organisms of increasing complexity, cells are able to "recognize" several hundreds of different messages, that is, transmitter molecules (Fig. 6). A given transmitter is generally recognized by several receptor types. Thus, the multiplicity of signals elicited by receptors is larger than that of extracellular messages. This multiplicity does not exist at the level of a single cell but does in organisms, which are continuously selected during evolution for adaptation to a given milieu.

The fact that receptors such as GPCRs form large families is the hallmark of the evolutionary origin of molecular multiplicity. It is necessarily the outcome of random processes of molecular diversification, of some degree of contingency and a part of real functional and adaptive necessity. These multiple forms of similar proteins are the result of many steps of gene duplications which that occurred at different times of species evolution. Obviously, the conservation of these duplicated genes and proteins reveals some functional requirements and constraints. Therefore, the strong and parsimonious logic of evolution has to be taken into account to understand receptor functions [Cardinaud et al., 1997; Vernier et al., 1995; Zuckerkandl, 1994].

In vertebrates, extracellular transmitters such as hormones, cytokines, chemoattractants or neurotransmitters are released in temporally and spatially organized ways which vary widely from one system to another. Requirements for receptor functioning are not the same for point-to-point fast synaptic transmission leading to ion channel activation as for the hormone-like, very diffuse and slow signaling displayed by many neuromodulatory or hormonal systems. Much of the molecular diversity of receptors and intracellular partners accounts for this necessity of anatomical organization. It is spectacularly illustrated in the central nervous system where most of the different subtypes of neurotransmitter receptors are localized in different areas, in different neurons, in different types of cells. For β-adrenoceptors as an example, β_1 receptors are found in the anterior olfactory nuclei, in the cerebral cortex, striatum, deep cerebellar nuclei to cite only a few, whereas β_2 receptors are found mainly in the olfactory bulb, and the piriform and cerebellar cortex. The β_3 receptor is not present in the brain [Nicholas et al., 1993]. Generally, various receptor subtypes of a given pharmacological class do not overlap in the brain and peripheral tissues [Nicholas et al., 1996; Sokoloff and Schwartz, 1995; Vernier et al., 1995]. Therefore, these different receptor subtypes, which in general share very similar functional characteristics, are not redundant, since they are not localized in the same cells. They ensure the necessary transduction of the extracellular transmitter or hormones in many different target cells. Even in organs other than the nervous system, a certain degree of spatial organization is displayed. In each type of cell expressing a different subtype of receptor, the expression of this receptor subtype is governed by the mechanisms which also determine the differentiation state of this cell. The logic of the differential distribution of GPCRs in vertebrates is that of the set-up of the organism which takes place during ontogeny, and allows the transmitters to fulfill their irregulatory functions both during development and adulthood. This anatomical or spatial organization of the transmitter systems corresponds to the bulk of the specificity of information transmission, which allows the whole range of fine regulation of the organic functions.

Is a similar degree of molecular diversity required at the cellular level? Certainly not, since the range of responses for a given cell in a metazoan organism is not extremely large. Most cells execute the phenotypic functions determined by their differentiation state. It is, indeed, generally observed that several different transmitters will trigger essentially similar responses in a single cell. Therefore, cells have to respond to a large number of different messages, but the types of responses elicited by these stimuli are rather limited. In other words, extracellular signals converge towards a few adaptative responses in each cell type. Accordingly, the number of proteins that comprise intracellular signaling pathways is much smaller than that of transmitters and receptors. Most, if not all of them (G proteins, effectors such as ion channels, metabolic enzymes, regulatory proteins such as GRK or arrestins), also belong to gene families generated by gene duplication. However, the logic that governs the building of cells is not exactly the same as that of organisms.

As is the case for membrane receptors, the different isoforms of a given transduction protein such as the α subunit of G proteins could be expressed in a strictly defined anatomical location (G_{olf} vs G_s, transducin vs G_i for example). The differentiation process that takes place during the development of organisms partially accounts for the molecular multiplicity of the components of signaling cascades, but it is not a general case. In most situations, intracellular signaling molecules have a very widespread distribution. The specificity of the cellular responses to different kind of signals depends on the biochemical properties of these intracellular signaling molecules, and on the nature of the very few effectors which ultimately determine phenotypic responses. Broadly speaking, if the incoming messages and the final responses are highly specific to a given cell type, the molecules which carry the signals between them do not need to be highly specific.

At the cellular level, the existence of sorting mechanisms that specifically address receptors and their interacting partners to membrane compartments is one essential part of the way functional specificity is achieved in cell signaling despite the apparent multiplicity and diversity of these molecular systems. For the same technical reasons as those which have hindered detailed knowledge of receptor trafficking, very few data are available on the precise nature of the components of receptor signaling modules. It is nevertheless very likely that specialized domains of the plasma membrane exist where these components are concentrated. Compartments such as caveolae could be an example of membrane domains specialized in signal transduction [Lisanti, 1994]. Clearly, dendritic spines, neuro-muscular junctions, or synapses in more general terms, are also specializations of the plasma membrane. A tremendous effort is still required to analyze in detail the composition of receptor modules in the "real world" of an organism.

An other way to a high degree of specificity in cell signaling is the temporal coherence of the messages that reach the cell. That has been called "coincident detection" [rev. in Bourne and Nicoll, 1993]. Examples such as adenylyl cyclase type II, whose activity is additively potentiated by both α_s and $\beta\gamma$ subunits, or phospholipase C, whose effect is affected by both α_q and $\beta\gamma$ subunits in highly integrated manner, highlight the way some signals emerge from the background noise.

The kinetics of the G protein cycle often dictates its rhythm to many biological events, and in this respect, too, the effect produced in cells by receptor activation is the result of the receptor-G protein-effector interactions, since at each of these protein interfaces regulation may occur. In addition, the cytoplasmic loops of the bioamine receptors do not interact solely with G proteins but also with other regulatory proteins such as arrestins, various kinases, the cytoskeleton and components of vesicular traffic. Therefore, the various receptor subtypes may also exhibit different properties with regard to corresponding cell functions. It has been shown that the β-adrenoreceptor subtypes desensitized at variable rates, and such observations are likely to be extended to other bioamine receptor classes. The recent discovery of RGS proteins (RGS for regulator of G protein signaling) such as GAIP or GOS8, which affect the rate of GTP hydrolysis by the α subunits of G proteins, is important in this respect and their place in GPCR transmission will be soon evaluated [Siderovski et al., 1996]. The nature of the components of the signalling pathways and of their interactions – either activatory or inhibitory – may change with the physiological status of the cell, explaining why a given stimulus can promote very different responses in the same cell. This is well illustrated by the prolactin cell of the anterior pituitary. In males or non-pregnant females, hormone release is efficiently inhibited by the tonic effect of low concentrations of dopamine, which enhances potassium channel permeability by D_2 receptor and $G\alpha_i$ protein activation, and thereby hyperpolarizes the cell [Lledo et al., 1992]. Thus at the resting state, membrane hyperpolarization is the primary mechanism that underlies inhibition of hormone release by D_2 receptors. On the other hand, during lactation many prolactin secreting cells display a completely different behavior with a low membrane resting potential and accordingly high and fluctuating levels of intracellular calcium, leading to a high level of spontaneous hormone release. In these cells, the D_2 receptor triggers $G\alpha_o$ activation and calcium channel blockade, promoting hormone release inhibition. Moreover, in lactating females, other prolactin cells with high membrane potentials can release prolactin only upon TRH receptor activation and become sensitive to dopamine only under this condition [Lledo et al., 1992, 1994]. Therefore, most of the apparent pleiotropy of GPCRs could be resolved when the various functional states of the cells and spatial distribution of the signaling systems are taken into account.

To summarize, we may state that specificity in cell signaling is essentially provided by cell differentiation (which governs the nature of the interacting components of GPCR signaling modules), by the specific localization and compartmentalization of molecular components in the cells, by their stochiometry and the precise timing of the recruitment of the interacting partners making the so-called signaling pathways.

5   Classification of the bioamine GPCRs

The diversity and modularity of the GPCRs represent a difficult challenge to receptor classification. Receptor classification is, however, an important aspect of theories about receptor activity and function. Not only does it provide the required framework for receptor nomenclature but also it represents a current and heuristic view of our knowledge and conceptions about these molecules.

Up to now, the dominant view of membrane receptors has been pharmacological, since pharmaceutical or natural ligands were for long almost the only available tools to study the receptors. This approach has led to the definition of many receptor classes or subtypes which have been later confirmed by other means. However, the diversity of the receptor molecules (the "real world" receptors) goes far beyond the pharmacological one.

Two difficult questions have been encountered by pharmacologists dealing with the molecular diversity of GPCRs. The first one relies upon the difficulty of describing receptor multiplicity with ligands only. The "circularity" of drug-receptor reciprocal discrimination has already been underscored by many authors [e.g. Kenakin, 1983], but the problem is even greater. Up to now, available drugs have not been able to fully differentiate between all the existing receptor subtypes for a given transmitter. In general, drug-based discrimination of receptor subtypes is better obtained by the "affinity profile" of several drugs than by the specific properties of a single "discriminating ligand". Indeed, since receptor sequences vary as a result of either gene duplication or speciation processes, ligands may behave in a rather unpredictable manner with these sequence variations. A single amino acid change can result in significant changes in binding and functional properties of the same receptor in different species. Alternatively, ligands of a single class may "recognize" receptors of completely different specificity [rev. in Vernier et al., 1995]. Finally, for animal species which have diverged from the ancestors of human from a very long time (such as fish or invertebrates), sequence divergence may be significant, and the ligands used for mammalian receptors could well be inefficient in these receptors, even if they are the true homologues of mammalian receptors. It has recently been suggested that receptor classification and nomenclature should follow that obtained for human receptors [Vanhoutte et al., 1996]. This position is perhaps too restrictive, since it denies the possibility for species other than human to have different receptor subtype diversity. For example, it is likely that most mammals, including humans, lack the D_{1C} or D_{1D} dopamine receptor subtype found in most other vertebrate species [Cardinaud et al., 1997; Demchyshyn et al., 1995] or that some serotonin receptor subtypes may be specific to primates

---

Fig. 7

A simplified phylogenic tree of monoamine G protein-coupled receptors. The sequences chosen for alignment and processing by a distance calculation method (Neighbor Joining Method, Saitou and Nei, 1987) were essentially the human sequences belonging to the main classes of bioamine receptors. Receptor classes and subtypes delineated by the phylogenic analysis in vertebrate species are indicated on the right part of the tree. All the other sequences are those of the non mammalian bioamine receptors. The branching included in the grey box have no robust position and cannot be used to infer the "true" relationships of the corresponding sequence group. Clearly, most of the invertebrate sequences cannot be assigned with confidence to any of the vertebrate receptor subtypes, but may correspond to classes which have homologues in vertebrate (dopamine D_1, serotonin $5HT_1$, muscarinic...). Contingency in the evolution of bioamine receptor sequences is examplified by the Drosophila dopamine DAMP receptor which sequence is in fact related to the vertebrate a1 adrenoreceptor. Classes of receptors binding the same ligand are not more closely related to each other than to the other classes of monoamine receptors ($\alpha 1, \alpha 2, \beta$ adrenoreceptors, D_1, D_2 dopamine receptors, $5HT_1, 5HT_2$, $5HT_5$... serotonin receptors...). The case of the dopamine D_1 receptor class is shown in more details to highlight the discrimination of the four subtypes (D_{1a}, D_{1b}, D_{1c} and D_{1d}) which are shared by most vertebrate species. Mammals are an exception since they have only D_{1a} and D_{1b} (also known as D_5) receptors. Heterogeneity in in the presently accepted receptor nomenclature is also easily apparent.

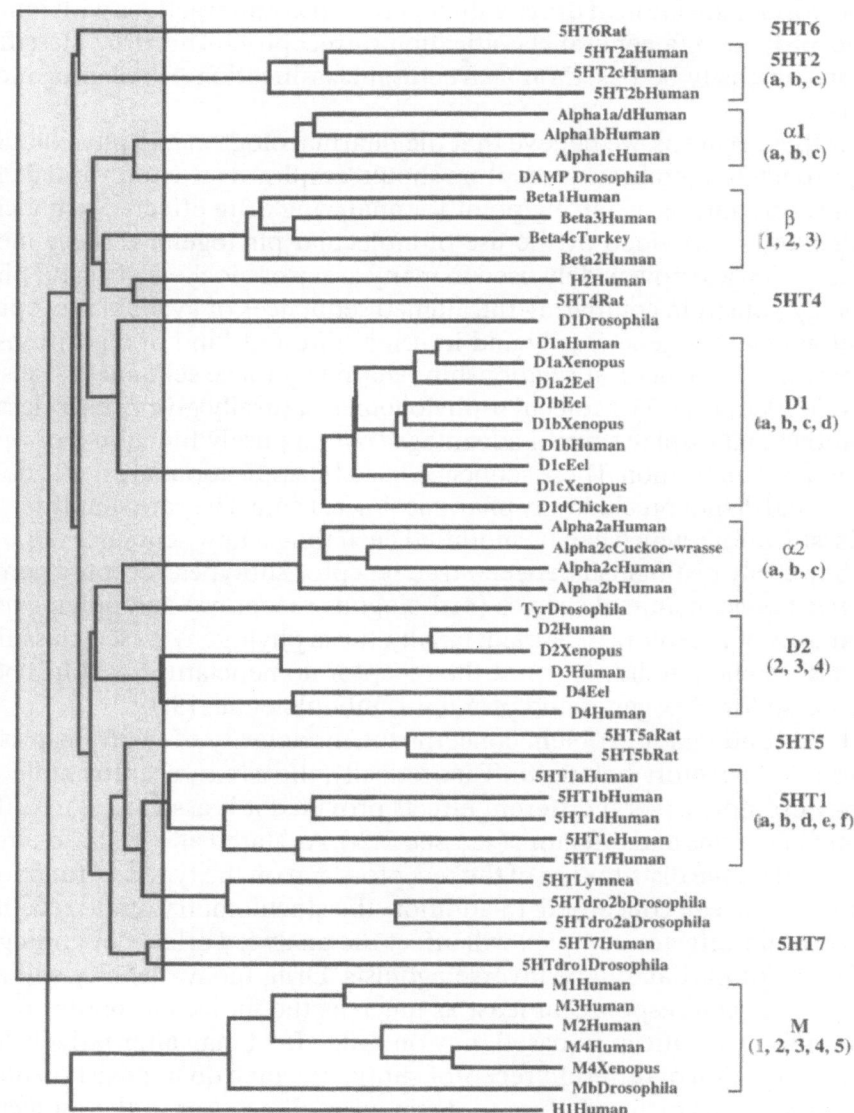

(some $5HT_5$ receptor subtypes). These findings are highly significant in terms of physiology for a given species and highlight important differences in their adaptive behavior. They need to be taken into account in receptor classification. Instead, what is required for human pharmacology is more a classification of drugs with regard to their interactions with human receptors than a general classification of receptors. This drug classification can easily be based on a structural classification of receptor molecules.

For these reasons, we believe that the pharmacological and physiological approach to membrane receptors should employ a structure-based classification only as a starting point for analyzing drug effects. Such a classification is provided by the use of molecular phylogenies. These methods, which are now widely used in many areas of biochemistry and physiology, consist in comparing the aligned sequences of available receptors belonging to a gene family and in using different kind of algorithms to describe the structural relationships shared by these sequences [Felsenstein, 1988] (Fig. 7). Molecular phylogenies naturally give rise to classifications that display several advantages over a purely functional or operational classification. These sequence-based classifications are never definitive and do not preclude any pharmacological data. They are simply factual classifications which can be modified each time a new sequence appears. They easily distinguish between true receptor subtypes, receptor homologies between animal species (orthologous receptors) and polymorphic variants of receptors in human. Finally, these phylogeny-based classifications also help to homogenize the receptor nomenclature, as it has been the case for Hox genes and proteins [Duboule et al., 1990].

The second major problem concerns the modularity of the transmission systems receptors belong to. Theoretically, the same receptor molecule may promote several different effects provided it is associated to different G proteins and effectors (see Sec. 3.2.). As stated above, these effects depend on the distribution of the receptors and on the type and functional state of the cell concerned. In addition, the stochiometry of the receptor-G protein-effector complex will affect the analyzed effect depending on the use of partial, full or inverse agonists. Drug bioavailability will also affect the cell response, at least as much as the molecular nature of the receptor. Classification based only on drug effect may alternatively lead to recognition of different receptor subtypes which do not exist on molecular grounds or to a failure to distinguish differences in the molecular nature of the receptors.

We have to keep in mind that G-protein coupled receptors are in fact modular entities requiring a set of interacting molecules to elicit a cellular response. Therefore, the relationship between pharmacological data in a broad sense (affinity, efficacy, potency of drugs) and receptor structures is unlikely to be direct. The hierarchical construction of an organism where cells are made of molecules, organs made of cells and organs assembled in a coordinate fashion impairs any simple prediction of the general phenotypic effect of the modulation of activity of a single molecule, as is often possible with receptor-specific drugs. Since robustness, reproducibility and confidence are important qualities for biological classification, a structural classification is the most logical choice. It seems more realistic to superimpose to a structural classification taken as primary framework, data obtained from the pharmacological, functional and anatomical analysis of receptors, as partly suggested by Humphrey et al. [1993].

To conclude this overview of the molecular and functional aspects of GPCRs, it is worth considering that the molecular approach to receptors that has dominated the last 10 years should serve as a reminder that, if molecular diversity exists, it is inside a whole organism. The large wealth of biochemical and structural data that have been accumulated underlines the logic which governs the construction of an organism, always building novelty from older things, modifying preexisting elements instead of creating new ones from scratch. In the end, the constraints imposed on molecules are always physiological, and the multiplicity and diversity of receptors, best exemplified in this review by the bioamine receptors, is essentially the visible consequence of these functional requirements.

Acknowledgments

This work is supported by grants from the CNRS, University Paris XI and EEC to P.V.

References

Abeijon, C. and Hirschberg, C.: Trends Biochem Sci *17*, 32–36 (1992).
Almaula, N., Ebersole, B., Zhang, D., Weinstein, H. and Sealfon, S.: J Biol Chem *271*, 14672–14675 (1996).
Applebury, M. and Hargrave, P.: Vision Res *26*, 1881–95(1986).
Arai, H., Hori, S., Aramori, I., Ohkubo, H. and Nakanishi, S.: Nature *348*, 730–2 (1990).
Arora, K., Sakai, A. and Catt, K.: J Biol Chem *270*, 22820–22826 (1995).
Arriza, J., Dawson, T., Simerly, R., Martin, L., Caron, M., Snyder, S. and Lefkowitz, R.: J Neurosci *12*, 4045–4055 (1992).
Attramadal, H., Arriza, J., Aoki, C., Dawson, T., Codina, J., Kwatra, M., Snyder, S., Caron, M. and Lefkowitz, R.: J Biol Chem *267*, 17882–17890 (1992).
Audigier, Y., Friedlander, M. and Blobel, G.: Proc Natl Acad Sci USA *84*, 5783–5787 (1987).

Avigan, J., Murtagh, J. J., Stevens, L., Angus, C., Moss, J. and Vaughan, M.: Biochemistry 31, 7736–7740 (1992).

Barak, L., Tiberi, M., Freedman, N., Kwatra, M., Lefkowitz, R. and Caron, M.: J Biol Chem 269, 2790–2795 (1994).

Barr, F.A., Leyte, A. and Huttner, W.B.: Trends Cell Biol 2, 91–94 (1992).

Bates, M., Senogles, S., Bunzow, J., Liggett, S., Civelli, O. and Caron, M.: Mol Pharmacol 39, 55–63 (1991).

Beltzer, J., Fiedler, K., Fuhrer, C., Geffen, I., Handschin, C., Wessels, H. and Spiess, M.: J Biol Chem 266, 973–978 (1991).

Benya, R., Fathi, Z., Battey, J. and Jensen, R.: J Biol Chem 268, 20285–20290 (1993).

Birnbaumer, L., Abramowitz, J. and Brown, A.: Biochim Biophys Acta 1031, 163–224 (1990).

Bluml, K., Mutschler, E. and Wess, J.: J Biol Chem 269, 18870–18876 (1994).

Boman, A. L. and Kahn, R. A.: Trends Biochem Sci 20, 147–150 (1995).

Bourne, H. R. and Nicoll, R.: Cell 72, 65–75 (1993).

Bouvier, M., Hausdorff, W., De, B.A., O'Dowd, B., Kobilka, B., Caron, M. and Lefkowitz, R.: Nature 333, 370–373 (1988).

Bouvier, M., Moffett, S., Loisel, T., Mouillac, B., Hebert, T. and Chidiac, P.: Biochem Soc Trans 23, 116–20 (1995).

Burstein, E., Spalding, T. and Brann, M.: J Biol Chem 271, 2882–2885 (1996).

Cali, J., Balcueva, E., Rybalkin, I. and Robishaw, J.: J Biol Chem 267, 24023–24027 (1992).

Campbell, P., Hnatowich, M., O'Dowd, B., Caron, M., Lefkowitz, R. and Hausdorff, W: Mol Pharmacol 39, 192–198 (1991).

Cardinaud, B., Sugamori, K.S., Coudouel, S., Vincent, J.D., Niznik, H.B. and Vernier, P.: J Biol Chem 272, 2778–2787 (1997).

Carty, D., Padrell, E., Codina, J., Birnbaumer, L., Hildebrandt, J. and Iyengar, R: J Biol Chem 265, 6268–6273 (1990).

Cavalli, A., Fanelli, F., Taddei, C., DeBenedetti, P. G. and Cotecchia, S.: FEBS Lett 399, 9–13 (1996).

Cerione, R.A., Staniszewski, C., Benovic, J.L., Lefkowitz, R.J., Caron, M.G., Gierschik, P., Somers, R., Spiegel, A.M., Codina, J. and Birnbaumer, L.: J Biol Chem 260, 1493–1500 (1985).

Chabre, O., Conklin, B., Brandon, S., Bourne, H. and Limbird, L.: J Biol Chem 269, 5730–5734 (1994).

Chen, J., DeVivo, M., Dingus, J., Harry, A., Li, J., Sui, J., Carty, D., Blank, J., Exton, J., Stoffel, R. et al.: Science 268, 1166–1169 (1995).

Cheung, A., Huang, R., Graziano, M. and Strader, C.: FEBS Lett 279, 277–280 (1991).

Chio, C.L., Lajiness, M.E. and Huff, R.M.: Mol Pharmacol 45, 51–60 (1994).

Chothia, C. and Finkelstein, A: Annu Rev Biochem 59, 1007–1039 (1990).

Chun, M., Lin, H., Henis, Y. and Lodish, H.: J Biol Chem 270, 10855–10860 (1995).

Clapham, D., Codina, J. and Birnbaumer, L.: Nature 379, 297–299 (1996).

Coleman, D., Berghuis, A., Lee, E., Linder, M., Gilman, A. and Sprang, S.: Science 265, 1405–1412 (1994).

Colombo, M.I., Inglese, J., D'Souza-Schorey, C., Beron, W. and Stahl, P. D.: J Biol Chem 270, 24564–24571 (1995).

Conklin, B., Chabre, O., Wong, Y., Federman, A. and Bourne, H.: J Biol Chem 267, 31–34 (1992).

Cotecchia, S., Exum, S., Caron, M. and Lefkowitz, R.: Proc Natl Acad Sci USA 87, 2896–2900 (1990).

Cotecchia, S., Ostrowski, J., Kjelsberg, M., Caron, M. and Lefkowitz, R.: J Biol Chem 267, 1633–1639 (1992).

Cox, B., Henningsen, R., Spanoyannis, A., Neve, R. and Neve, K.: J Neurochem 59, 627–635 (1992).

Dahl, S., Edvardsen, O. and Sylte, I.: Therapie 46, 453–459 (1991).

Dalman, H. and Neubig, R.: J Biol Chem 266, 11025–11029 (1991).

Degtyarev, M., Spiegel, A. and Jones, T: J Biol Chem 268, 23769–23772 (1993).

Demchyshyn, L.L., Sugamori, K.S., Lee, F.J., Hamadanizadeh, S.A. and Niznik, H.B.: J Biol Chem 270, 4005–4012 (1995).

Denker, B.M., Schmidt, C.J. and Neer, E.J.: J Biol Chem 267, 9998–10002 (1992).

Dixon, R., Sigal, I., Candelore, M., Register, R., Scattergood, W., Rands, E. and Strader, C.: EMBO J 6, 3269–3275 (1987).

Dixon, R., Sigal, I. and Strader, C: Cold Spring Harb Symp Quant Biol 53 Pt 1, 487–97 (1988).

Dohlman, H., Bouvier, M., Benovic, J., Caron, M. and Lefkowitz, R.: J Biol Chem 262, 14282–14288 (1987).

Dohlman, H., Caron, M., DeBlasi, A., Frielle, T. and Lefkowitz, R.: Biochemistry 29, 2335–2342 (1990).

Dohlman, H., Thorner, J., Caron, M. and Lefkowitz, R: Annu Rev Biochem 60, 653–688 (1991).

Donnelly, D., Findlay, J. and Blundell, T.: Receptors Channels 2, 61–78 (1994).

Duboule, D., Boncinelli, E., DeRobertis, E., Featherstone, M., Lonai, P., Oliver, G. and Ruddle, F.H.: Genomics 7, 458–459 (1990).

Eason, M. and Liggett, S.: J Biol Chem 270, 24753–24760 (1995).

Eason, M. and Liggett, S.: J Biol Chem 271, 12826–12832 (1996).

Ehrlich, P., In: Readings in Pharmacology (1962), L. Schuster, ed. (Boston: Little Brown & Co), pp. 231–244.

Ehrlich, P: Lancet 2, 445–451 (1913).

Engelman, D., Steitz, T. and Goldman, A.: Annu Rev Biophys Biophys Chem 15, 321–353 (1986).

Felsenstein, J.: Annu Rev Genet 22, 521–565 (1988).

Ferguson, S., Downey, W.R., Colapietro, A., Barak, L., Menard, L. and Caron, M.: Science 271, 363–366 (1996).

Ferreira, P.A., Nakayama, T.A. and Travis, G.H.: Proc Natl Acad Sci USA 94, 1556–1561 (1997).

Fishburn, C.S., Elazar, Z. and Fuchs, S.: J Biol Chem 270, 29819–29824 (1995).

Fraser, C., Wang, C., Robinson, D., Gocayne, J. and Venter, J.: Mol Pharmacol 36, 840–847 (1989).

Galas, M.C., Helms, J.B., Vitale, N., Thierse, D., Aunis, D. and Bader, M.F.: J Biol Chem 272, 2788–2793 (1997).

Gantz, I., DelValle, J., Wang, L., Tashiro, T., Munzert, G., Guo, Y., Konda, Y. and Yamada, T.: J Biol Chem 267, 20840–20843 (1992).

Goldman, P., Schlador, M., Shapiro, R. and Nathanson, N: J Biol Chem 271, 4215–4222 (1996).

Green, S. and Liggett, S.: J Biol Chem 269, 26215–26219 (1994).

Groblewski, T., Maigret, B., Larguier, R., Lombard, C., Bonnafous, J.C. and Marie, J.: J Biol Chem 272, 1822–1826 (1997).

Gruenberg, J. and Clague, M.J.: Curr Opin Cell Biol 4, 593–599 (1992).

Gudermann, T., Kalkbrenner, F. and Schultz, G: Annu Rev Pharmacol Toxicol 36, 429–459 (1996).

Guiramand, J., Montmayeur, J., Ceraline, J., Bhatia, M. and Borrelli, E.: J Biol Chem *270*, 7354–7358 (1995).

Hasegawa, H., Negishi, M. and Ichikawa, A.: J Biol Chem *271*, 1857–1860 (1996).

Hausdorff, W., Bouvier, M., O'Dowd, B., Irons, G., Caron, M. and Lefkowitz, R.: J Biol Chem *264*, 12657–12665 (1989).

Hausdorff, W., Hnatowich, M., O'Dowd, B., Caron, M. and Lefkowitz, R.: J Biol Chem *265*, 1388–1393 (1990).

Hawes, B., Luttrell, L., Exum, S. and Lefkowitz, R.: J Biol Chem *269*, 15776–15785.

Hebert, T., Moffett, S., Morello, J., Loisel, T., Bichet, D., Barret, C. and Bouvier, M.: J Biol Chem *271*, 16384–16392 (1996).

Henderson, R., Baldwin, J., Ceska, T., Zemlin, F., Beckmann, E. and Downing, K.: J Mol Biol *213*, 899–929 (1990).

Henderson, R. and Unwin, P.: Nature *257*, 28–32 (1975).

Hermans, E., Octave, J. and Maloteaux, J: Mol Pharmacol *49*, 365–372 (1996).

Hibert, M., Trumpp-Kallmeyer, S., Bruinvels, A. and Hoflack, J.: Mol Pharmacol *40*, 8–15 (1991).

Hibert, M., Trumpp-Kallmeyer, S., Hoflack, J. and Bruinvels, A.: Trends Pharmacol Sci *14*, 7–12 (1993).

Higashijima, T., Uzu, S., Nakajima, T. and Ross, E.: J Biol Chem *263*, 6491–6494 (1988).

High, S. and Dobberstein, B.: Curr Opin Cell Biol *4*, 581–586 (1992).

Hill-Eubanks, D., Burstein, E., Spalding, T., Brauner-Osborne, H. and Brann, M.: J Biol Chem *271*, 3058–65 (1996).

Ho, B.Y., Karschin, A., Branchek, T., Davidson, N. and Lester, H.A.: FEBS Lett *312*, 259–262 (1992).

Hogger, P., Shockley, M., Lameh, J. and Sadee, W.: J Biol Chem *270*, 7405–7410 (1995).

Hsu, W., Rudolph, U., Sanford, J., Bertrand, P., Olate, J., Nelson, C., Moss, L., Boyd, A., Codina, J. and Birnbaumer, L: J Biol Chem *265*, 11220–11226 (1990).

Humphrey, P. P., Hartig, P. and Hoyer, D.: Trends Pharmacol Sci *14*, 233–236 (1993).

Hwa, J., Graham, R. and Perez, D.: J Biol Chem *270*, 23189–23195 (1995).

Hwa, J., Graham, R. and Perez, D.: J Biol Chem *271*, 7956–7964 (1996a).

Hwa, J. and Perez, D.: J Biol Chem *271*, 6322–6327 (1996b).

Inglese, J., Freedman, N., Koch, W. and Lefkowitz, R.: J Biol Chem *268*, 23735–23738 (1993).

Javitch, J., Fu, D. and Chen, J.: Biochemistry *34*, 16433–16439 (1995a).

Javitch, J., Fu, D., Chen, J. and Karlin, A.: Neuron *14*, 825–831 (1995b).

Jensen, A.A., Pedersen, U.B., Kiemer, A., Din, N. and Andersen, P.H.: J Neurochem *65*, 1325–1331 (1995).

Johannes, F., Prestle, J., Dieterich, S., Oberhagemann, P., Link, G. and Pfizenmaier, K.: Eur J Biochem *227*, 303–307 (1995).

Kahlert, M., Konig, B. and Hofmann, K.: J Biol Chem *265*, 18928–18932 (1990).

Kawate, N. and Menon, K.: J Biol Chem *269*, 30651–30658 (1994).

Kenakin, T.P.: Trends Pharmacol Sci *4*, 291–295 (1983).

Kjelsberg, M., Cotecchia, S., Ostrowski, J., Caron, M. and Lefkowitz, R.: J Biol Chem *267*, 1430–1433 (1992).

Kleuss, C., Hescheler, J., Ewel, C., Rosenthal, W., Schultz, G. and Wittig, B.: Nature *353*, 43–48 (1991).

Kleuss, C., Scherubl, H., Hescheler, J., Schultz, G. and Wittig, B.: Nature *358*, 424–426 (1992).

Kleuss, C., Scherubl, H., Hescheler, J., Schultz, G. and Wittig, B.: Science *259*, 832–834 (1993).

Kobilka, B., Kobilka, T., Daniel, K., Regan, J., Caron, M. and Lefkowitz, R.: Science *240*, 1310–1316 (1988).

Koenig, J. and Edwardson, J.: Mol Pharmacol *49*, 351–359 (1996).
Kubo, T., Bujo, H., Akiba, I., Nakai, J., Mishina, M. and Numa, S.: FEBS Lett *241*, 119–125 (1988).
Kuipers, W., Van, W.I. and Ijzerman, A.: Drug Res Discov *11*, 231–249 (1994).
Lambright, D., Noel, J., Hamm, H. and Sigler, P.: Nature *369*, 621–628 (1994).
Lambright, D., Sondek, J., Bohm, A., Skiba, N., Hamm, H. and Sigler, P.: Nature *379*, 311–319 (1996).
Lameh, J., Philip, M., Sharma, Y., Moro, O., Ramachandran, J. and Sadee, W.: J Biol Chem *267*, 13406–13412 (1992).
Langley, J.N.: J Physiol (London) *33*, 374–413 (1905).
Lattion, A., Diviani, D. and Cotecchia, S.: J Biol Chem *269*, 22887–22893 (1994).
Laugwitz, K.L., Allgeier, A., Offermanns, S., Spicher, K., Van Sande, J., Dumont, J.E. and Schultz, G.: Proc Natl Acad Sci USA *93*, 116–120 (1996).
Lechleiter, J., Hellmiss, R., Duerson, K., Ennulat, D., David, N., Clapham, D. and Peralta, E.: EMBO J *9*, 4381–4390 (1990).
Lee, C., Katz, A. and Simon, M.: Mol Pharmacol *47*, 218–223 (1995).
Leyte, A., Barr, F.A., Kehlenbach, R.H. and Huttner, W.B.: EMBO J *11*, 4795–4304 (1992).
Liggett, S., Ostrowski, J., Chesnut, L., Kurose, H., Raymond, J., Caron, M. and Lefkowitz, R.: J Biol Chem *267*, 4740–4746 (1992).
Linder, M., Ewald, D., Miller, R. and Gilman, A.: J Biol Chem *265*, 8243–8251 (1990).
Lisanti, M., Scherer, P.E., Tang, Z.L. and Sargiacomo, M.: Trends Cell Sci *4*, 231–235 (1994).
Liu, X., Davis, D. and Segaloff, D. L.: J Biol Chem *268*, 1513–1516 (1993).
Liu, J., Powell, K., Sudhof, T. and Robinson, P.: J Biol Chem *269*, 21043–21050 (1994).
Liu, J., Blin, N., Conklin, B. and Wess, J.: J Biol Chem *271*, 6172–6178 (1996).
Lledo, P.M., Homburger, V., Bockaert, J., Vincent, J.D., Lledo, P.M., Homburger, V., Bockaert, J. and Vincent, J.D.: Neuron *8*, 455–463 (1992).
Lledo, P.-M., Vernier, P., Kukstas, L. A., Vincent, J.-D., Homburger, V. and Bockaert, J., In: Dopamine receptors and transporters, H.B. Niznik, ed. (New York: Marcel Dekker Inc.), pp. 59–88 (1994).
Logothetis, D., Kurachi, Y., Galper, J., Neer, E. and Clapham, D.: Nature *325*, 321–326 (1987).
Lohse, M. Andexinger, S., Pitcher, J., Trukawinski, S., Codina, J., Faure, J., Caron, M. and Lefkowitz, R.: J Biol Chem *267*, 8558–8564 (1992).
Lohse, M., Benovic, J., Caron, M. and Lefkowitz, R.: J Biol Chem *265*, 3202–3211 (1990a).
Lohse, M., Benovic, J., Codina, J., Caron, M. and Lefkowitz, R.: Science *248*, 1547–1550 (1990b).
Luttrell, L., Ostrowski, J., Cotecchia, S., Kendall, H. and Lefkowitz, R.: Science *259*, 1453–1457 (1993).
Luttrell, L.M., Hawes, B.E., van Biesen, T., Luttrell, D.K., Lansing, T.J. and Lefkowitz, R.J.: J Biol Chem *271*, 19443–19450 (1996).
Maggio, R., Vogel, Z. and Wess, J.: FEBS Lett *319*, 195–200 (1993a).
Maggio, R., Vogel, Z. and Wess, J.: Proc Natl Acad Sci USA 90, 3103–3107 (1993b).
Mansour, A., Meng, F., Meador-Woodruff, J., Taylor, L., Civelli, O. and Akil, H.: Eur J Pharmacol *227*, 205–214 (1992).
Moffett, S., Mouillac, B., Bonin, H. and Bouvier, M.: EMBO J *12*, 349–356 (1993).
Montmayeur, J., Guiramand, J. and Borrelli, E.: Mol Endocrinol 7, 161–170 (1993).
Moro, O., Lameh, J., Hogger, P. and Sadee, W.: J Biol Chem *268*, 22273–22276 (1993a).
Moro, O., Lameh, J. and Sadee, W.: J Biol Chem *268*, 6862–6865 (1993b).
Moro, O., Shockley, M., Lameh, J. and Sadee, W.: J Biol Chem *269*, 6651–6655 (1994).

Munro, S.: EMBO J *10*, 3577–3588 (1991).

Namba, T., Sugimoto, Y., Negishi, M., Irie, A., Ushikubi, F., Kakizuka, A., Ito, S., Ichikawa, A. and Narumiya, S.: Nature *365*, 166–170 (1993).

Neer, E.J.: Cell *80*, 249–257 (1995).

Nicholas, A.P., Hokfelt, T. and Pieribone, V.A.: Trends Pharmacol Sci *17*, 245–255 (1996).

Nicholas, A.P., Pieribone, V.A. and Hokfelt, T.: Neuroscience *56*, 1023–1039 (1993).

Noel, J., Hamm, H. and Sigler, P.: Nature *366*, 654–663 (1993).

O'Dowd, B., Hnatowich, M., Caron, M., Lefkowitz, R. and Bouvier, M.: J Biol Chem *264*, 7564–7569 (1989).

O'Dowd, B.F., Hnatowich, M., Regan, J.W., Leader, W.M., Caron, M.G. and Lefkowitz, R.J.: J Biol Chem *263*, 15985–15992 (1988).

Ohta, K., Hayashi, H., Mizuguchi, H., Kagamiyama, H., Fujimoto, K. and Fukui, H.: Biochem Biophys Res Commun *203*, 1096–1101 (1994).

Okamoto, T., Murayama, Y., Hayashi, Y., Inagaki, M., Ogata, E. and Nishimoto, I.: Cell *67*, 723–730 (1991).

Parent, J., Le Grouill, C., de Brum-Fernandes, A., Rola-Pleszczynski, M. and Stankova, J.: J Biol Chem *271*, 7949–7955 (1996).

Parma, J., Duprez, L., Van, S.J., Cochaux, P., Gervy, C., Mockel, J., Dumont, J. and Vassart, G.: Nature *365*, 649–651 (1993).

Pelham, H.R. and Munro, S.: Cell *75*, 603–605 (1993).

Perez, D., Hwa, J., Gaivin, R., Mathur, M., Brown, F. and Graham, R.: Mol Pharmacol *49*, 112–122 (1996).

Perez, D.M., Hwa, J., Gaivin, R., Mathur, M., Brown, F. and Graham, R.M.: Mol Pharmacol *49*, 112–122 (1997).

Pimplikar, S.W. and Simons, K.: J Cell Sci Suppl *17*, 27–32 (1993).

Piomelli, D., Pilon, C., Giros, B., Sokoloff, P., Martres, M.P. and Schwartz, J.C.: Nature *353*, 164–167 (1991).

Pitcher, J.A., Inglese, J., Higgins, J. B., Arriza, J.L., Casey, P. J., Kim, C., Benovic, J.L., Kwatra, M.M., Caron, M.G. and Lefkowitz, R.J.: Science *257*, 1264–1267 (1992).

Pollock, N., Manelli, A., Hutchins, C., Steffey, M., MacKenzie, R. and Frail, D.: J Biol Chem *267*, 17780–17786 (1992).

Popot, J. and Engelman, D.: Biochemistry *29*, 4031–4037 (1990).

Premont, R., Koch, W., Inglese, J. and Lefkowitz, R.: J Biol Chem *269*, 6832–6841 (1994).

Premont, R., Inglese, J. and Lefkowitz, R.: FASEB J *9*, 175–182 (1995).

Premont, R., Macrae, A., Stoffel, R., Chung, N., Pitcher, J., Ambrose, C., Inglese, J., MacDonad, M. and Lefkowitz, R: J Biol Chem *271*, 6403–6410 (1996).

Prezeau, L., Gomeza, J., Ahern, S., Mary, S., Galvez, T., Bockaert, J. and Pin, J.: Mol Pharmacol *49*, 422–429 (1996).

Pronin, A. and Gautam, N.: Proc Natl Acad Sci USA 89, 6220–6224 (1992).

Rands, E., Candelore, M.R., Cheung, A.H., Hill, W.S., Strader, C.D. and Dixon, R.A.: J Biol Chem *265*, 10759–10764 (1990).

Raposo, G., Dunia, I., Delavier–Klutchko, C., Kaveri, S., Strosberg, A. and Benedetti, E.: Eur J Cell Biol *50*, 340–52 (1989).

Ren, Q., Kurose, H., Lefkowitz, R. and Cotecchia, S.: J Biol Chem *268*, 16483–16487 (1993).

Roth, N., Campbell, P., Caron, M., Lefkowitz, R. and Lohse, M.: Proc Natl Acad Sci USA *88*, 6201–6204 (1991).

Saitou, N. and Nei, M.: Mol Biol Evol *4*, 406–425 (1987).

Sakurai, T., Yanagisawa, M., Takuwa, Y., Miyazaki, H., Kimura, S., Goto, K. and Masaki, T.: Nature *348*, 732–735 (1990).

Samama, P., Cotecchia, S., Costa, T. and Lefkowitz, R.: J Biol Chem *268*, 4625–4636 (1993).

Schatz, G. and Dobberstein, B.: Science *271*, 1519–1526 (1996).

Scheer, A., Fanelli, F., Costa, T., De, B.P. and Cotecchia, S.: EMBO J *15*, 3566–3578 (1996).

Scheer, A., Fanelli, F., Costa, T., DeBenedetti, P.G. and Cotecchia, S.: Proc Natl Acad Sci USA *94*, 808–813 (1997).

Schertler, G., Villa, C. and Henderson, R.: Nature *362*, 770–772 (1993).

Schwartz, T.W., Gether, U., Schambye, H.T. and Hjorth, S.A.: Current Pharmaceutical Design *1*, 355–372 (1995).

Senogles, S.: J Biol Chem *269*, 23120–23127 (1994).

Senogles, S. E., Spiegel, A.M., Padrell, E., Iyengar, R. and Caron, M.G.: J Biol Chem *265*, 4507–4514 (1990).

Shapiro, R., Palmer, D. and Cislo, T.: J Biol Chem *268*, 21734–21738 (1993).

Shaw, G.: Bioessays *18*, 35–46 (1996).

Shenker, A., Laue, L., Kosugi, S., Merendino, J.J., Minegishi, T. and Cutler, G.J.: Nature *365*, 652–654 (1993).

Sibley, D., Strasser, R., Benovic, J., Daniel, K. and Lefkowitz, R: Proc Natl Acad Sci USA *83*, 9408–9412 (1986).

Siderovski, D. P., Hessel, A., Chung, S., Mak, T. W. and Tyers, M.: Curr Biol *6*, 211–212 (1996).

Simon, M., Strathmann, M. and Gautam, N.: Science *252*, 802–808 (1991).

Smrcka, A.V. and Sternweis, P.C.: J Biol Chem *268*, 9667–9674 (1993).

Sokoloff, P. and Schwartz, J.C.: Trends Pharmacol Sci *16*, 270–275 (1995).

Sondek, J., Bohm, A., Lambright, D., Hamm, H. and Sigler, P.: Nature *379*, 369–374 (1996).

Spalding, T., Burstein, E., Brauner-Osborne, H., Hill-Eubanks, D. and Brann, M.: J Pharmacol Exp Ther *275*, 1274–1279 (1995).

Spengler, D., Waeber, C., Pantaloni, C., Holsboer, F., Bockaert, J., Seeburg, P. and Journot, L.: Nature *365*, 170–175 (1993).

Stoffel, R., Randall, R., Premont, R., Lefkowitz, R. and Inglese, J.: J Biol Chem *269*, 27791–27794 (1994).

Strader, C., Candelore, M., Hill, W., Sigal, I. and Dixon, R.: J Biol Chem *264*, 13572–13578 (1989).

Strader, C., Dixon, R., Cheung, A., Candelore, M., Blake, A. and Sigal, I.: J Biol Chem *262*, 16439–16443 (1987b).

Strader, C., Gaffney, T., Sugg, E., Candelore, M., Keys, R., Patchett, A. and Dixon, R.: J Biol Chem *266*, 5–8 (1991).

Strader, C., Sigal, I., Blake, A., Cheung, A., Register, R., Rands, E., Zemcik, B., Candelore, M. and Dixon, R.: Cell *49*, 855–863 (1987a).

Strader, C., Sigal, I., Candelore, M., Rands, E., Hill, W. and Dixon, R.: J Biol Chem *263*, 10267–10271.

Strange, P.G., In: Advances in Drug Research, Vol. 28, B. Testa and U. A. Meyer, eds. (24–28 Oval Road, London, England NW1 7DX: Academic Press Ltd), pp. 313–351 (1996).

Sullivan, K.A., Miller, R.T., Masters, S.B., Beiderman, B., Heideman, W. and Bourne, H. R.: Nature *330*, 758–760 (1987).

Sunahara, R.K., Dessauer, C.W. and Gilman, A.G.: Annu Rev Pharmacol Toxicol *36*, 461–480 (1996).

Thomas, W., Thekkumkara, T., Motel, T. and Baker, K.: J Biol Chem *270*, 207–213 (1995).

Tiberi, M. and Caron, M.: J Biol Chem *269*, 27925–27931 (1994).

Tomic, M., Seeman, P., George, S. and O'Dowd, B.: Biochem Biophys Res Commun *191*, 1020–1027 (1993).

Touhara, K., Inglese, J., Pitcher, J., Shaw, G. and Lefkowitz, R.: J Biol Chem *269*, 10217–10220 (1994).

Tsuga, H., Kameyama, K., Haga, T., Kurose, H. and Nagao, T.: J Biol Chem *269*, 32522–32527 (1994).

Tsukamoto, T., Toyama, R., Itoh, H., Kozasa, T., Matsuoka, M. and Kaziro, Y.: Proc Natl Acad Sci USA *88*, 2974–2978 (1991).

Vallar, L., Muca, C., Civelli, O. and Meldolesi, J.: Neurochem Int *20*, 197S–200S (1992).

van Biesen, T., Hawes, B.E., Luttrell, D.K., Krueger, K.M., Touhara, K., Porfiri, E., Sakaue, M., Luttrell, L.M. and Lefkowitz, R.J.: Nature *376*, 781–784 (1995).

Vanhoutte, P.M., Humphrey, P.P. and Spedding, M.: Pharmacol Rev *48*, 1–2 (1996).

Vernier, P., Cardinaud, B., Valdenaire, O., Philippe, H. and Vincent, J.D.: Trends Pharmacol Sci *16*, 375–381 (1995).

von Heijne, G. and Gavel, Y.: Eur J Biochem *174*, 671–678 (1988).

von Heijne, G. and Manoil, C.: Protein Eng *4*, 109–112 (1990).

von Zastrow, M. and Kobilka, B.: J Biol Chem *267*, 3530–3538 (1992).

Vuong, T. and Chabre, M.: Nature *346*, 71–74 (1990).

Wall, M., Coleman, D., Lee, E., Iniguez–Lluhi, J., Posner, B., Gilman, A. and Sprang, S.: Cell *83*, 1047–1058 (1995).

Wang, C., Buck, M. and Fraser, C.: Mol Pharmacol *40*, 168–179 (1991).

Wang, C., Gallaher, T. and Shih, J.: Mol Pharmacol *43*, 931–940 (1993).

Wang, H., Lipfert, L., Malbon, C. and Bahouth, S.: J Biol Chem *264*, 14424–14431 (1989).

Watson, A., Katz, A. and Simon, M.: J Biol Chem *269*, 22150–22156 (1994).

Wess, J., Bonner, T., Dorje, F. and Brann, M.: Mol Pharmacol *38*, 517–523 (1990).

Wess, J., Gdula, D. and Brann, M.: EMBO J *10*, 3729–3734 (1991).

Wess, J., Maggio, R., Palmer, J. and Vogel, Z.: J Biol Chem *267*, 19313–19319 (1992).

Whitehead, I., Kirk, H., Tognon, C., Trigo–Gonzalez, G. and Kay, R.: J Biol Chem *270*, 18388–18395 (1995).

Wong, S., Parker, E. and Ross, E.: J Biol Chem *265*, 6219–6224 (1990).

Woodward, R., Coley, C., Daniell, S., Naylor, L. and Strange, P.: J Neurochem 66, 394–402 (1996).

Yoon, H., Hajduk, P., Petros, A., Olejniczak, E., Meadows, R. and Fesik, S.: Nature *369*, 672–675 (1994).

Yu, S., Lefkowitz, R. and Hausdorff, W.: J Biol Chem *268*, 337–341 (1993).

Zhang, J., Ferguson, S., Barak, L., Menard, L. and Caron, M.: J Biol Chem *271*, 18302–18305 (1996).

Zuckerkandl, E.: J Mol Evol *39*, 661–678 (1994).

Progress in Drug Research, Vol. 49 (E. Jucker, Ed.)
© 1997 Birkhäuser Verlag, Basel (Switzerland)

Antifungal therapy, an everlasting battle

By Annemarie Polak

Spitzenrainweg 45, 4147 Aesch, Switzerland

Glossary

Amorolfine	Amor
Amphotericin B	Amph B
Flucytosine	5-FC
Fluconazole	Flu
Granulocyte-colony-stimulating-factor	G-CSF
Granulocyte-macrophage-stimulating-factor	GM-CSF
Itraconazole	Itra
Ketoconazole	Keto
Minimal inhibitory concentration	MIC
Terbinafine	Ter
once daily	q.d.
twice daily	b.i.d.

1   Introduction

- Superficial mycoses: Antifungal therapy is winning.
- Deep mycoses: An everlasting battle is on-going with an interactive triangle among fungus, patient and drug.

In the early 1990s [1], A. Polak and P. Hartman had some hope that we would be able to win the fight for an effective antifungal therapy in dermatology as well as in deep mycoses. Seemingly, the old gold standard amphotericin B (Amph B) with its broad antifungal efficacy but its package of frequent and severe side effects would be replaced by well-tolerated, efficacious triazoles. Six years later, Amph B is still fully alive and is even getting new clothes. The use of the new triazoles has indeed significantly increased, and they are now better established; however, they are by no means the powerful "wonder weapon" we once hoped for. Despite the recent, heightened interest in antifungals within the pharmaceutical industry and the increased efforts of basic researchers to fill in knowledge gaps regarding fungal biochemistry, the fungus cell seems to be winning the battle. The fungus always seems to be one step ahead of the imaginative researcher. Fungal diseases fall into three major classes: superficial, subcutaneous and invasive mycoses. Throughout this book the author will adhere to this division not for microbiological reasons but because the problems associated with the three classes are completely distinct. No overwhelming problems remain in the field of dermatomycoses and gynecological infections, and indeed, high success rates are now obtainable because of the recent development of highly active, fungicidal compounds with special pharmacokinetic properties. We will summarize the most recent innovations in this important field and show that we may be winning the battle in this era. By contrast, in therapy for deep mycoses, we are still struggling with the same problems we had 6 years ago, while new problems are emerging with disturbing speed. In this field, the battle will likely go on for some years, and it is by no means certain that scientists will win in the end.

The problems encountered in antifungal therapy can be described as an interactive triangle or, more picturesquely, as a devil's circle between the fungus, the patient and the drug (see Fig. 1).

The ability of fungi to colonize and invade human organs is impressive, and the list of fungi causing fungal diseases continue to grow: an increasing number of fungi once thought to be harmless for humans are nowadays recognized as being human pathogens. The difficulty of killing an eukaryotic fungal cell invading host cells without damaging the host

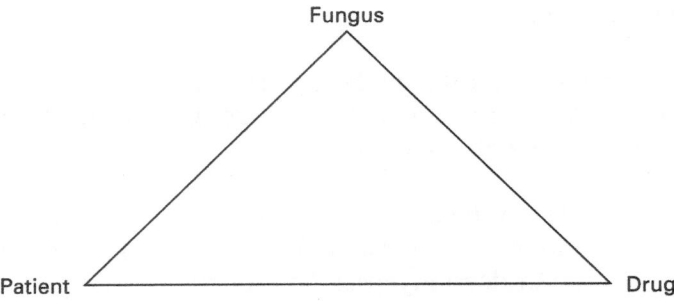

Fig. 1

proved to be a nearly non-bridgeable task for research and human chemotherapy.

Patients with invasive fungal infections often have to fight against underlying malignant disease or general immunological/physiological disorders. The list of predisposing risk factors is long, and the mycosis is very often set against the complex background of an underlying disease and its treatment. This phenomenon is not only true for established opportunistic fungal infections like candidosis, cryptococcosis and aspergillosis; even the pathogenic fungus *Histoplasma capsulatum* behaves like an opportunistic fungus, especially in patients with acquired immunodeficiency syndrome (AIDS). An increasing number of cancer, leukaemia, transplant, surgical and AIDS patients are keeping their disease under control, only to become victims of opportunistic fungal infections because of their weakened immune status. The situation is complicated because the host defense against fungal infections varies. Some fungal infections, like aspergillosis or deep candidosis, are granulocyte-dependent; others, like cryptococcosis or oral candidosis, are T-cell dependent.

The wonder drug to prevent or cure all invasive fungal infections does not yet exist; all drugs available have benefits and drawbacks. Amph B, the agent with the broadest spectrum, unfortunately is associated with a toxicity that would rule out its use were there a genuine alternative. Similarly, the narrow spectrum and resistance problem of flucytosine reduce its use to combination therapy. The new generation of triazoles enthusiastically welcomed 6 years ago as the hope of a new era in the antifungal chemotherapy has not yet reached its goal of replacing Amph B in the antifungal field. The new triazoles have clearly gained respect, and they are now the treatment of choice for maintenance therapy; however, a truly safe, fungicidal triazole does not yet exist.

This chapter is not intended as a general overview on all the antifungal drugs available on the market, already well covered by P.D. Hoeprich in this series in 1995 [2]. Rather, this chapter summarizes the progress made in the last 6 years to help patients suffering with fungal disease, praises the efforts that the pharmaceutical industry and universities have made in the antifungal field and highlights the difficulties still to be overcome.

2   Superficial mycoses

• Superficial mycoses are not life-threatening, but they are irritating.

2.1   Dermatomycosis

• A large choice of effective topical and systemic treatments exist.

The treatment of infections of the skin or hair is no longer a problem. The era of dyes is past, and griseofulvin, the first antifungal available, is losing its place in the arsenal of antidermatophytic drugs, as allylamines and triazoles have revolutionized the therapy of dermatomycosis.

Not only is an enormous, still increasing palette of agents at hand, but numerous and varied galenical forms are available: tablets, creams, tinctures, sprays, powder, shampoos, nail lacquers. For topical use, a variety of chemical classes (azoles, allylamines, tolnaftate, tolciclate, amorolfine, ciclopirox etc.) are in wide use and have become well established. All show high efficacy and a low incidence of adverse events.

The choice is less for systemic treatment of dermatomycoses. Two agents are highly recognized, itraconazole (Itra, triazole) and terbinafine (Ter, allylamine), the latter being the most efficacious agent for infections caused by dermatophytes [2–5]. Fluconazole (Flu), a compound that is highly efficacious against yeasts, is still struggling for a well-established place in the field of dermatomycoses.

Treatment schedules have become easier and even shorter: once-daily treatment replaced twice-daily treatment 6 years ago; the duration of therapy, originally as long as 6 months, is now often as short as 2 weeks. Attempts are ongoing to reduce the duration even more; however, a dose larger than that for the usual period will be required. The rationale for this treatment reduction is based on the properties of the new agents: both Ter and Itra have a high affinity to keratinous tissues, where they remain for a long time. Therefore, higher drug levels are found in these tissues than in plasma. Ter also exerts a strong fungicidal activity against dermatophytes and, thus, is generally more efficacious than Itra.

The strategy for the treatment of dermatomycosis has changed drastically in recent years. Traditionally, fungal skin infections were treated for several days after complete disappearance of clinical signs and symptoms. Since the new agents reach high and long-lasting tissue levels in skin and hair, the treatment can be stopped long before the clinical symptoms disappear, because the antifungal, curative effect is continually nourished from the tissue levels of the agent long after therapy has stopped.

Ter was highly effective (93% cure rate) in the treatment of children with tinea capitis even when administered with a shorter duration of treatment (4 weeks) than the one used with the old standard drugs. Ter was also highly efficacious in children with other dermatophytic infections after short-duration treatment. Ter was generally well tolerated in children [6].

Ter also showed high cure rates in tinea imbricata, a chronic, recurrent *Trichophyton concentricum* infection characterized by concentric rings of papulosquamous plaques endemic in village populations of Indonesia [7]. Thus, even recurrent dermatophytic infection may be under control in the near future.

2.2   Onychomycosis

- Nail infections with whole plate and matrix involvement respond to treatment with oral antifungals or to treatment with topical and oral agents administered according to a combination schedule.
- Nail infections without matrix involvement respond to topical treatment.

Onychomycosis is a non-life-threatening, non-aesthetic-appearing, chronic fungal infection of the nail, slowly destroying the whole nail plate and matrix. Dermatophytes (mainly *T. rubrum*) are by far the most common nail pathogens, accounting for 80–90% of all infections. Toenails are more frequently affected than fingernails. Until recently, pedal onychomycosis was considered an incurable disease. Therapy was lengthy, usually unsuccessful and perceived to be mainly for cosmetic purposes.

Griseofulvin, discovered in 1958, traditionally was the only antifungal agent prescribed for this infection. Topical therapies became available 10 years ago; however, their clinical efficacy was not sufficient, especially when a significant proportion of the nail plate or matrix was diseased. Until recently, the only curative alternative to griseofulvin was the surgical avulsion of the infected nail followed by application of an antifungal cream. In the last 6 years, however, significant progress has been made not only in systemic treatment but also in topical treatment of nail infection; it would be a mistake today for a doctor to remove an infected nail as therapy.

Three entities are mainly responsible for revolutionizing the treatment of onychomycosis: Ter, amorolfine (Amor) and Itra.

Ter and Amor, mainly used for dermatophytic infections, will be discussed in detail later in this section, whereas Itra, with a broader clinical spectrum, will be considered in the section on deep-seated mycosis.

2.2.1   Terbinafine

• Ter has fungicidal activity and is the most efficacious antifungal against dermatomycosis.

Ter possesses a broad antifungal spectrum against a wide variety of pathogenic fungi. The antifungal effect is especially strong against dermatophytes (minimal inhibitory concentration [MIC] 0.003–0.2 µg/ml) [1, 2]. Besides this strong fungistatic effect, Ter also exerts a strong fungicidal activity, the minimal fungicidal concentrations being in the same range as the MIC. This property makes Ter an outstanding antifungal agent, since most of the antifungals (excluding Amor) either have only fungistatic activity or a degree of fungicidal activity that is significantly lower than the fungistatic one.

Ter is a sterol biosynthesis inhibitor that interferes with the ergosterol pathway at the level of squalene epoxidase. This interaction leads to depletion of ergosterol and accumulation of squalene. A clear correlation exists between growth inhibition and degrees of sterol biosynthesis inhibition. The fungicidal effect is not directly related to the depletion of ergosterol, but instead seems to correlate with the high intracellular accumulation of squalene. Changes in the lipid content are known to disrupt chitin synthesis. The cell walls of dermatophytes contain higher amounts of chitin than the walls of yeast cells. Thus, this sequaelae of the mode of action may explain the greater sensitivity of dermatophytes to Ter [8].

Generally, Ter is well tolerated in adults and children [9]. Gastrointestinal adverse events are the most frequently observed (3.9%). Skin side-effects are reported in 6% of cases; central nervous system (CNS) and respiratory adverse effects are found in 2% of cases. Pregnancy with a successful outcome was reported in three patients. Taste loss or taste disturbance, a reversible event, is the only new side-effect to emerge post marketing. The incidence of this side-effect, however, is rare. A low body mass index, history of taste loss and aging are risk factors for developing taste loss [9a].

Several clinical studies have revealed that the fungicidal and pharmacokinetic properties of Ter have an important impact on the efficacy of the agent and on the rapid onset of mycological cure in dermatophytic infections: the drug accumulates to high concentrations in adipose tissue, skin and nails and is only slowly metabolized and released from these sites. Ter reaches the nail plate rapidly and persists there for several months after cessation of active treatment. It is detectable in the distal nail within 1 week of starting therapy and reaches concentrations well above the MIC for dermatophytes. Whereas plasma levels decrease rapidly after termination of treatment, Ter was detected in the nails as long as 30 weeks after termination of treatment [10].

Treatment duration in all dermatophytic infections including onychomycoses could be drastically shortened as a result of its high fungicidal activity and its pharmacokinetic properties [11–13]. Disappearance of symptoms is ongoing even after therapy has been stopped. Ter was also used to treat some invasive fungal infections. Successful compassionate use of Ter was reported for pulmonary aspergillosis [13a].

Itra has pharmacokinetic properties comparable to Ter, and it is just as effective therapy in nail infections [5]. Based on advances in our understanding of the pharmacokinetics of Ter and Itra, new, innovative dose regimens have been studied [14, 15]. For Ter, the optimal correlation between duration of treatment and clinical outcome is not yet established, but there is a trend among clinicians to decrease further the already short treatment [16–18]. The future direction for Itra, which is less fungicidal than Ter, lies in an intermittent pulse-dosing therapy (1 week each month for 3–4 months) [15].

Overall, Ter and Itra are both highly effective treatments for onychomycosis, but treatment with Ter has been proven to be more cost-effective for the two reasons: the relapse rate is lower with Ter, and therapy with Itra has to be repeated more often [19].

2.2.2   Amorolfine

- Amor has a broad spectrum, is fungicidal and highly efficacious in treating onychomycosis.

The morpholine derivative amorolfine possesses a broad antifungal spectrum including dermatophytes, yeasts, dimorphic fungi, dematiaceae and non-dermatophytic molds causing onychomycosis such as *Alternaria* spp., *Scopulariopsis brevicaulis, Hendersonula, Acremonium* sp. and so on. However, it is inactive against aspergilli. The highest degree of activity is seen against dermatophytes (geometric mean MIC 0.02 µg/ml) [1, 2, 20, 21]. Amor exerts both fungistatic and fungicidal activity against most fungal species, including especially dermatophytes *and* yeasts. The high degree of fungicidal effectiveness against dermatophytes is important, the MFC being very close to the MIC [22]. The same observation was made with Ter. Thus, both Amor and Ter are highly suitable for treating dermatophytic infections, whereas Amor is more effective against skin infections caused by yeasts because of its essential fungicidal activity against yeasts. Like all sterol biosynthesis inhibitors, Amor causes depletion of ergosterol and accumulation of an unplanar sterol, ignosterol [1, 21, 23, 24]. The agent interferes at two levels in the essential ergosterol biosynthesis pathway, the (Δ_{14}-reductase and the Δ_7-Δ_8-isomerase, with IC_{50} of 2.39 µM and 0.0018 µM, respectively [1, 24]. Thus, a natural synergistic effect is built into the molecule so that the risk of appearance of resistant mutants is low, and the efficacy of Amor is high.

The fungistatic activity of Amor is clearly correlated with the depletion of ergosterol and not with the accumulation of ignosterol [24]. Although the basis of the fungicidal effect is not fully understood, two hypotheses have been suggested to explain its mode of action: at high doses of Amor, squalene is accumulated in dermatophytes, and this accumulation may lead, as with Ter, to a fungicidal effect. Electron microscopy studies [25], on the other hand, have revealed an extreme accumulation of chitin in the membrane. Thus, severe chitin synthesis disturbance may be the cause of the distinct fungicidal effect.

Due to its favorable pharmacokinetic properties, Amor has fulfilled its great promise as an agent for topical treatment of onychomycosis. In the past, topical therapy has met with little success, mostly due to poor penetration of the antifungal into nail tissue.

Amor (from 5% lacquer) penetrates rapidly into the nail. As expected, the kinetics of the penetration follow an exponential law; the level of Amor measured in the upper levels of the nail already exceeds the MIC of most fungi causing onychomycosis after 24 h of contact. Even the lower part of the nail shows measurable microbiological activity within 24 h [20, 26]. Penetration into the deepest nail slice is also observed in patients with severe onychomycosis treated for 4 weeks with Amor nail lacquer. The level of Amor obtained in the deepest layer ranged in the same order as in the upper levels; thus, a steady state concentration – well in excess of the MIC against most dermatophytes and yeasts – is reached after this treatment period [27]. Amor applied topically is detectable in the nail earlier than Ter or Itra after oral application.

Amor should be used only in cases of onychomycosis characterized by less than 80% of affected nail surface and an intact matrix and lunula. In patients treated with Amor nail lacquer once weekly for 6 months, clinical cure or improvement was achieved in 77.6% of all toenails and in 83.7% of nail infections by three months after the end of therapy [20,

28]. Generally, eradication rates for *T. rubrum* were slightly lower than for *T. mentagrophytes*; the same phenomenon also has been observed with Ter and Itra. Local adverse events have been recorded in less than 1% of patients.

2.2.3   Combination therapy in onychomycosis

It has always been a matter of contention whether one should burden the body with an oral drug when an effective topical treatment is available. Until recently, no equivalent topical therapy existed in onychomycosis; nowadays, however, we have that choice. Both treatment schedules – systemic and topical – still have their drawbacks. Thus, it has always been of interest to investigate whether a combination of the two would prove advantageous, especially in difficult cases with extensive diseased areas and matrix involvement.

Amor has shown an additive or even synergistic *in vitro* effect with several antifungals, including Keto, Itra, Ter and griseofulvin [29]. The beneficial effect was seen not only when the fungistatic activity was measured but also when the fungicidal effect was studied. The synergy between Amor and other sterol biosynthesis inhibitors was predictable, but the positive effect with griseofulvin is surprising from a biochemical viewpoint. The synergy observed *in vitro* also translates into chemotherapeutic activity, the degree of synergy being even more pronounced *in vivo* than *in vitro*. In murine trichophytosis, combination therapy of Amor with griseofulvin, Ter, Itra and Flu is always more efficient than monotherapy [29, 30]. In extensive onychomycosis, the beneficial effect of local treatment with Amor combined with a short oral treatment of griseofulvin has been proven in clinical studies [31, 32]. In an open comparative study, 339 patients with severe onychomycosis (affecting lunula or matrix) received either a combined treatment with Amor nail lacquer (twice weekly for 12 months) and griseofulvin (500 mg b.i.d. for 2 months) or griseofulvin alone (500 mg b.i.d. for the first 2 months and q.d. for the remaining 10 months). Three months after the end of the treatment, the clinical cure and improvement rate was more than 90% in both groups. Mycological cure was quicker and better in the combination group than in the griseofulvin group (78% vs 61%). The most common adverse events were headache, nausea and vomiting, all attributed to griseofulvin and not Amor. The results of this study show that by combining Amor with griseofulvin, the duration of griseofulvin treatment can be drastically shortened with the same clinical response but a quicker mycological cure.

The combination of Ter [250 mg q.d.] for 12 weeks plus Amor lacquer (once per week for 15 months) showed a clear beneficial effect over the

control group, which received Ter monotherapy [250 mg q.d. for 12 weeks).
After 15 months, 64% of the patients treated with the combination therapy were cured, whereas only 42% of the patients treated with the monotherapy were cured [33]. A cost-effective analysis additionally showed that
the combination of Amor plus Ter (12 weeks) is the most cost-effective
way to treat severe onychomycosis with matrix involvement [34].

A study comparing the combination therapy of Itra (200 mg q.d. for 6
weeks or 3 months) plus Amor lacquer (once weekly for 6 months) with
Itra monotherapy (200 mg q.d. for 3 months) shows the same trend: a clear
advantage of combination therapy over monotherapy (the study is ongoing in Spain).

In conclusion, combination therapy may be particularly helpful for very
severe nail infections. Above all, the duration of the oral therapy may be
significantly reduced, and consequently the risk to the patients of lengthy
oral therapy may be minimized. This would be a real step forward in the
treatment of extensive onychomycosis.

2.3 Pityriasis versicolor

• Keto in various galenical forms is the new standard therapy.

Pityriasis versicolor and seborrhoeic dermatitis are the most widespread
superficial infections. They are both benign but cause unpleasant aesthetic
disorders and show a strong tendency to relapse. The epidemiology of seborrhoeic dermatitis is not yet fully understood, but the lipophilic, kera-
tinophilic yeast *Malassezia furfur* seems to play an important role in the
course of seborrhoeic dermatitis as it clearly does in pityriasis.

Due to the high relapse rate, pityriasis and seborrhoeic eczema have not
been curable with one single treatment. Recently, significant progress has
been made in winning the battle against these unaesthetic diseases. Azoles
and especially ketoconazole (locally applied in form of gel, cream or sham-
poo) have shown high cure rates and significantly reduced the relapse rates.
One single application of 20 g of Keto gel moussant on affected skin during 5 min (while taking a shower) has proven to be curative in several
studies [35]. Itra and Flu, orally applied, were also efficacious in this clinical setting and reduced relapses [5].

Ter, the most efficacious drug against superficial infections caused by dermatophytes, is ineffective in the treatment of pityriasis or seborrhoeic
eczema after oral application. Although topical treatment with Ter cream
showed some activity, it is still too early for a definitive statement regarding the place of Ter in the therapy of pityriasis [36, 37].

2.4   Vaginal candidosis

- Therapy for acute disease is unproblematic, since efficacious topical or oral treatment is available.
- Recurrent disease is still a problem, since it remains incurable.

Vaginal candidosis is a common gynaecological complaint. Indeed, estimates show that up to 75% of women experience at least one episode of vaginal candidosis during their lifetime. *Candida albicans* is the typical causative agent; however, *C. glabrata* is increasingly isolated. This organism is associated with a lower clinical response to standard therapy and with a higher relapse rate. Various risk factors may predispose women to vaginal candidosis: pregnancy, oral contraceptives, diabetes, antibiotic therapy (especially with cotrimoxazole) and human immunodeficiency virus (HIV) infection [38].

The choice for a successful therapy is extensive; a broad spectrum of pharmaceuticals similar to those used for the treatment of dermatomycosis is available with the two chemical classes azoles and polyenes. Various galenical forms are at the patient's convenience: vaginal tablets, ovula, creams, lotions and normal tablets.

Both topical and systemic treatment have proven high efficacy in acute vaginal candidosis. Improvements in recent years have not so much been in the improvement of efficacy (clotrimazole, the first azole available back in 1970, achieved a cure rate of more than 80%), but in decreasing the duration of therapy. A 1-day treatment period is the standard today. A single dose of Flu or a daily dose of 2 x 200 mg of Itra has shown the same degree of efficacy as topical treatment with a single dose of clotrimazole [5, 39, 40].

Scientific discussions today deal mainly with the potential benefits and liabilities of topical versus oral therapy [41]. As a rule, it is preferable to treat topical disorders with topical therapy. Most women, however, prefer systemic treatment in spite of the increased risk of interactions or adverse events. Topical therapy is clearly safer, since the drugs are only poorly absorbed and scarcely reach the circulation, and is advisable during pregnancy and breast feeding. Women receiving therapy with other drugs that could interact with oral azoles should also be treated with topical agents.

In summary, the therapy for acute vaginal candidosis is unproblematic and highly efficient. However, some women suffer from chronic recurrent vaginal candidosis over periods of months and years and endure associated physical and psychological stress. The pathogenesis of the disease remains obscure, although the condition has been recognized for a very long time. Intensive studies have not yet revealed distinct predisposing factors, though the early stages of HIV infection, for example, may constitute such a predisposing factor.

The optimal treatment for recurrent vaginal candidosis has not yet been established. Several approaches have been tried, including treatment with transfer factor and immunotherapy with *Candida* vaccines [1]. In recent years, so-called maintenance therapy or prophylaxis has been promoted as a successful approach. Generally, vaginal candidosis is treated topically or orally until the infection disappears; then a maintenance therapy is initiated for a certain period of time. The drug of choice is given weekly or monthly, locally or orally. The efficacy of this regimen is measured in terms of reduction in recurrence. During maintenance therapy the rate of relapses is generally significantly reduced; however, many patients experience a relapse after the treatment ends. Thus, a proper cure has not yet been achieved.

A recent study [42] showed that chronic suppressive therapy with Itra was more effective than suppressive therapy with clotrimazole. The recurrence was, however, common in both regimens after stopping maintenance therapy. Flu, administered as a single dose every 28 days, was highly effective in reducing the incidence of recurrent episodes of vaginal candidosis: during the 12-month phase of prophylaxis, recurrence was seen in 68% of the placebo-treated patients but in only 42% of the Flu-treated patients. Two months after discontinuation of therapy, more patients 94% vs 84%) remained disease-free in the Flu group [39].

Thus, there is some hope for future success based on the promising results with suppressive therapy; however, the disease is not yet curable, and the pathology and risk factors for this condition remain unknown.

3   Subcutaneous mycoses

• Subcutaneous mycoses are not life-threatening diseases, but associated morbidity is high.
• Progress has been made in successful therapy by Itra or combination therapy in chromomycosis.
• Itra is the drug of choice for lymphocutaneous sporotrichosis.

The three fungal infections – Madura feet (mycetoma), chromomycosis and sporotrichosis – fall into the category of subcutaneous mycoses. The distribution of the three infections is mainly in tropical and subtropical areas. Skin trauma is the portal of entry for the fungal spores of all three infections, and most cases of Madura feet and chromomycosis occur in male agricultural workers working barefoot.

3.1   Madura feet (mycetoma)

The term "mycetoma" is used to denote any tumor due to fungal infection. This group of infections is caused by a variety of unrelated fungi found on plants or in the soil. Subcutaneous infections of this type are not common but are difficult to treat and tend to be very chronic. In those parts of the world in which the infections are endemic, the morbidity of the condition can pose a problem for the patient as well as for the community. Mycetoma can be caused by filamentous bacteria (actinomycetes) or by a fungus. The infection is classified according the appearance of "grains" which are composed of microcolonies of the causative fungus or actinomycete filaments found within the lesions [43]. The therapy for both types of mycetoma differs depending on the causative agent: if the infection is due to a bacterial strain of actinomycetes, then antibacterial therapy must be used. Treatment with cotrimoxazole (Bactrim) or penicillin is often successful.

Therapy for fungal infection is more difficult. Surgery or even amputation has been the standard therapy for a long time and is still in use. In recent years Keto or Itra have been successfully used for some cases of mycetoma. More successful than monotherapy with an antifungal is the combination of surgery or of curettage plus antifungal therapy [44, 45]. The ideal treatment regimen for mycetoma has not yet been found, but there is evidence that the azoles (Keto, Itra and Flu) [46, 47] are of some benefit.

3.2   Chromomycosis

Chromomycosis is a chronic fungal infection of the subcutaneous tissues caused by a group of dematiaceous fungi. Direct examination of a biopsy or a potassium hydroxide preparation show the deeply pigmented, thick-walled sclerotic cells typical of dematiaceous fungi. The course of the disease is chronic, the time of inoculation often being years before the symptoms are apparent.

The treatment of choice for early localized lesions is surgical removal by excision or destruction by means of cryotherapy, cautery or diathermy. In more chronic cases systemic amphotericin therapy was not curative; however, combination therapy of flucytosine plus Amph B or Keto was in some cases beneficial [48, 49]. Itra alone was successful in many cases of chromomycosis especially caused by *Cladosporium carrionii*. Combination therapy of Itra with 5-FC or 5-FC with thiabendazole is needed for infection caused by *Fonsecaea pedrosoi* [48–52]. Therefore, in the field of chromomycosis real progress can be seen in the introduction of Itra and the use of combination therapy.

Compassionate long-term oral Ter was highly curative in a pilot study of 42 patients with chromomycosis due to *F. pedrosoi* or *C. carinii* [52a]. Recently, a rare case of chromomycosis due to an unidentified species of *Phialophora* has been reported which was eventually cured by topical Amor and local hyperthermia after recurrence following initially successful Itra and local Amph B and then retreatment with Itra and ciclopirox olamine cream [52b]. Thus, new therapeutic approaches including the systemic Ter or the topical Amor may be used successfully for this chronic disease.

3.3   Sporotrichosis

This fungal infection involves the lymphatics and subcutaneous tissues and is caused by the dimorphic fungus *Sporotrix schenckii*. The sporotrichosis lesions spread via the lymphatics from the original wound and form nodules or postules that quickly ulcerate. In some cases, sporotrichosis disseminates to organs and bones.

Potassium iodide has been the therapy of choice for many years. Amph was and is still used in the more disseminated cases. In recent years, Itra has been set up as standard therapy for cutaneous and lymphatic sporotrichosis [52–54]. The trade name of Itra, Sporanox, is based on its efficacy in this indication.

Treatment of pulmonary sporotrichosis with Amph B or Itra has been disappointing, with low response rates of 30–50%. Some patients may need lifelong suppression therapy with Itra. Itra has proven to be at least as effective as Amph B in this difficult setting and in disseminated sporotrichosis in HIV patients [53]. It also has produced responses in antifungal-refractory forms of sporotrichosis [55]. Flu seems to be only moderately active in sporotrichosis and will never replace Itra in this indication [56].

4   Systemic mycoses

- Systemic mycoses are life-threatening infections that must always be treated.

- Pathogenic fungi, endemic in distinct areas, cause infections in immuno-competent patients.
- Opportunistic fungi cause disseminated infections in non-immunocompetent patients.

4.1   The causative agents

Fungi are eukaryotic cells, structurally and biochemically similar to human cells. Biochemical studies have identified a number of potential targets for antifungal chemotherapy, including cell wall synthesis (the only fungus-specific target), membrane sterol biosynthesis, nucleic acid synthesis, metabolic inhibition and macronuclear biosynthesis. However, most antifungal drugs interfere with the enzymatic steps of sterol biosynthesis that are common for fungi and human cells.

Sterol biosynthesis seems to be the Achilles' heel of the fungus cell, since ergosterol, the essential component of the fungal membrane, exerts two functions: it is the bulk membrane component and it regulates growth and proliferation. Up to now no antifungal drugs interfering with the sole specific target, the synthesis of chitin or glucan needed for the structure of the fungal cell wall, are on the market.

Agents of deep mycoses can be divided into two groups according to their ability to infect a healthy immunocompetent host. Those that are able to do so are known as primary pathogens; these include *Coccidioides immitis*, *Histoplasma capsulatum*, *Blastomyces*, *Paracoccidioides*, and *S. schenckii*. Opportunistic pathogens, such as *Candida*, *Aspergillus*, *Cryptococcus*, *Trichosporon* and Zygomycetes, cause invasive deep infection only if specific predisposing risk factors (immune deficiency, antibacterial therapy, underlying severe disease etc.) are present.

Although in the past most fungi have been clearly placed into one of the two categories, the borders have recently been effaced. The primary pathogen *H. capsulatum*, which causes outbreaks in endemic areas, behaves like an opportunistic fungus in patients with AIDS. The old, seemingly cured infection suddenly flares up when AIDS has weakened the patient's immune system. This phenomenon happens in non-endemic areas and is therefore entirely dependent on the immune status of the host and not on the environment.

Classifying some rare fungi as primary pathogens or opportunists has always been difficult. No clear correlation between pathogenicity and immunological state has been demonstrated for dematiaceous fungi, which cause chronic subcutaneous infections as well as acute brain infections.

Primary dimorphic pathogens cause serious systemic fungal infections in normally immunocompetent hosts. Epidemics are often observed in endemic areas. These species are to a large extent resistant to the defense mechanisms of the host. Their spores, inhaled by the host, overcome the alveolar macrophages that play the main role in the primary defense mechanism against parasites. Converting into their invasive tissue form, the fungi also seem to be resistant to human neutrophils.

The phenomenon of recurrent histoplasmosis in AIDS patients may be explained by the fact that a functional, active population of T cells is needed to control the overtly cured disease. In case of a disturbance of the T-cell function, the latent fungal infection causes a secondary severe invasion. Many questions regarding the nature of the immunological defense mechanisms towards primary pathogenic fungi still remain unsolved.

The opportunistic pathogen is only a danger if the immune defense has been weakened. Observations of which infections are associated with which form of immune adequacy have contributed significantly to our understanding of the natural defense mechanism against mycoses. The scarce knowledge regarding the host defense towards *Cryptococcus neoformans* has increased significantly in the last years since this fungal species has become prominent among opportunistic pathogens causing invasive disease in HIV patients. It has become clear that the main defense against *Cryptococcus* must be based on T cells and not on neutrophils. Which fungal species can cause a systemic infection in an immunocompromised patient is not something that can be stated with confidence, but all are potential candidates. Besides the typical opportunistic fungi (*Candida*, *Aspergillus*, *Cryptococcus*, Zygomycetes), the primary pathogenic fungi, usually causing little sickness in a healthy individual, can be devastating in the immunocompromised patient. Other fungi that have always been regarded as non-pathogenic and harmless for humans are now causing life-threatening mycoses. It is necessary to look closer at a few of the "newer" pathogens, as doing so it gives some indication of the problems the physician faces when trying to determine the most probable diagnosis.

4.1.1   Emerging pathogens

As mentioned earlier, it is slowly becoming impossible to find a fungal species that has not been reported in the literature to cause severe infections in humans, but certain fungi have made themselves more visible than others.

Saccharomyces cerevisiae could be considered the least dangerous of the fungi; nevertheless, several cases of invasive life-threatening infection have been caused by this harmless baker's yeast [1]. *Rodotorula* has generally been regarded as having low pathogenicity; however, several cases of bloodstream infections related to use of indwelling central catheters have recently been reported [57, 58]. A successful therapy should include removal of the catheter plus antifungal therapy [59]. The antifungal flucytosine (alone or in combination with Amph B) should be chosen, since *Rodotorula* is highly susceptible to 5-flucytosine (5-FC) but only moderately to Amph B [57].

In recent years, it has become apparent that *Fusarium*, a well-known plant pathogen, is able to cause severe infections in humans, mainly in leukaemic patients [60–63]. These infections are difficult to control in the neutropenic patients since most *Fusarium* species are relatively resistant to all antifungals used in human chemotherapy. Amph B or liposomal Amph B therapy proved to be successful in some rare cases [64, 64a]; however, in many other cases, the therapy failed [65, 65a]. Concomitant therapy of Amph B and immunomodulators (e.g. GM-CSF or GCSF) may become the therapy of choice for this life-threatening disease in the near future [66].

Another unusual pathogen is *Trichosporon beigelii*, which has been shown to cause sepsis in premature infants [67]. A cluster of sepsis cases has been observed in a neonatal intensive care unit [68]. Other known risk factors for this fungal infection are neutropenia [1], valve replacement [69], ambulatory peritoneal dialysis [70] and AIDS [71]. *T. beigelii* has been found to be resistant to Amph B; however, successful treatments with Amph B alone or in combination with rifampicin or flucytosine recently have been reported [69, 72, 73]. The combination of high-dose Amph B plus flucytosine may be more active than Amph B alone [65a]. Flu proved to be active in murine trichosporonosis. Furthermore, Flu showed activity in *Trichosporon* infection refractory to a therapy that combined Amph B plus flucytosine [65a].

Penicillium marneffei, a fungus endemic in Southeast Asia and Japan, causes disseminated fungal infections, especially in HIV-positive patients [71, 74, 75]. About 550 cases of *P. marneffei* infections were diagnosed in Japan up to 1995. Most patients responded to appropriate antifungal therapy (such as Amph B, Keto, Flu and Itra). In HIV-infected children, Keto was successfully used as prophylactic therapy to prevent relapses [75]. Disseminated *P. marneffei* infections in AIDS patients have also been diagnosed in Europe in subjects returning from a visit to certain areas of Southeast Asia [76, 77]. *P. marneffei* is highly susceptible *in vitro* to Itra, Keto, and flucytosine, but appears to be less susceptible to Amph B and Flu. In AIDS patients, mild to moderately severe infections should be treated with Itra or Keto, and severely ill patients should be treated with Amph B.

However, a substantial failure rate is observed in AIDS patients. Maintenance therapy should be considered in advanced AIDS patients, since relapses are common after the treatment has been stopped.

Hansenula anomala is another emerging fungal species causing fungaemia in children and neutropenic adults. This infection is often associated with a central catheter and total parenteral nutrition [78, 79]. Removal of the catheter is essential for successful therapy. Some patients recovered without antifungal therapy, but only because the catheter was removed [78]. Amph B or Flu therapy (always with concomitant removal of the catheter) seems to be successful in this clinical setting [78–80]. However, a breakthrough fungaemia due to *H. anomala* in a leukaemic patient under Flu prevention has been observed [81]. The patient responded favorably to Amph B treatment.

Malassezia pachydermatis, a skin habitant, is another fungus able to cause bloodstream infection in premature infants or in neutropenic adults who receive parenteral nutrition and/or intravenous lipids. Recently, a nosocomial outbreak in a neonatal intensive care unit was studied epidemiologically; the transmission occurred most likely from person to person via the hands of the medical staff [82].

Treatment consists of discontinuing the parenteral lipid emulsion and removal of central venous catheter. Non-immunocompromised patients seldom require antifungal therapy once the catheter is removed and the lipid emulsion is discontinued. If antifungal therapy is necessary, systemic azoles (such as Keto, Itra or Flu) are to be preferred to Amph B, since they are considered to be more efficacious.

Pseudoallescheria boydii infections are known to be resistant to Amph B treatment; however, miconazole has been the therapy of choice for this disease for many decades despite the fact that miconazole has severe safety liabilities. Recently, successful treatment has been reported with Keto [83], Itra alone [83a] or in combination with debridement [84]. In the future, the less toxic triazoles may replace miconazole therapy for *Pseudoallescheria* infections.

During recent years, all of the above-mentioned fungal species have been observed to cause fatal infections in immunocompromised patients with a disquieting, increasing frequency. Certain other fungi are still rarely seen but are nevertheless causing deep concern in the medical world.

Scedosporium prolificans (*inflatum*) caused deadly disseminated infections in four neutropenic patients. The isolated strain was resistant – *in vitro* – to all available systemic antifungals (Amph B, flucytosine, imidazoles and triazoles) [85].

For the first time, a case of fatal dissemination due to *Myceliophthora thermophila* [86] has been diagnosed *post mortem*. *Trichoderma pseudokonigii* in a bone marrow transplant patient proved to be resistant to Amph B, Flu and liposomal Amph B plus flucytosine [87]. A liver transplant recipient developed a fatal infection due to *T. viride* [88]. A fungal infection caused by *Chaetomium* spp was detected in a drug user [89]. Disseminated infection due to *Scytalidium dimidiatum* in a granulocytopenic child responded well to Amph B [90]. *Pythium insidiosum* caused fatal arteritis in six patients with thalassaemia. Early recognition and radical amputation are at present the only chance for surviving [91].

4.2   The patient

The major factor in the increase in systemic mycoses is undoubtedly immunodeficiency. There is an expanding community of people with weakened or even non-existent immune systems due to underlying diseases, medical treatment, surgical invention or transplantation (especially bone marrow transplantation). Although travel to endemic areas is becoming more common, and disease caused by primary pathogens is more often diagnosed, it is the increase in opportunistic infections that has completely changed the significance and necessity of antifungal therapy.
The fungi have not changed their habitat, but the factors that turn a saprophyte into a virulent pathogen have become more varied and more common. For instance, immune suppression in organ transplant patients and antitumor therapy in cancer patients have become rather common; however, it is the AIDS pandemic that changed the whole picture of opportunistic infections. The division between primary and opportunistic pathogens is blurred, as colonization or asymptomatic infections can flare up into life-threatening diseases in a host whose immune system is weakening from day to day.
HIV-positive patients are at the highest risk of falling ill with infections caused either by traditionally recognized opportunistic fungi, an emerging new pathogen or a recognized primary pathogen. In AIDS patients, all fungal infections, superficial or deep mycoses, display a more severe clinical course with frequent therapy resistance in comparison to normal or less strictly immunocompromised patients.
Seborrhoeic dermatitis, which in normal patients can be kept under control by an array of compounds active against *Malassezia furfur*, is a clinical problem in HIV-infected patients. Dermatophytic infections need a longer treatment duration, and relapses are common. The recurrent form,

not the acute form, of vaginal candidosis is observed in HIV-positive females.

Before the emergence of AIDS, oropharyngeal candidosis was seen only in patients of extreme age (babies or very old people). Today, oropharyngeal candidosis is the commonest infectious disease in HIV patients, affecting about 90% of the patients, with a 60% recurrence rate within 3 months [92]. Oropharyngeal candidosis appears at an early stage of HIV infection, whereas oesophagal infections are seen in those with more advanced disease. Eradication of the clinical manifestations of candidosis is the major goal in treating mucosal candidosis of HIV-positive patients. As follow-up action, suppression of recurrence becomes the ultimate goal.

Cryptococcus meningitis is the most frequent manifestation of a systemic mycosis caused by an opportunistic fungus. The disease takes a more severe course, and lifelong maintenance therapy is mandatory, since the prostate and meninges act as nidi of infection despite successful therapy. Optimal initial treatment should aim to immediately stop the fungal infection in order to prevent further immunosuppression of the host by the cryptococcal polysaccharide, which is known to be immunosuppressive. Additionally, it has been shown that cryptococcal polysaccharide significantly enhances HIV-1 infectivity, further depleting the residual CD4 cells [93]. Two of the four major endemic mycoses of America, histoplasmosis and coccidioidomycosis, have increasingly appeared as HIV-associated opportunistic infections. Penicillosis (caused by *P. marneffei*) is known to be one of the most frequent opportunistic fungal infections of AIDS patients in Southeast Asia.

In a setting of neutropenia, severe diabetes mellitus or use of broad spectrum antibacterials the main opportunistic infections are caused by *Candida* and *Aspergillus*. Treatment is often ineffective unless the underlying disease can be controlled. As soon as this control is working, antifungal therapy is successful and no maintenance therapy is necessary.

In recent years, more knowledge has accumulated about the way the human body defends itself against fungal infections and about the particular risks of specific groups of patients. Oropharyngeal candidosis is seen in T-cell disturbance, whereas *Candida* infection of organs is mainly observed in neutropenic patients. *C. tropicalis* and *C. krusei* have an affinity for leukaemic patients and are increasingly isolated from AIDS patients in the late stage of the disease. *Mucor* has an affinity for diabetes mellitus and *Fusarium* for neutropenic patients. Despite increased understanding regarding host-fungus interactions, there is still a long way to go until we understand the host defense mechanism towards fungi in detail. Until our knowledge regarding the immunology of fungal diseases becomes more detailed, the most important advance will remain the increased awareness of the medical world of the power and danger of fungal infections in the ever-growing population of the immunocompromised.

In conclusion, AIDS patients are at a very high risk of contracting severe fungal infections, of experiencing a relapse or even of dying from opportunistic fungal infections. Thus it is of importance to initiate maintenance therapy for all deep fungal infections after the first therapy has proven successful, even if the niche of the fungus is not known, since relapses are extremely frequent as soon as antifungal therapy is stopped. The detailed recommendation for antifungal therapy in neutropenic and AIDS patients will be discussed in the section for each drug.

4.3   The drugs on the market

Six years ago, only three established drugs for the treatment of systemic mycoses existed; today this number has increased at least to five: Amph B (with the new formulations taken as one single entity), flucytosine (5FC), Keto, Flu and Itra.

4.3.1   Amphotericin B, the old drug
- Amph B is the most efficacious antifungal; the only drawback is its infusion-related toxicity and its negative influence on renal function.

Although hundreds of macrolide polyenic antibiotics are synthesized by actinomycetes, only one, Amph B, is used in systemic antifungal therapy. It is produced by *Streptomyces nodosus* [2]. Amph B has a very broad spectrum of antifungal activity (fungistatic and fungicidal), including the established opportunistic fungi (*Candida* spp., *Cryptococcus neoformans*, *Aspergillus* spp, *Mucoraceae*) and the primary pathogens (*H. capsulatum*, *Coccidioides immitis*, *Paracoccidioides brasiliensis*). Dermatophytes, the dematiaceous fungi and species of *Madurella*, are considered to be resistant [1].

4.3.1.1   Resistance
It was always easy to isolate resistant mutants in the laboratory. These mutants are generally distinguished from parent strains by an altered lipid composition. However, secondary resistance to Amph B has remained a rare event despite its extensive use in chemotherapy for more than 40 years. This may be explained by the fact that the changes in the sterol composition of the membrane leading to *in vitro* resistance will reduce viru-

lence and slow cell growth rate. No resistance or increased MICs to Amph B has been observed in 43 isolates of a surveillance study on bone marrow transplant recipients treated prophylactically with Amph B [94].

It seems, however, that Amph B-resistant bloodstream infections are increasing during chemotherapy in highly immunodeficient patients [1, 95, 96].

4.3.1.2   Mode of action

The current model for the mechanism of action of Amph B is based on the formation of a 1:1 Amph B/sterol aggregate, which associates into a transmembrane barrel with a large –OH-lined aqueous pore down the middle [97, 98]. The result of the interaction between Amph B and the sterols is a disturbance of the ergosterol function leading to increased permeability, disruption of the proton gradient and leakage of potassium ions. The fungistatic effect of Amph B was thought to be related to the efflux of potassium; the fungicidal effect, however, has been linked to irreversible inhibition of the membrane of ATPase.

The complete mechanism of action of Amph B is still not fully understood. New hypotheses are being framed, and many researchers, studying the interaction of Amph B at the cellular level with natural membranes or artificial bilayers, are trying to prove them. Conflicting membrane permeability data suggest a multiplicity of Amph B channel structures and modes of action [98]. Oxidative damage to the cells seems to be involved, and the drug appears to induce a cascade of oxidative reactions linked to its own oxidation. The fungistatic activity seems to be related to the permeability changes; the lethal activity is more dependent on the oxidative challenge [97, 99].

4.3.1.3   Toxicity

Amph B has a higher specificity for ergosterol than for cholesterol, the mammalian sterol; this is considered the key to the relatively low toxicity of Amph B to the human host in comparison with other polyenes like nystatin or candicidin. Nevertheless, the major drawback for broader use of Amph B is the frequent occurrence of adverse events. Amph B does induce reversible and chronic side-effects that are unpleasant and, in many cases, menacing [1, 2, 100].

Acute reactions to Amph B – usually fever, chills, rigor or nausea – can be ameliorated by concomitant administration of meperidine, acetominophen or hydrocortisone. There is, additionally, the possibility of tailoring time and duration of the infusion to the individual patient, since the acute reactions vary significantly. The incidence of side-effects and adverse reactions is dependent on the infusion rate, being higher under rapid infusion. Reversible anaemia develops in 75% of patients. The potential value of coadministration of eythropoietin has not yet been fully evaluated [2]. Chronic toxicity of Amph B is mostly due to renal damage. Hypokalaemia, hypomagnesaemia and increased creatinin are common and troublesome. Nephrotoxicity does not appear to be strictly dose-dependent and can occur with standard therapy. In recent years, the knowledge regarding this chronic adverse event has significantly increased [1, 101], and prevention of the chronic tubular injury seems feasible. Making certain that the patient is eunatraemic appears to mitigate nephrotoxicity. The reversal of sodium depletion by salt loading gained its full acceptance in clinical practice. This can be achieved either by a special salt diet or by combination therapy with 5-FC infusion, which contains 0.9% saline. Using this combination therapy avoids not only the nephrotoxic effects of Amph B but coincidentally improves efficacy against several opportunistic fungal infections based on the proven synergism between Amph B and 5-FC (see detail in Sec. 4.3.7). An interesting phenomenon related to the nephrotoxicity of Amph B was recently observed. Patients with higher serum LDL cholesterol concentrations were more susceptible to Amph B-induced renal toxicity than patients with lower LDL cholesterol levels [101a]. In AIDS patients, a combination of Amph B and foscarnet (an antiviral agent) should be avoided, since this combination rapidly induces renal insufficiency [102].

The attitude towards the use of Amph B has drastically changed in recent years. Most clinicians have lost their fear of prescribing Amph B, and they now use the drug, despite its toxicity, with confidence. Courageous medics have successfully treated AIDS patients with *Candida* endophthalmitis with i.v. Amph B at home. Renal function deterioration was observed, but all side-effects were reversible [103]. These authors conclude that patients requiring i.v. Amph B therapy can be treated at home under hospital supervision, with considerable financial savings to the hospital.

Research has detected another way to avoid the major side-effects of Amph B. The adverse event rates are drastically reduced if Amph B is embedded in liposomes or associated with lipids (see Sec. 4.3.2).

4.3.1.4   Therapy

Despite its toxicity, Amph B is still used as superior therapy for a wide range of systemic mycoses: its fungicidal effect makes it irreplaceable for disseminated infections in immundeficient patients at least as initial therapy (e.g. example histoplasmosis and cryptococcal meningitis in AIDS). It must, however, be mentioned that even after more than 30 years of clinical use, no general agreement exists regarding the optimal dose, the duration of therapy or method of administration. The therapeutic or pharmacokinetic rationale for optimal Amph B dosing is still lacking [104].

In the last 6 years Amph B has kept and will in the near future keep its leadership role in the area of severe fungal infections in highly immunocompromised patients, including HIV-infected patients. Amph B monotherapy remains the drug of choice for initial treatment in disseminated histoplasmosis [92,105,106] and coccidioidomycosis of AIDS patients [92, 107]. The optimal initial treatment for cryptococcal meningitis aiming to rapidly halt the infection in order to prevent further immunosuppression remains a combination therapy of Amph B with flucytosine [92,108,109] (detailed description under Sec. 4.3.6). Amph B prevails in the therapy of mucormycosis (zygomycosis), since all Zygomycetes are resistant to azoles. Amph B is the drug of choice for candidemia, hematogenously disseminated *Candida* infection and *Candida* meningitis; 5-FC should be administered concurrently with Amph B in patients whose condition is not improving under monotherapy [101].

The crude mortality and rate of response to Amph B therapy of invasive aspergillosis has recently been reviewed in 1223 immunocompromised patients [110]. The response rate of pulmonary aspergillosis was not overwhelming, and was dependent on the underlying disease and the duration of treatment. Only patients treated for more than 134 days had any real chance of being cured. Pulmonary aspergillosis responded in 33% of the bone marrow transplant patients, 54% of the leukaemic cases and 83% of the heart or renal transplant patients. *Aspergillus* sinusitis cases responded with 49%; cerebral aspergillosis with 33%. Thus, Amph B is in no way the "wonder drug" for aspergillosis therapy, but it is not yet clear whether Itra or one of the new Amph B formulations is superior to Amph B.

4.3.2   Amph B in new clothes

• Encapsulation of Amph B into liposomes or complexing of the drug with other lipid carriers brings a major reduction in toxicity.

The first publication of clinical experiments with liposomal Amph B appeared by Lopez-Bernstein in 1984 [111]. Three lipid-associated forms are now on the European market. These include liposomal Amph B (AmBisome), Amph B lipid complex (ABLC, Abelect) and Amph B colloidal dispension (ABCD, Amphocil, Amphotec). Amphocil has been recently received marketing approval in the United States from the Food and Drug Administration (FDA).

The properties of these three marketed lipid formulations differ in terms of the amount of Amph B and lipids used, as well as in their physical form, serum clearance and acute infusion-related toxicity; however, they are similar in that they permit Amph B to bypass the kidney and to concentrate in the liver, spleen and lungs. The *in vitro* activity, mode of action, toxicity and efficacy will be reviewed in this section. Most published data are available for AmBisome, which was the first on the market for salvage therapy in patients experiencing toxicity with the normal Amph B.

Anecdotal reports of the use of Amph B mixed with fat emulsions used for parenteral nutrition are increasing [112–120a]. Several researchers are studying and evaluating their own mixtures in laboratories and hospitals. Patients treated with Amph B/fat emulsion mixture seem to have a significant reduction in infusion-related toxicity, as well as in renal dysfunction, without losing the high efficacy of Amph B. A drawback of these individual mixtures is the fact that Amph B does not mix well with fat emulsions and that no standardized methods exist to prepare these mixtures [121].

4.3.2.1   Mode of action

The *in vitro* antifungal activities of AmBisome and Amphocil (ABCD) were found to be comparable to that of Amph B [121, 122].

Much work has been done investigating the physical biochemistry of Amph B liposomal complexes and the mechanism by which toxicity is reduced. The details of these investigations are beyond the scope of this review, but more information can be found in refs. 2, 121 and 123–127. The essentials are that Amph B in any formulation consists of complexed and free substance in equilibrium, and it is only the latter that is active. The job of the liposomes is to bring the drug into close contact with sterol-containing membranes in tissue, where the greater affinity of ergosterol ensures better transfer of active substance to the fungal cell. Less free Amph B is available to cause toxic side-effects.

In vitro and *in vivo* studies have clearly demonstrated that AmBisome accumulates at sites of infections [128]. Empty and drug-containing liposomes bind to the surface of the fungal cell, but only Amph B-containing liposomes interact with the fungal cells. This interaction results in the disruption of the liposomes, releasing Amph B and causing the death of the cell within 2 to 4 hours.

As with free Amph B, not every detail of the mode of action of liposomal or lipid complexed Amph B is understood, but some aspects of the interactions became clear from the intensive study of AmBisome. Amph B is anchored in the liposome so that no dissociation of free Amph B from

AmBisome takes place in aqueous medium. AmBisome remains intact in circulation for a prolonged period of time [128], whereas lipid-based formulations are more rapidly cleared from the circulation and accumulate very quickly in the tissues [129]. AmBisome as well as the lipid-complexed formulations accumulate in infected tissues. Liposomal Amph B interacts directly with the fungal cell and only minimally with the mammalian membrane.

4.3.2.2   Toxicity

All three marketed new formulations of Amph B have a better safety profile than the conventional formulation (Fungizone). This is truly a beneficial achievement [121, 123–125].

The safety of AmBisome has been studied in patients with AIDS, hematological malignancy (bone marrow transplants) and in patients receiving liver or heart/lung transplants [123, 130–141]. Rapid administration [30–60 min) of a high daily dose of AmBisome is feasible without the well-known acute adverse events of traditional Amph B. The influence on renal function is also significantly reduced. No change of serum creatinine levels was seen in 99 of 121 (81%) patients. However, 11 (15%) episodes were associated with increased creatinine concentrations, evenly distributed among the various cumulative doses of AmBisome. It should be stressed, however, that in 17 (34%) episodes the initially high creatinine level was reduced to normal during AmBisome therapy.

The safety of liposomal Amph B has also been evaluated in 187 transplant patients who were concomitantly treated with cyclosporin [132]. The major problem using Amph B in these patients is the synergistic nephrotoxic effect between Amph B and cyclosporin. Dramatic increases in serum creatinine have been seen in transplant patients treated with Amph B plus cyclosporin. Furthermore, Amph B as well as AmBisome cause a significant increase of the cyclosporin level in blood. When Amph B was replaced by AmBisome in transplant patients, an improvement in renal function was observed. However, AmBisome is not free of nephrotoxic effects in this clinical setting. In 31% of the patients a mild increase (average 20%) of serum creatinine was observed, which could be attributed to AmBisome or to other nephrotoxic drugs, concomitantly applied. In this study, all side-effects caused by AmBisome (at doses of 3 to 4 mg/kg/day) were mild, manageable and reversible. This result positively contrasts to the experience gathered over years with conventional Amph B.

ABCD (Amphocil) was safely applied in doses up to 7.5 mg/kg/day over 6 weeks to bone marrow transplant patients without any renal toxicity. The major toxicities associated with Amphocil (only at high doses) were the typical fevers, rigors, chills and hypotension also seen with conventional Amph B [133]. Thus, Amphocil is another new formulation with a better safety profile (especially without renal toxicity) compared with traditional Amph B.

The safety and efficacy of ABLC has been evaluated in AIDS patients with *Cryptococcus* meningitis. The total number of adverse events, infusion-related or renal impairment, was identical to that with conventional Amph B, but ABLC caused milder and reversible events. Transfusion requirements, mean decrease in hemoglobin level and mean increase in creatinine level were significantly greater with conventional Amph B (Fungizone) than with ABLC [142].

In summary, all three marketed formulations have the advantage of a better safety profile over conventional Amph B; this is a major step forward in the battle against fungal diseases.

4.3.2.3   Efficacy

The three marketed formulations of Amph B have primarily been developed using an emergency use protocol: the new formulations were only allowed to be given to patients who did not respond to conventional antifungal therapy or who showed severe side-effects to Amph B therapy or who suffered from renal impairment [121, 123, 125]. This principle has to be kept in mind if one evaluates the clinical data of the various studies. Most patients will have been treated before with conventional therapy (in most of the cases this was Amph B). Therefore, the beneficial efficacy seen under the new therapy may not be entirely attributable to the new formulations, since the first standard treatment could still have had a positive input to the final outcome.

The efficacy of AmBisome was first evaluated in a multicenter open trial with 126 patients. Of the 108 episodes that were clinically evaluable, 52 were caused by *Candida* spp. and 34 by *Aspergillus* spp. The patients have been treated for at least 8 days with doses of 0.7to 5 mg/kg/day. Among 64 cases with proven invasive fungal infections, 58% were cured. Among 24 cases with presumptive invasive fungal infection, 58% were cured [136]. Schneeman [123] has summarized the early clinical experience with AmBisome in great detail. AmBisome was curative in 37 of 52 (71%) candidosis cases, in 12 of 35 [34%] aspergillosis cases and in 7 of 8 (88%) cryptococcosis cases. It was efficacious in one case of *Mucor* infection, one case of madura feet and 2 *Trichosporon* infections. The efficacy and safety of AmBisome were evaluated in a retrospective study of 116 neutropenic patients [137]. Overall, there was a successful outcome in 81 of 133 (61%) episodes, 13 having aspergillosis and 39 candidosis. The outcome was fatal in 25 (19%) episodes. However, the diagnosis was equivocal in most, and in 20% of the episodes there was subsequent evidence of non-mycotic pathogenesis.

Another study [138] demonstrated some efficacy in lung transplant recipients with aspergillosis. AmBisome was also successfully applied to children with candiduria [136]. Liposomal Amph B yielded favorable results in eight AIDS patients with cryptococcosis; the initial response to the therapy occurred rapidly [140]. The authors of a summary on the compassionate use data of AmBisome, gathered during 1990–1992 in 30 patients in the United Kingdom, conclude that AmBisome is efficacious in the treatment of invasive fungal infections and provides an alternative therapy for those who fail to respond or become intolerant to conventional Amph B [141].

The beneficial effect of ABLC for invasive fungal infections has been studied in various emergency use studies [125, 142].

The first clinical efficacy results with ABLC were not highly impressive; ABLC was not more efficacious than modest doses of conventional Amph B [125]. However, newer data show equal or even better cure rates under ABLC treatment than with Amph B. ABLC proved to be efficacious in candidosis and aspergillosis. Clinical response rates of 69 and 67% have been observed in patients with candidosis and aspergillosis, respectively [142, 143]. A case of rhinocerebral mucormycosis involving the cavernous sinus was cured with ABLC. This is the first well-documented case of rhinocerebral mucormycosis with intracranial involvement responsive to antifungal therapy [144]. In the United States, 151 patients with aspergillosis have been treated with the ABLC in an emergency use program. Overall, these patients showed higher response rates (40 vs 23% $p = 0.002$) than the historical control group treated with conventional Amph B [145]. In another study, 12 high-risk immunocompromised patients were treated for various invasive fungal infections. The overall response rate was 70% [146].

In a phase I study [133], ABCD proved to be efficacious in patients with invasive fungal infections after bone marrow transplantation. The complete or partial response across dose levels and infection types was 52%. For fungaemia the curative rate was 55%, for pneumonia 37%. ABCD was also effective in another open-labeled compassionate trial [134]. Complete clinical response was observed in 49% of the patients after a mean treatment period of 18.5 days.

All three new formulations of Amph B are more expensive than conventional Amph B, and this fact may cause some concern about the cost-effectiveness of this newer treatment form. The therapeutic role and cost outcome cannot be defined at present since randomized clinical trials are lacking [147].

In conclusion, the use of all three new formulations of Amph B results in an overall improvement of the therapeutic index. This step forward is of greatest importance for all patients with fungal infections of known or unknown pathogens. The possibility of reducing the toxic side-effects of Amph B has given new life to the old standard, which still has the broadest antifungal spectrum. The positive finding with lipid-complexed Amph B has prompted investigations into whether other active but highly toxic polyenes embedded in liposomes or complexed with lipids could be used for systemic treatment of fungal infections. Nystatin could only be used orally to eradicate *Candida* from the gastrointestinal tract, since its systemic toxicity was extremely high. However, positive interim results from a recent multicenter phase II/III study of nystatin in its lipid i.v. form for candidosis has been reported (Prous weekly essential online, November 1996).

4.3.3   Flucytosine
• 5-FC is a true antimetabolite.
• 5-FC should only be used for therapy as a combination partner.

5-FC, a mock pyrimidine, is the only antifungal drug that acts as true antimetabolite. Its antifungal spectrum is limited to species of *Candida* and *Cryptococcus*, which are highly sensitive (MIC 0.1–2 μg/ml) and *Aspergillus* and *Dematiaceae*, which are only moderately sensitive (MIC 1–25 μg/ml). 5-FC shows fungistatic *and* fungicidal activity against yeasts and *Dematiaceae*, but it is only fungistatic against aspergilli. [1, 2].

4.3.3.1   Mode of action
Exposure of sensitive fungi to 5-FC almost immediately induces inhibition of the synthesis of DNA and RNA. In yeasts and dematiaceous fungi, cell growth continues with carbohydrate and protein overproduction; this unbalanced growth is defined as thymineless death. In aspergilli the inhibition of nucleic acid causes immediate inhibition of growth, and the lack of overproduction of proteins and carbohydrates is probably the reason why 5-FC is not fungicidal in this species [148].

The metabolic pathway of 5-FC has been carefully studied using various mutants resistant to the drug. 5-FC is taken up actively by a cytosine permease which is normally responsible for the uptake of adenine, guanine, hypoxanthine and cytosine [148, 149] and is therefore antagonized by these natural substrates. Inside the cell 5-FC is immediately deaminated to

5-fluorouracil (5-FU) which is the active principal responsible for killing the fungal cell. This step is essential for the antifungal activity of 5-FC, since fungi lacking the cytosine deaminase are resistant to the drug. The low toxicity of 5-FC in humans is due to the absence of the cytosine deaminase in mammalian cells [150]. Normal enteric bacteria, however, are capable of deaminating 5-FC [151]; the resulting 5-FU is fortunately poorly absorbed from the normal colon.

5-FU acts along two different pathways. It is converted by uridine monophosphate pyrophosphorylase into 5-FUMP, which is finally incorporated into the RNA (a step which is antagonized by uridine). Simultaneously, it is converted to 5-fluorodeoxyuridine monophosphate, a potent inhibitor of thymidylate synthetase; this step leads to inhibition of DNA synthesis. 5-FU itself cannot be used for antifungal therapy, since its uptake by the fungal cell is poor, and its toxicity for mammalian cells forbids systemic use of the high doses necessary to kill a fungal cell. The details of the mode of action of 5-FC were reviewed in 1990 [152].

What is remarkable about the action of 5-FC is that the fungal cell itself produces the fungicidal principle from an inert compound by internal metabolization and further metabolizes it to cause its own death, a situation unique in medical mycology. However, the length of the metabolic pathway and the several different enzymes involved are also the reason for the frequent appearance of 5-FC-resistant mutants.

4.3.3.2   Resistance

Primary and acquired resistance to 5-FC may result from absence, dysfunction or deletion of one or more enzymes not essential to fungal survival. In every normally sensitive population of fungi, there is a minority that is resistant to 5-FC. The absolute number of primary resistant cells is species dependent, the lowest resistance frequency is seen in *Candida albicans* (2.7×10^{-7}) and the highest in aspergilli (3.5×10^{-5}). A highly significant correlation has also been found between the incidence of primary resistance to 5-FC and the serological type of *C. albicans*, the incidence being significantly greater in *C. albicans* of serotype B [1, 153, 154]. During lengthy monotherapy with 5-FC, the proportion of resistant cells can so increase that the population as a whole becomes resistant [1,2]. As there is a clear correlation between therapy failure and the appearance of secondary (acquired) resistance, 5-FC monotherapy is no longer used in long-term chemotherapy, but is always used in combination with another antifungal (see Sec. 4.3.7).

Most mutants isolated (clinically or in laboratory) lack uridine monophosphate pyrophosphorylase. However, resistance may also be due to changed cytosine permease or deaminase or to overproduction of pyrimidine. A clear segregation between highly resistant and partially resistant mutants has been observed [155] in experiments showing that *C. albicans* is a diploid organism. It was clearly demonstrated that the mutation in partially resistant strains is only located on one allele, whereas totally resistant strains have the mutation on both alleles.

It is not clearly proven whether the appearance of 5-FC resistance does or does not influence the virulence of the strains. The degree of virulence may be dependent on the enzyme altered. Dysfunction of the cytosine deaminase and uridine transport seems to induce loss of virulence [156]; however, the uridine monophosphate pyrophosphorylase dysfunction seems to have a minor effect on virulence [1, 157]. The loss of virulence is at any rate less pronounced than that seen with Amph B- or azole-resistant isolates.

4.3.3.3   Toxicity

The actual clinical relevance of 5-FC toxicity is controversial. Some clinicians emphasize it and speak of it as if it were a major problem. Others have a different opinion, stating clearly that adverse effects are uncommon and rarely severe or irreversible.

It was assumed that the toxicity of 5-FC was related in some way to the internal production of 5-FU; yet no direct correlation was ever found to the 5FU-levels measured in serum. The frequency of adverse events is, however, directly correlated with 5-FC concentrations above 100 μg/ml for a sustained time period [1, 2, 158]. This correlation has been observed for all patients suffering from side-effects during controlled studies with combination therapy [159, 160]. Most important, since 5-FC is entirely excreted by the kidneys, even a minor impairment of renal function (e.g. by combination with the nephrotoxic drug Amph B) leads to elevated 5-FC levels. Thus it is important to monitor 5-FC levels and adapt the dose to actual kidney function. This reduces the toxic effects of 5-FC to acceptable levels [160].

Anorexia, nausea, vomiting, diarrhoea and/or abdominal pain occur in 6% of treated patients. Hepatic disturbance (liver enzyme elevation) may occur with or without hepatomegaly in about 5% of patients. Of greater concern is the potential for bone marrow depression (seen in 5% of cases, all with elevated 5-FC levels), which is not always reversible, especially if not recognized early enough. This aspect of 5-FC toxicity is often overplayed, and more careful monitoring would decrease fears.

5-FC was temporarily abandoned after a warning that it has a potential for myelotoxicity in AIDS patients. However, a retrospective analysis of the clinical outcome of cryptococcal meningitis suggested that 5-FC is tolerated in AIDS patients as least as well as it is in cancer patients [107, 161]. As with Amph B, exact evaluation of toxicity is complicated by the fact that patients are invariably suffering from an underlying disease that disturbs metabolic function and that all patients are treated concomitantly with other potentially toxic drugs [1, 2].

4.3.3.4   Efficacy
Despite its narrow spectrum and resistance problems, 5-FC remains a useful agent for the treatment of opportunistic fungal infections in combination with Amph B or another antifungal (see Sec. 4.3.7).

4.3.4   Old imidazole derivatives: Miconazole and ketoconazole
- Keto was the first oral, broad spectrum azole for deep mycoses.
- Keto's drawback is its significant interactions with other drugs and endocrinopathies or hepatopathies.

4.3.4.1   Mode of action
The imidazoles and triazoles appear to operate via a common mechanism of action. They disturb the function of the cell membrane by interfering with cytochrome P450-dependent lanosterol C_{14} demethylase, leading to depletion of ergosterol and accumulation of lanosterol in the membrane. At the molecular level, one of the nitrogen atoms of the azole ring binds to the haeme moiety of cytochrome P450. Only compounds with higher specific binding to the fungal cytochrome than to the human one can be used as antifungal drugs. Compared with the imidazoles, the triazoles have a much higher affinity for fungal cytochrome than for human cytochrome P450 enzyme steps [2].

The fungistatic action of all azoles is related to inhibition of lanosterol C_{14} demethylase, leading to depletion of ergosterol. Ergosterol has two fundamental functions in the fungal cell membrane: it is the major bulk material, giving the membrane its essential structure, and it has an important regulatory function [24]. The depletion of ergosterol alters fluidity, thereby reducing the activity of membrane-bound enzymes (e.g. chitin synthetase, lipid metabolism and oxidative enzymes) and initiating increased permeability. Depletion of ergosterol also reduces cell membrane sites for the interaction of polyenic antifungal agents leading to antagonism with Amph B (see Sec. 3.7).

In addition to the main interaction with the P450 cytochrome, azoles may inhibit cytochrome C oxydase and peroxidative enzymes; they may also interact with phospholipids and inhibit the transformation of yeasts to mycelial form. The fact that miconazole and Itra are fungicidal is thought to be the result of a direct membrane interaction, leading to the loss of cytoplasmic constituents [24, 162].

The mode of action of azoles has been intensively studied; a detailed review of all the accumulated knowledge is beyond the scope of this paper (for more information, see refs. 24, 162 and 163).

Intravenous miconazole was the first imidazole derivative used for the treatment of invasive fungal infection. It was soon followed by oral Keto. Both drugs had shown efficacy and have opened a new era in research, as well as in human chemotherapy. However, they have been or are going to be replaced soon by the more specific, less toxic and more efficacious triazoles Flu and Itra.

Miconazole retains its niche indication treating the invasive infections caused by *Pseudoallescheria boydii*.

Neither primary nor secondary resistance seems to be a great problem with Keto. However, the necessity of using a high dosage of Keto for various indications has led to crucial toxic problems. Nausea and vomiting are the most frequent adverse reactions; they increase in severity with increased doses. Endocrinopathies – manifested in males as gynaecomastia and in females as irregular menses – were seen. Hepatotoxicity is rare, usually reversible, but some lethal cases have been observed [2, 164, 165]. These adverse reactions limit the broad use of oral Keto in dermatology.

A number of meaningful interactions between Keto and other drugs has already been found, and new ones are continually observed. Most interactions occur by means of one of two basic mechanisms:

– inhibition of absorption of the azole leading to lower bioavailability or
– interference with the activity of hepatic microsomal enzymes, which alters the metabolism and plasma levels of the azole, the interacting drug or both.

Keto significantly prolongs the elimination half-life of cyclosporin A by inhibition of cytochrome P450 enzymes. It also increases the levels of warfarin, digoxin, terfenadine, astemizole and tulbutamide. Absorption of Keto is influenced by H_2-receptor antagonists and sucralfate. The serum levels of Keto are significantly decreased with concomitant administration of rifampicin, isoniazid and phenytoin. Tirilazad mesylate levels are significantly increased in the presence of Keto [2, 164–166].

Keto was, and is still, highly useful in chronic mucocutaneous candidosis. However, Keto should only be used for fungal infections in non-immunosuppressed patients. Keto has shown its beneficial value in all endemic fungal infections like paracoccidioidomycosis, blastomycosis and histo-plasmosis, provided the patients are not immunosuppressed.

Amph B remains the standard treatment for all these infections in patients with decreased host defenses. All meningeal infections are excluded due to the poor penetration of Keto into the cerebrospinal fluid. Keto is also not recommended for empirical antifungal therapy for suspected candidosis, since Amph B proved to be more efficacious in a randomized trial [164, 167].

4.3.5   Fluconazole

- Flu is significantly better tolerated than Amph B and has fewer interactions than Keto with other drugs.
- Oral Flu is well established as a first-line therapy for oropharyngeal candidosis and *Candida* oesophagitis.
- Emergence of resistant strains or species may become a problem in the future.
- Flu is the drug of choice for maintenance therapy in AIDS patients with meningeal cryptococcosis or histoplasmosis.

Flu has some properties that are unique among azoles. It is highly soluble in water or saline; it shows a high bioavailability and is distributed in all body water. No CNS or ocular barrier exists, it is scarcely metabolized and is primarily excreted by the kidneys as unchanged mother drug.

Flu is active *in vitro* against a variety of molds and yeasts including *Cryptococcus neoformans* and *Candida* spp. The species cluster of *Candida albicans*, *C. tropicalis* and *C. parapsilosis* has distinctly higher susceptibility than *C. krusei* or *C. glabrata*. *Aspergillus* spp. are resistant to the drug. Generally all fungal species tested show a higher sensitivity in animal models or in the clinic than *in vitro*. Most fungi showed high MICs when in use with conventional standard culture media. However, recent advances in susceptibility testing of *Candida* spp. have improved the reproducibility of these tests, which now show low MICs and lead to a better correlation with animal data or with the actual clinical responses [2, 39, 164, 165].

4.3.5.1   Resistance

Until the late 1980s, the development of clinically important resistance to azoles was rare. However, during the last 6 years treatment failures and appearance of resistant isolates have increasingly been reported, especially in AIDS patients who are receiving intermittent or continuous Flu therapy for oropharyngeal candidosis [165, 168, 169]. Risk factors predisposing resistance to azoles, particularly Flu, are HIV infection, advanced stage of immunosuppression (low number of CD4 T cells), recurrent oral candidosis and prior azole use [168, 170].

Therapeutic failure of antifungal therapy is based either on microbiological resistance due to the fungus or on clinical resistance due to host factors. The clinical resistance may be seen in extremely immunosuppressed patients who fail to respond to therapy despite high susceptibility of the fungus and adequate concentrations of the drug or in patients with unfavorable drug interactions. Microbiological resistance is based on two mechanisms: the originally sensitive fungus has become resistant, or a new agent has appeared with a lower susceptibility to the drug. In this section only the appearance of microbiological resistance is discussed.

Microbiological resistance of *Candida* to Flu has been appearing surprisingly fast in AIDS patients with recurrent oropharyngeal candidosis. In France, an increase in MICs combined with the first clinical failures have already been observed only 4 years after the first clinical trials with Flu. Before 1987 all *C. albicans* strains isolated from AIDS patients were highly sensitive: however, in the period 1990–91 roughly 40% of the isolated strains showed an MIC >12.5 µg/ml [168]. Gradual increase in MIC values, together with therapeutic unresponsiveness, has also been observed in other parts of the world after intermittent or continuous use of Flu for oral candidosis in AIDS patients [169, 171–173].

Oropharyngeal candidosis may also be caused by a mixed population of sensitive and resistant yeasts, and under Flu therapy the resistant species may become dominant [169, 172, 174]. An AIDS patient suffering simultaneously from oral candidosis and from Candida meningitis was found to harbor two different but resistant strains of *C. albicans*; one caused the oral, the other the disseminated candidosis [175].

Transmission of strains between HIV-positive partners can occur [172, 176], but it remains unclear whether azole-resistant strains of *C. albicans* can persist if transmitted to HIV-negative persons. Not only *Candida* strains, but also other yeasts, may become resistant to Flu. To date, three cases of resistant *Cryptococcus* strains have been diagnosed under prolonged maintenance therapy with Flu [172]. It seems that the acquisition of resistance to Flu causes a major problem in AIDS patients with relapsing oral candidosis and less so in other immunosuppressed patients who received Flu therapy only for a short term. Only a few reports describe the appearance of resistance to Flu in HIV-negative patients [172]. Infections with *C. krusei*, an organism with intrinsic resistance to Flu have been diagnosed in conjunction with Flu prophylaxis. Primary Flu-resistant *C. albicans* strains could be isolated from non-HIV-infected patients who were never before exposed to Flu; this finding is of concern for the future [177].

There is not yet clear evidence that the pattern of strains causing invasive infections has changed since the introduction of Flu. A. Kunova and colleagues [178] claim that use of Flu is not associated with a higher incidence of *C. krusei* or other non-*albicans C.* species. M.F. Price and collaborators [179] studied the distribution of species isolated from blood over a 5-year period and found a clear change in the pattern. The susceptibility to Flu remained the same, but the number of isolated *C. albicans* decreased, whereas *C. glabrata, C. tropicalis* and *C. parapsilosis* increased. The emergence of new, non-*C. albicans* strains was also observed in a prospective study of patients with candidemia. *C. krusei* and *C. parapsilosis* were isolated more frequently from patients with prior prophylactic Flu than either *Candida* spp. C. krusei is innately resistant to Flu, but also 40% of the isolated *C. parapsilosis* strains showed resistance to the drug [180].

Three major mechanisms of resistance to Flu have been identified: decreased binding affinity to the P450 cytochrome enzyme, increased production of the drug target cytochrome P450 [181] and, most important, decreased accumulation of Flu in the fungal cell due to reduced uptake or increased efflux [168, 182–185]. The mechanism of Flu efflux can be inhibited by compounds (like Azid) blocking the active metabolism of ions. Other mechanisms of action have been identified on the level of the ergosterol pathway [186].

The presence or absence of cross-resistance between azoles may be explained on the basis of these different mechanisms causing resistance. Fungal isolates have been observed with a 10-fold increase of MIC for both Flu and Itra; other isolated strains were found to be resistant to Flu but remained more or less sensitive to Itra. This phenomenon may be explained as a different mechanism of resistance related to the hydrosolublility or liposolubility of the two drugs [171, 187, 188].

Sensitivity to Flu seems to correlate with adherence capacity. Flu-resistant *C. albicans* showed slightly less adherence to buccal epithelial cells than did sensitive ones. 5-FC resistant mutants have also shown lower virulence than the sensitive *C. albicans* [157]. It may be that Flu-resistant fungal cells are less virulent. This would explain why rapid appearance of resistance to Flu is only seen in severely immunosuppressed AIDS patients and not yet so often in more immunocompetent cancer patients, and why transmission of resistant strains to HIV-negative persons has not yet been described.

4.3.5.2   Safety
Flu is generally better tolerated than Keto. Nausea, vomiting, rash and asymptomatic elevations of plasma aminotransferases occur in less than

5% of the patients [2, 164, 165]. The adverse effects on levels in the liver and the endocrine system are significantly lower and less severe than with Keto; hepatoxicity is rare, and inhibition of the steroidogenesis has not yet been detected. However, Flu has been reported to worsen liver function in case of an antecedent hepatitis [189]. The risk of hepatotoxicity is reported to be increased in HIV-positive patients.

A short course of Flu seems to have no influence on the outcome of pregnancy. Flu was taken by 289 women for vaginal candidosis before or during pregnancy with no harmful effects [190]. However, prolonged treatment with Flu for coccidioidomycosis induced congenital abnormalities in three infants; only one of them survived [191].

4.3.5.3   Drug interactions

In contrast to Keto, only a minimal number of interactions between Flu and other agents have been described [164, 165, 192]. H_2-receptor antagonists have no effect on the absorption of Flu [193]. Coadministration of rifampicin reduces the plasma level of Flu [194]. The major interaction is seen with phenytoin, in which Flu causes a rise of the plasma level and increased toxicity of the phenytoin [195]. In addition, Flu occasionally increases the level of cyclosporin, tolbutamide and other sulfonylurea drugs. Flu also strongly influences the metabolism of warfarin, leading to a change in prothrombin time [196–198].

4.3.5.4   Therapeutic indications in opportunistic mycoses
Candidosis
Oropharyngeal candidosis is the most frequent complication of HIV infection, affecting 80–90% of patients at some point during the disease. Symptomatic oesophagal candidosis becomes common as the CD4 count drops below 100/ml [168, 169]. During recent years, the relative good safety of oral azoles has led to their widespread use as a first-line treatment for this indication. Flu at doses of 50–100 mg/day has become the first choice, since it has proven to be superior to Keto [92, 107, 164]. Oral Flu administered for 7–21 days cured 71% and improved 16% of 103 HIV-infected patients with oral candidosis [199]. Short-term Flu treatment for 5 days showed favorable clinical success in 85% of oral candidosis episodes [171].

Flu also proved its beneficial effect in oesophagal candidosis; the long-term efficacy has been proven in 1105 AIDS patients [200]. Flu was already curative in more than 80% of the cases 2 weeks after the treatment started. At months 6 and 12, endoscopic and clinical cures were observed in 97% of patients. High clinical response with Flu was also reported in cancer patients. The efficacy of Flu appears to be equivalent to that of Amph B, but with the advantage of fewer side-effects [201, 202, 202a].

A new galenical formulation – a Flu suspension – brings the advantage of higher concentration in the saliva than the conventional capsules, leading to an additional local effect against *Candida* oropharyngitis or oesophagitis. A prospective study showed that Flu suspension achieved a faster clinical response than the old Flu capsules [203, 204].

It may be argued whether prevention therapy for symptomatic recurrence of thrush is advisable. In 1994 [205], a study clearly showed that the probability of recurrent oral candidosis was significantly decreased in patients continuing long-term therapy with Keto or Flu. Some authors even claim that empirical Flu treatment would be a more cost-effective strategy than one that starts treatment only after confirmation of the disease [206]. However, neither prevention nor empirical treatment with Flu is yet fully established for oral candidosis.

The development of clinical resistance combined with decreased *in vitro* susceptibility in AIDS patients is a new challenge. It may be that in the near future alternative treatment schedules will have to be developed. Up to now, Flu-resistant oral candidosis was found to respond to high doses of Flu, which can be safely administered to HIV-positive patients, or to Itra [207–209]. However, with increasing Flu-resistant oral candidosis, clinicians may choose to use the new oral Amph B suspension which was recently approved by the FDA [169].

Flu was as effective but better tolerated than Amph B in the treatment of candidemia without neutropenia [193, 210]. Similar efficacy of Flu compared with Amph B was also reported for haematogenous candidosis in cancer patients, in surgical patients or in patients under treatment for haematological malignancy [193, 211–212a]. Systemic candidosis in neutropenic or otherwise severely immunocompromised patients should still be treated with the fungicidal Amph B combined with 5-FC [213].

Flu has become the first choice for the treatment of neonatal candidosis, since Flu showed a high clinical response without severe adverse effects in contrast to Amph B, which is poorly tolerated in neonates [193, 214–216]. Even a case of *Candida* meningitis was cured by Flu therapy in a premature infant [217].

The syndrome of hepatosplenic candidosis is rather slow in responding to therapy. The best regimen seems to be an initial therapy with Amph B with or without 5-FC followed by Flu [213, 218].

Ocular fungal infections respond favorably to treatment with Flu, since this drug is evenly distributed in all body fluids, including ocular fluid. Flu has been successfully used for *Candida* endophthalmitis in heroin addicts

[219]. Flu as sole long-term therapy achieved a 94% cure rate in 15 affected eyes, including five infections complicated by vitreitis [220].

Flu is also of value in treating complicated and uncomplicated fungal urinary tract infections. The observed high efficacy is based on the pharmacokinetic properties of Flu, which is mainly excreted as unchanged drug by the kidneys, and thus high concentrations are achieved in the urine [192]. Flu has proven to be a safe and more efficacious alternative to Amph B bladder irrigation [221, 222]. A short course of Flu has resulted in a prolonged clearance of yeasts, whereas intermittent bladder irrigation with Amph B has resulted in prompt but short-lived clearance [223]. We note, however, that appearance of Flu-resistant species has been observed, and these cases must of course be treated with Amph B [224].

Cryptococcosis

Overall, Flu has proven to be as effective as Amph B monotherapy for primary therapy of cryptococcal meningitis in patients with AIDS. The sterilization of the cerebrospinal fluid was, however, more rapid under Amph B treatment than with Flu [192, 193, 225, 226]. Thus, Amph B in combination with 5-FC remains the standard therapy for meningeal cryptococcosis in AIDS patients [107, 213]. Flu may be useful as initial therapy in mild cases of cryptococcosis in AIDS patients, since in one study non-meningeal cryptococcosis of 15 HIV-positive patients responded favorably to Flu monotherapy [227]. Chronic maintenance therapy is essential for all AIDS patients to avoid relapses of meningeal cryptococcosis. The prostate and meningen act as nidi of infection, inducing frequent relapses despite successful primary therapy. Flu has become the agent of choice for chronic maintenance therapy in AIDS-related cryptococcal meningitis [92, 107, 165, 192, 193].

Chronic prophylactic treatment with Flu for recurrent oral candidosis is described to influence the incidence of meningeal cryptococcosis in AIDS patients. Under weekly Flu maintenance therapy, only 4% of treated patients developed disseminated cryptococcosis compared with 14% of untreated patients [228]. However, long-term, low-dose therapy with Flu does not invariably prevent a clinical manifestation of severe cryptococcosis. In France, two fulminate cryptococcal infections have been diagnosed in AIDS patients on Flu [229].

Flu was found to be as effective as Amph B against cryptococcosis in HIV-negative patients [230, 231], but only a prospective large trial will determine the best treatment regimen for cryptococcosis in non-AIDS patients. Combination therapy with Amph B plus 5-FC is still the standard.

Aspergillosis and other mold infections
Flu is not recommended for invasive mold infections, since its therapeutic value is limited, even at extremely high doses (1600 mg/day) [232].

4.3.5.5 Therapeutic indications in endemic mycoses
The addition of Flu and itraconazole to the antifungal armamentarium has clearly been of benefit in the treatment of endemic deep mycoses, both drugs being less toxic and easier to handle than Amph B. Flu seems to be less active than Itra in the area of endemic mycoses and should, therefore, be considered as second-line therapy.
Favorable responses have been observed in immunocompetent patients with histoplasmosis, coccidioidomycosis, sporotrichosis and/or paracoccidiomycosis [54, 192, 193, 233]. Flu seems to be only moderately efficacious against blastomycosis; relatively high doses are needed to see a positive clinical effect [234]. In histoplasmosis, Flu is less efficacious than itraconazole and should, therefore, be used only for those infections that do not respond to itraconazole [234a].
Flu has been reported as efficacious as itraconazole for non-meningeal coccidioidomycosis. Thus, Flu has become the drug of first choice for non-meningeal coccidioidomycosis [54]. Unfortunately, an extremely high relapse rate has been observed after azole therapy is stopped, and lifelong suppression therapy is needed for this indication [233]. No curative therapy exists for meningeal coccidioidomycosis; new therapeutic approaches are urgently needed.
Amph B therapy remains the standard for all endemic infections in severely immunocompromised patients. In AIDS patients, maintenance therapy is always necessary after an initial successful therapy with Amph B. Flu has proven to be effective in preventing relapses of disseminated histoplasmosis in AIDS [193, 235].

4.3.6 Itraconazole
- Itra is the first choice in sporotrichosis, histoplasmosis and blastomycosis in non- AIDS patients.
- Itra is fungicidal against *Aspergillus* spp.
- Itra shows promising results in aspergillosis.
- Itra is used as maintenance therapy in histoplasmosis in AIDS patients.

In contrast to Flu, Itra is highly lipophilic and has a broader antifungal spectrum, including dematiaceous fungi and molds, especially *Aspergillus* spp. Itra has a unique characteristic among the azoles: it is fungicidal against aspergilli. This fungicidal effect is not associated with the typical mode of action, the inhibition of sterol biosynthesis, but is due to direct interaction of the molecule with the fungal membrane [1, 236, 236a].

Itra is available as an oral formulation only. Because the drug needs an acid pH in the stomach for good absorption, higher plasma levels are achieved when it is administered with a meal. Significant, unpredictable variation of plasma levels in patients often causes problems, and monitoring to assure adequate plasma levels is essential, especially in neutropenic patients [237].

Itra poorly penetrates into body fluids such as eye fluid, cerebrospinal fluid, sputum, tracheobronchial secretion and urine; however, it is well distributed into the tissues, reaching significantly higher levels in tissues than in plasma. Itra is especially accumulated in pus, fat and keratin; it is excreted in sebum and sweat [2, 164]. It is strongly protein-bound without losing its antifungal activity [238].

Itra is extensively metabolized by the liver and mainly excreted in the bile. Hydroxy-itraconazole, the major metabolite, is antifungally active and accounts for antifungal effects in the blood. Less than 1% of the mother compound and 34% of the inactive metabolites are excreted in the urine [2, 164, 193].

4.3.6.1   Resistance

Development of resistance to Itra has not yet caused the same level of concern as with Flu. The lower incidence of resistance may be due to the less widespread use of Itra for prevention or therapy of *Candida* infection. A survey in Spain, however, found a relatively high degree of resistance in clinical isolates: 8.5% of *C. albicans*, 34.3% of *C. tropicalis*, 4.4% of *C. glabrata* and 1.5% of *C. parapsilosis* were resistant to Itra [5].

4.3.6.2   Safety

Like Flu, Itra is relatively well tolerated with a significantly better safety profile than Amph B. Nausea is the most common side-effect (2.4–10.6%); less frequent are vomiting, abdominal pain, diarrhoea, headache and skin rashes. No effect on steroidal hormones has been observed. There have been reports on hypertension and hypokalaemia. Asymptomatic abnormalities of hepatic function occur in less than 3% of the patients. Reversible, apparently idiosyncratic hepatitis is rare. The use of Itra is, however, limited to 30 days in many countries, and periodic liver function tests may be necessary if Itra is given over a prolonged period of time [2, 164, 193, 239].

4.3.6.3 Drug interactions

Clinically significant interactions with other drugs are less frequent and less severe than with Keto, but they are more significant than with Flu [193]. H_2 antagonists, ormeprazole and all drugs increasing intragastric pH, including those formulations with buffering agents such as didanosine, significantly decrease the absorption of Itra. Combination with these drugs should be avoided in order not to hamper the already poor absorption of Itra [193, 240].

Coadministration of rifampicin reduces the plasma concentration of Itra to undetectable levels [241]. Interactions are also seen with phenytoin, isoniazid, carbamazepine and phenobarbital. Itra significantly increases the plasma concentration and the pharmacodynamic effect of midazolam and triazolam, but not of temazepam [193, 242, 243]. The same potentiation is seen with digoxin [244], lovastatin [245], terfenadine [246], warfarin and cyclosporin. The plasma levels of all these coadministered drugs have to be monitored and the dose adjusted accordingly [2, 193].

4.3.6.4 Therapeutic indications in opportunistic mycoses

Candidosis

The role of Itra for the therapy of muccosal or disseminated candidosis is still open. Itra showed clinical response in oropharyngeal and oesophageal candidosis. In a comparative trial, Itra achieved marginally better clinical response than did Keto [247], but Flu is still the first choice of treatment for these indications. In a study of 2213 AIDS patients with *Candida* oesophagitis, Itra compared favorably with Flu: after 2 weeks of treatment the response rate was higher under Flu than under Itra therapy (81.2 vs 65.6%), but after long-term follow-up, both agents achieved a success rate of 96% [202a]. Itra also showed promising results in Flu-resistant *Candida* oropharyngitis or oesophagitis [168, 172, 248].

In two studies, Itra has been reported to be as effective as Amph B for candidosis in neutropenic patients [249, 250]. The widespread use of Itra for disseminated candidosis in neutropenic patients is, however, not recommended because of its erratic bioavailability in neutropenic patients [237] and the lack of large clinical trials.

Cryptococcosis

Itra was found to be active in murine cryptococcosis, but its role for therapy or prevention of human cryptococcosis is not clear; the drug is neither fully accepted as first-line treatment nor as maintenance therapy for cryptococcosis in AIDS patients. Flu has become the first choice for maintenance therapy in this indication.

Itra alone – or in combination with 5-FC – has achieved clinical response as first-line therapy for cryptococcal meningitis in AIDS patients despite its low level in the cerebrospinal fluid [1, 54, 193, 251–253, Sec. 3.7]. The agent was also successfully used for prevention of relapses, although the available data suggest inferior efficacy compared with Flu. For patients at risk for aspergillosis, Itra may be the better choice [92, 193].

Aspergillosis

Invasive aspergillosis remains a devastating opportunistic infection despite Amph B therapy. An overall response rate to Amph B of 55% has been observed in all host groups at all sites of the disease [254]. The outcome of antifungal therapy in aspergillosis strongly depends on the immunological status of the host; no cure can be achieved if the immunosuppression is not overcome.

Itra represents a real step forward in the battle against various forms of aspergillosis, including pulmonary, disseminated aspergillosis, aspergilloma and allergic bronchopulmonary aspergillosis. It is the first oral and safe agent active against aspergillosis. Early non-comparative trials suggested that the efficacy of Itra is similar to that of Amph B with the advantage of lower toxicity and the possibility of treating outpatients for a prolonged period of time (for details, see Suppl. 1 of Chemotherapy 38, 1992, and [255–257]).

In a thorough, well-controlled multi-center study [258], Itra proved to be a useful alternative therapy for invasive aspergillosis with response rates apparently similar to Amph B. The overall response rate at the end of the treatment was 39%, and the failure rate attributable to Itra therapy was 26%. In this kind of aspergillosis, the clinical response to antifungal therapy varies widely according to the site of infection and the underlying disease. Itra failure was seen in 14% of the pulmonary or tracheobronchial disease, in 50% of the sinus cases and in 63% of the CNS cases. The highest failure rate was seen in AIDS patients (44%) compared with 14% in those with prolonged granulocytopenia and 29% in allogeneic bone marrow transplants. Post-treatment follow-up showed a relatively high relapse rate in patients who were still immunocompromised. Thus, Itra clearly is of benefit in treating invasive aspergillosis, but the underlying immunosuppression should simultaneously be resolved; otherwise relapses may occur.

Invasive aspergillosis is recognized as a major cause of morbidity and mortality after lung transplantation. Itra was reported to be safe and highly efficacious in preventing dissemination of *Aspergillus* infection if it was promptly used for non-invasive bronchitis after lung transplantation [259].

One case of chronic (over 10 years) invasive paranasal aspergillosis was cured with Itra despite an initial poor prognosis [260].

Itra at a high dose of 800 mg/day has been reported to be effective in a case of cerebral aspergillosis that did not respond to conventional Amph B therapy. The authors suggest that high doses of Itra may improve the prognosis for refractory cerebral aspergillosis [261].

Itra is clearly a breakthrough for the therapy of aspergilloma. Before the appearance of Itra, surgery offered the only possibility of eradicating an aspergilloma. Nowadays Itra therapy replaces surgery in all cases where there is no danger of hemoptysis [1].

The standard therapy for allergic bronchopulmonary aspergillosis is corticosteroid therapy without addition of antifungals. Addition of Itra to steroid therapy seems to improve the clinical outcome and lowers the requirement for steroids. In patients with cystic fibrosis, Itra may even be curative as monotherapy [262, 263].

Phaeohyphomycosis

Phaeohyphomycosis is a new classification for a diverse group of previously known entities grouped together on the basis of finding dematiaceous fungi in tissue. Tissue involvement may be superficial, cutaneous, subcutaneous, corneal or systemic. The infections occur both in immunocompetent and immunocompromised patients.

Itra has been dramatically successful in individual patients [264, 264a]. Cutaneous infections caused by *Alternaria* sp. in normal and immunosuppressed patients were successfully cured with Itra [265, 266]. Itra rapidly cleared subcutaneous phaeohyphomycosis due to *Exophiala jeanselmei* in a diabetic patient and in three cardiac transplant recipients. None of these patients had evidence of dissemination [267, 268]. Sinonasal *Alternaria* infection refractory to Amph B treatment markedly improved in response to Itra therapy. Itra therapy was, however, unsuccessful in one case of cerebral phaeohyphomycosis caused by *Dactylaria* [269].

The number of patients with phaeohyphomycosis is so small that no comparative trials are likely ever to occur. Thus, changes in therapy will be based on individual reports. The optimal duration of therapy with Itra is not yet determined. Relapses seem to occur if Itra is stopped too early. Despite all these unknowns, it is clear that Itra has a definite place in this rare but sometimes dangerous indication.

4.3.6.5   Therapeutic indications in endemic mycoses

Itra is of greatest benefit in endemic mycoses; histoplasmosis, blastomycosis, paracoccidiodomycosis, coccidioidomycosis and sporotrichosis all respond favorably to Itra therapy [54, 165, 193].

Histoplasmosis

Before the advent of azoles, Amph B was the drug of choice in patients with chronic pulmonary and disseminated histoplasmosis. Keto and especially Itra became safe and effective alternatives to Amph B. The response rate among patients with chronic pulmonary histoplasmosis treated for at least 2 months was 86% [54]. Patients with disseminated histoplasmosis responded even better.

Disseminated histoplasmosis is an increasingly recognized opportunistic fungal infection in AIDS patients [54,165]. It is currently standard to initiate maintenance therapy after successful primary therapy with Amph B or Itra. (Itra was found to be effective for both primary and maintenance therapy.) Wheat et al. [270] found a cure rate of 85% among AIDS patients with mild to moderate histoplasmosis; Amph B is recommended for severe histoplasmosis in AIDS patients. A total of 93% of the AIDS patients remained relapse-free when Itra was given as maintenance therapy [271].

Blastomycosis

In recent years, Itra has replaced Amph B in the treatment of blastomycosis in non-AIDS patients and has become the agent of choice. A response rate of 90–95% has been achieved [272].

Paracoccidioidomycosis

Based on positive clinical results, Itra is also recommended as therapy in paracoccidioidomycosis [273].

Coccidioidomycosis

The appearance of azoles has markedly changed the approach to the treatment of coccidioidomycosis. A prolonged course of therapy is still needed, but this is much easier to handle with a safe oral drug than with the parenteral Amph B. Itra appears to be effective in meningeal and non-meningeal coccidioidomycosis [54]; however, the response rates are lower than the ones seen in histoplasmosis and blastomycosis. Flu and Itra achieve the same degree of efficacy in chronic coccidioidomycosis in contrast to histoplasmosis and blastomycosis, where Itra is superior to Flu. Flu may be the better choice for meningeal coccidioidomycosis based on its pharmacokinetic properties.

Sporotrichosis
Itra is clearly the agent of first choice for the treatment of all forms of sporotrichosis. It achieved a higher efficacy than Keto or Flu against this disease, reaching response rates of 90-100%. For lymphocutaneous sporotrichosis, treatment duration is usually 3–6 months with doses of 100–200 mg per day. Osteoarticular sporotrichosis is more problematic; higher doses (400 mg/day) and a prolonged treatment period is necessary (>1 year) to achieve good clinical response. Pulmonary sporotrichosis is refractory to all therapies. Neither Amph B nor Itra achieve high cure rates; lifelong therapy may be needed for this form of the disease. Lengthy treatment is easier to handle with the oral than with the parenteral drug [54, 274].

4.3.7   Combination therapy
* Combination therapy broadens spectrum, increases efficacy and reduces appearance of resistant strains.
* Combination of 5-FC plus Amph B is still the gold standard for the acute phase of cryptococcal meningitis.
* Triple combinations of 5-FC plus Amph B plus Flu are used in Europe for cryptococcal meningitis in AIDS patients.
* Combination therapy of 5-FC plus Itra broadens the spectrum in chromomycosis.

Combination therapy has found its place in the antifungal field since the first detection of the synergistic effect of 5-FC plus Amph B by Medoff and co-workers in 1971 [275]. Studies *in vitro* and particularly in animal models have shown that a real increase in efficacy can be achieved with certain combinations in some indications, but that others should be avoided, as they are antagonistic. Based on these preclinical studies, drug combinations have increasingly been used in clinical situations. For years the combination of 5-FC plus Amph B was considered the gold standard for meningeal cryptococcosis.

4.3.7.1   Pre-clinical studies
The results of combination studies *in vitro* and *in vivo* strongly depend on the fungal strain, the methodology, the animal species and last but not least on the antifungal drug used. The published *in vitro* data show a great variability and are rather controversial; however, the following general conclusion can be drawn: 5-FC plus Amph B is additive or synergistic against most of the opportunistic fungal strains, especially against 5-FC-resistant strains. Amph B and the azoles act as antagonists when added simultaneously or when an azole is added first, but synergy has been ob-

served in cases where the azole was added to cells that were pre-treated with sub-inhibitory concentrations of Amph B. Azoles and 5-FC are usually indifferent, occasionally additive and never antagonistic [1, 276–278]. Combination therapy has been and is still studied in animal models of a variety of infections in normal and neutropenic animals. The results of the animal models vary to a greater extent than those of the *in vitro* studies. The outcome strongly depends on the dose, the application route, the type of infection and the end-points. Most animal work has been done with the combination of 5-FC plus Amph B, but other combinations have also been examined.

5-FC plus Amph B improved activity in murine candidosis, cryptococcosis, wangiellosis and to a lesser extent in aspergillosis. With this combination a real microbiological cure can be achieved in *Candida*-infected mice which is never achieved with realistic doses of single antimycotics in this model [276, 279].

Additionally, in neutropenic rabbits only this combination was able to eradicate renal candidosis, which neither Flu nor Itra was able to achieve [280]. The combination of 5-FC with azoles has a beneficial effect in most cases, and no antagonism is apparent. The degree of interaction is weak with Keto, but strong with Flu and Itra. The synergism was most impressive in murine wangiellosis [277, 279]. However, a study recently proved that in cryptococcosis in hamsters the combination of 5-FC plus Itra was less effective than a high dose of Itra [281].

The situation with a combination of Amph B and an antifungal belonging to the class of azoles is more controversial and strongly dependent on the fungal species. No interaction was seen between Amph B and Keto in histoplasmosis and blastomycosis. Synergy was apparent with Amph B combined with Keto, Flu or Itra in murine cryptococcosis, but antagonism or indifference was observed in murine candidosis or aspergillosis. In neutropenic, *Aspergillus*-infected mice, pre-treatment with Keto for 24–48 h completely abolished the curative effect of Amph B therapy [279, 282]. In a similar aspergillosis study, Itra also showed antagonism, but to a lesser degree [283]. In histoplasmosis prophylactic treatment with Keto had no effect on the outcome of Amph B therapy [279]. Results of a recent study combining Amph B with Flu in murine candidosis indicated that this combination was not antagonistic *in vivo*, in contrast to the *in vitro* findings [284]. In trichosporonosis, the combination of Amph B plus Flu proved to be more active in prolonging survival and reducing fungal burden in the kidney than either drug alone [285].

The triple combination of Amph B plus 5-FC and Flu or Itra was tested in various animal models. This triple combination was the optimal therapy for murine cryptococcosis, while a slight antagonism was seen in *Candida* and *Aspergillus* infections [49].

These pre-clinical results of antifungal combinations have not remained in a vacuum but have shown themselves to be predictive for clinical use.

Cryptococcosis

For years the combination of 5-FC plus Amph B has been the optimal treatment for cryptococcal meningitis. The rationale was to accelerate killing of the organism and prevent emergence of 5-FC resistance. The superiority of this combination over monotherapy with Amph B was proven in non-AIDS patients by two randomized prospective clinical trials [286, 287]. Faster sterilization of the cerebrospinal fluid was seen as well as a more rapid clinical response and an overall higher cure rate.

Encouraged by the positive clinical results of Flu monotherapy and the proven synergism of 5-FC plus Flu in animal cryptococcosis [279, 288], a study was launched by the Mycosis Study Group of the National Institute of Allergy and Infectious Diseases (NIAID) to evaluate the beneficial value of this combination in cryptococcal meningitis of non-AIDS patients. This study was terminated, however, because of the progression of the disease in several patients [121].

Thus, despite search for alternative treatment schedules and despite occasional safety problems, which can be overcome by serially monitoring the 5-FC level, the combination of 5-FC plus Amph B remains the optimal treatment for cryptococcosis in non-AIDS patients [289].

The situation with *Cryptococcus* in AIDS is more confused. The illness proceeds more aggressively and is far more difficult to eradicate, as reservoirs of infection seem to remain especially in the prostate even after the therapy has apparently succeeded. A high relapse rate is the rule if maintenance therapy with Flu or Itra is not installed. The optimal therapy for cryptococcosis in AIDS patients has not yet been found, and a great variety of different treatment schedules exist in this difficult clinical setting.

In the United States alternative regimens to the standard combination of 5-FC plus Amph B have been sought, especially since Americans fear the myelosuppressive adverse effects of 5-FC. However, neither Amph B nor Flu monotherapy showed high cure rates in the acute phase of cryptococcal meningitis in AIDS patients. Flu proved to be as efficacious as Amph B monotherapy, with a 34–40% successful outcome [290].

Yet in a retrospective study by White and co-workers [291], an aggressive combination therapy regimen with 5-FC [100 mg/kg/day) plus Amph B [1.0 mg/kg/day) cured 78% of patients with AIDS and 43% of patients with neoplastic diseases. Based on these results, the combination of 5-FC plus Amph B was revived and is still used for all high-risk patients, at least for the acute phase of the disease. Based on these positive findings, a randomized, double-blind clinical trial of the Mycosis Study Group-AIDS Clinical Trial Group (MSG-ACTG) was initiated. After a 2-week initiation phase with the combination of 5-FC plus Amph B, a consolidation phase follows with either Flu or Itra monotherapy for another 8 weeks. The final results of this study are not yet published, but results of the initial therapy look encouraging [107].

A Californian study group was interested in evaluating the combination of 5-FC plus Flu for therapy of cryptococcal meningitis in AIDS patients [292]. The rate of clinical success was significantly greater than that previously reported for Amph B or Flu monotherapy. A total of 75% of the patients had negative culture in the cerebrospinal fluid 10 weeks after initiation of the therapy; only 35–40% of the cultures became negative under monotherapy. The overall clinical success was 63% with the combination. However, toxic side-effects that were sufficiently severe to lead to withdrawal of 5-FC were observed in 28% of the patients. Thus, additional trials have to be performed to define the future place of this combination in the treatment of cryptococcal meningitis in AIDS patients.

Another problem regarding Flu treatment deserves mention; the appearance of Flu-resistant *Cryptococcus* strains is drastically increasing. In 1987 10% of the strains were resistant to Flu, whereas in 1992 50% of the strains were Flu-resistant. The emergence of resistant strains may be enhanced by the use of Flu as primary prophylaxis. It does not look as if the combination of 5-FC plus Flu will replace the standard combination of 5-FC plus Amph B in the near future.

In Europe Flu and Itra monotherapy have been successfully used, but the combination of 5-FC plus Itra works faster and better [293]. In Germany the triple combination of 5-FC plus Amph B plus Flu proved to be highly efficacious [294, and Habilitation work of G. Just-Nübling], and this triple combination is now routinely used in several German and Swiss hospitals, as well as in tropical areas [295, 296].

The large number of variations employed in just one narrow area, cryptococcosis in AIDS, clearly demonstrates that combination therapy opens up many possibilities, but it also demonstrates that this fungal disease is rather difficult to eradicate.

Candidosis

Combination therapy has also proven its worth in deep-seated *Candida* infection [49, 213]. Response to therapy is strongly dependent on both the location of infection and the underlying disease. In some cases monotherapy is sufficient to eradicate the mycosis; in others combination therapy with 5-FC plus Amph B is needed to win the battle.

Candida fungaemia may resolve spontaneously after removal of the catheter, but it also may cause endophthalmitis. *Candida* endophthalmitis has been found in 28–37% of non-neutropenic patients with *Candida* fungaemia. Endophthalmitis has to be treated aggressively with prolonged therapy (preferentially a combination of 5-FC and Amph B), to minimize visual impairment and to effect a complete cure of the infection, which in most cases has disseminated to other organs, too [297].

In neutropenic patients the need for fungicidal chemotherapy is paramount, and the combination of 5-FC plus Amph B has achieved the best results here. Bone marrow recovery is, however, necessary to achieve cure. A recent study in 28 neutropenic patients showed an extremely poor clinical outcome under Amph B monotherapy, as well as under combination therapy with 5-FC plus Amph B, because the mycoses were too far advanced at the time therapy was started, and the recovery of neutrophils was achieved in only half of the patients [298]. The combination of 5-FC plus Amph B showed its highest degree of success in infections due to *Candida tropicalis*, a species that is regularly more resistant to Amph B than *C. albicans* [213]. In the future other combinations, like 5-FC plus Flu or 5-FC plus Itra, may be successful in these clinical situations; however, no results of clinical trials are yet available.

The syndrome of hepatosplenic candidosis or chronic progressive candidosis is increasingly recognized in patients recovering from neutropenia. This form of *Candida* infection, which responds very slowly to therapy, is another candidate for an initial combination therapy with 5-FC plus Amph B followed by Flu monotherapy if cure is not rapidly achieved.

Candida meningitis or encephalitis, as well as *Candida* endocarditis, initially has to be treated with a combination therapy of 5-FC plus Amph B. *Candida* osteomyelitis or arthritis should be treated with a combination, since the efficacy of Flu monotherapy in these types of infections is not known. The combination of 5-FC plus Amph B is recommended by Filler and Edwards [297]; however, 5-FC plus Flu or 5-FC plus Itra may also be successful if the osteoarthritis is a sequel of the *Candida* syndrome in heroin addicts. *Candida* endocarditis is also preferentially treated with combination therapy. Recently, a successful treatment of fungal prosthetic valve endocarditis with 5-FC plus Flu was reported [299].

Candida peritonitis can lead to complications and interruption of dialysis treatment. Monotherapy does not achieve cure without removal of the catheter, according to most authors [300]. However, combination therapy with 5-FC plus Amph B, 5-FC plus Keto and 5-FC plus Flu have all given high cure rates (>93%) without removal of the catheter [300, 301].

The *Candida* syndrome peculiar to heroin addicts [302] responds well to monotherapy with Keto or newer triazoles if the infection is restricted to the skin. However, combination therapy is needed as soon as other localizations are additionally involved. In the case of concomitant endophthalmitis, combination therapy eradicates the fungal infection sufficiently quickly to save the patient's sight, whereas under monotherapy the fungal disease is cured, but the eyesight is lost.

Aspergillosis

Aspergillosis responds so poorly to antifungal therapy that more emphasis is put on prevention or empirical therapy than in other indications. For therapy, the combination 5-FC plus Amph B also seems to be superior to monotherapy, especially when the diagnosis is made early and high doses of Amph B are used. Burch and co-workers [303] reported 90% survival in granulocytopenic patients, but they used an unusually high dose of Amph B (1.5 mg/kg/day). Walsh and Pizzo [304] are likewise recommending the combination of 5-FC plus Amph B for aspergillosis, especially at the beginning of the therapy. The combination of 5-FC plus Itra may lead to higher success rates, but no results from clinical trials are yet available.

Phaeohyphomycosis

Phaeohyphomycosis is defined as an invasive infection due to Dematiaceae, a family of fungi characterized by the production of brown pigment. All dematiaceous fungi are highly sensitive to 5-FC and Itra; a combination of 5-FC plus Itra may become the most beneficial treatment for this rare infection. 5-FC plus Itra proved to be the therapy of choice in chromomycosis cases caused by *Fonsecaea pedrosoi* [49]. A case of disseminated phaeohyphomycosis due to Exophilia spinifera responded well to combination therapy with 5-FC plus Itra [305]. Controlled clinical trials are not feasible, because the patients are so scattered; therefore, anecdotes are likely to become the basis for any future change in the therapy of phaeohyphomycosis.

4.3.8   Immunomodulators
• Cytokines will become important adjuncts to conventional antifungal therapy in severely immunosuppressed patients.

There is, of course, more than one way to fight opportunistic fungal infections. The classical approach is chemotherapy with an effective, preferably fungicidal, antifungal. However, one could also use compounds that influence the virulence of the fungi or the host defenses. Knowledge concerning virulence is increasing, but at present the overall information is still too scarce to be of practical use in drug design. The ability to influence the host immune system, however, has become a reality. Knowledge of the host defense against fungal infections is steadily accumulating, and research in immunology has characterized much of the body's diverse armament of interleukins, interferons, colony-stimulating factors, tumor necrosis factor etc. Various cytokines have been isolated, and several have been produced using biotechnological methods [1, 306].

In the last 6 years, most of these factors have been thoroughly investigated *in vitro* and in animal models to define their role in the defense against fungal infections. Some were found to show a deteriorating capacity, increasing the acute course of fungal infection. For example, circulating levels of interleukin-4 accelerate the death of *Candida*-infected mice. The survival time of such mice could be significantly prolonged by treatment with a recombinant soluble interleukin-4 receptor, leading to persistent ablation of circulating interleukin-4 [307].

Most immunomodulators, however, have the capacity to increase host defense. Interleukin-1α and -1β prolonged survival in lethal *Candida* infection. Histoplasmosis in mice is associated with depression of cellular immune response due to a deficiency in the production of interleukin-2. This cytokine is able to enhance natural killer cell activity through induction of interferon γ. Treatment with interleukin-2 has, however, no influence on the course of histoplasmosis. Interferon γ stimulates the antifungal activity of macrophages and/or polymorphonuclear neutrophils (PMNs). The growth of several fungi, including *C. albicans*, *Histoplasma capsulatum* and *Blastomyces dermatitidis*, was significantly more inhibited in the presence of interferon-γ-stimulated macrophages and/or PMNs than unstimulated ones [1, 306]. Interferon γ was found to be a very important component of normal defenses against systemic cryptococcosis [308]. The most promising immunomodulators for fungal infections appear to be granulocyte-, granulocyte-macrophage- and macrophage-colony stimulating factors (G-CSF, GM-CSF, M-CSF). G-CSF treatment results in significant protection against systemic infections caused by *C. albicans* or *Aspergillus fumigatus* in neutropenic (cyclophosphamide-treated but not cortisone-treated) mice [309]. It was clearly of interest to investigate whether a synergistic effect exists when cytokines are added to conventional antifungal therapy. The available animal data and *in vitro* data with macrophages clearly show that addition of various immunomodulators augments the beneficial effect of conventional antifungals.

Interferon-γ has been found to act *in vitro* synergistically with Amph B, increasing the intracellular killing of *Cryptococcus neoformans* in murine macrophages [310]. The combination of interferon-γ and Amph B also proved beneficial in murine cryptococcosis. The reduction of the *Cryptococcus* load in the brain was significantly faster and more efficacious than with either regime alone [311, 312]. However, no synergistic activity was seen when Flu was used instead of Amph B.

The addition of G-CSF to antifungal therapy clearly augments the beneficial effect of the antimycotic drug in candidosis and aspergillosis, but not so in cryptococcosis [313, 314]. GM-CSF exerts effects broadly similar to those of G-CSF, but there are fewer data available on this cytokine. M-CSF, known to enhance the anticryptococcal activity of macrophages and PMNs, showed a clear synergistic effect with Flu, drastically increasing the killing capacity [315, 316]. M-CSF in combination with Flu also significantly increased the median survival time of rats infected with *C. albicans* [317].

Thus, the role of cytokines alone or in combination is better understood now than 6 years ago, and the confidence in using cytokines in human chemotherapy for fungal infections has grown significantly.

Large clinical trials are not yet available, but literature on the use of cytokines alone (as prevention) or combined with an antimycotic drug (as an adjunct to therapy) is accumulating. No guidelines concerning the appropriate dose and duration of therapy are yet available, but the adjunct therapy with cytokines has become more accepted.

The data from preliminary human studies combining cytokines with traditional antifungal therapy generally suggest that augmentation of the immune response complements the effect of antifungal therapy. For example, reversal of immunodeficiency is essential to successful recovery from invasive aspergillosis. The depth and duration of granulocytopenia can be decreased by addition of G-CSF or GM-CSF to conventional antifungal therapy, leading to more rapid and complete recovery [65a]. Interferon-γ proved of benefit in the treatment of CNS aspergillosis in a patient with chronic granulomatous disease. The patient recovered after combination therapy with interferon-γ plus Amph B followed by a combination of interferon-γ plus Itra [318]. A case of *Aspergillus* sinusitis refractory to conventional therapy was successfully cured under a combination therapy of interferon-γ plus Amph B, Itra and 5-FC [319].

Most clinical work has been done with the various colony stimulating factors (G-CSF, GM-CSF, M-CSF). Several encouraging reports exist describing the use of G-CSF in patients with fungal infections and underlying conditions that cause neutrophilic deficiency, such as aplastic anaemia or chronic granulomatous disease [121]. Promising results have been seen combining miconazole and G-CSF for the treatment of deep-seated mycoses in patients with gynaecological cancers [320]. Recently, the beneficial role of G-CSF in the management of two cases of unusual fungal infections caused by *Fusarium* or *Trichosporon* have been described. Both patients died from the underlying disease, but the fungal infections had been cured [321, 322].

GM-CSF has been used successfully as adjuvant therapy for various fungal infections in cancer patients [323]. A case of disseminated *Fusarium* infection has been described which was successfully treated with a concomitant therapy of granulocyte transfusion, GM-CSF and Amph B [324]. Bone marrow transplant recipients treated with M-CSF for proven aspergillosis fared better than did historical controls [121]. M-CSF was evaluated in a phase II study as adjuvant therapy in 15 transplant and 10 cancer patients with *Candida* or *Aspergillus* fungal infections. The patients treated with the combination of M-CSF plus Amph B survived longer than did those with Amph B alone. Long-term mortality was reduced by 19% [325].

In conclusion, even though the clinical data accumulated up to now are still limited, in the future these modulators will become important adjuncts to conventional antifungal therapy of established fungal infections in severely immunosuppressed patients. Additionally, these cytokines will find a permanent place in the prevention of fungal infections. The success in reducing the rate of infections in immunosuppressed patients has in some cases been remarkable, and awakens real hope for the future [326]. The costs of cytokines are unfortunately still rather high, preventing widespread use in patients at risk of developing fungal infections.

4.4   The methodology: Empirical and prophylactic therapy

4.4.1   Empirical therapy
- Empirical antifungal therapy should be initiated in patients who remain febrile despite broad antibacterial therapy.
- Amph B remains the agent of choice.
- The milieu in which empirical therapy is initiated is rapidly changing.

Patients receiving intensive cytotoxic chemotherapy or ablative radiation carry a high risk of acquiring invasive fungal infections, which are the major cause of morbidity and mortality in neutropenic patients. In these patients fever is initially managed with empirical broad spectrum antibiotic therapy; however, not all patients respond to this therapy. The probability that patients who remain febrile under antibiotic therapy have developed an invasive, not-yet-diagnosed fungal infection is extremely high. Empirical antifungal therapy with Amph B is usually initiated in these patients. The value of this approach was documented in the 1980's in two randomized clinical trials [326, 327]. These studies proved that the use of empirical Amph B in persistently or recurrently febrile neutropenic patients decreased the frequency, morbidity and mortality of invasive fungal infections. Amph B used empirically clearly reduces the occurrence of a broad spectrum of fungal infections, including aspergillosis, but it does not have the capacity to completely prevent the development of severe fungal infections. Under empirical Amph B breakthrough due to non-*albicans Candida*, *Aspergillus*, *Trichosporon*, *Fusarium* and *Blastoschizomyces* have been observed [65a, 328, 329].

In recent years a number of new developments have changed the environment in which empirical Amph B therapy was traditionally practiced. First, the azoles have appeared with their potential to be used as empirical antifungal therapy. They are generally better tolerated and easier to handle than is Amph B. Keto was not considered to be an appropriate alternative to Amph B, but Flu showed promising results. In a multicenter prospective study with granulocytopenic patients, Flu was found to be safer and as efficacious as Amph B [330]. Similar beneficial value of empirical Flu therapy was observed in a Japanese study [331]. However, in another study, Flu was less effective than Amph B: Flu took longer to achieve defervescence, and the frequency of fatal fungal infections was higher under Flu than under Amph B. Flu is, of course unable to prevent aspergillosis. Thus Flu is an interesting alternative for Amph B in some cases, but its definite place in empirical therapy is not yet defined.

The appearance of haematopoietic factors is another new development with an important impact on the use of empirical therapy. Immunomodulators such as G-CSF are able to reduce the duration of neutropenia, and as a consequence fewer patients will be at risk to attire deep fungal infections. Furthermore, reasonably effective antifungal prophylactic regimens exist nowadays which in many centers form a part of the routine care of neutropenic patients. Both new developments (introduction of growth factors and prevention therapy) have changed the conditions in which empirical Amph B is used. Several questions have newly to be addressed. The place of empirical Amph B therapy in patients already benefiting from the new treatments mentioned above has to be investigated, and the criteria to initiate an empirical antifungal therapy have to be defined anew. For example, at what point empirical Amph B should be started remains controversial; the answer most probably depends on local experience. If aspergillosis is the main problem, an aggressive approach with an early start of empirical Amph B is imperative; however, in centers where aspergillosis is a minor problem, a more liberal approach appears more appropriate, with a longer observation period under antibiotic therapy [332]. Recently J.S. Fraser and D.W. Denning [333] reappraised the empirical use of Amph B considering all new developments, and they have suggested that use of empirical Amph B be based on risk factors and prophylaxis.

4.4.2   Prophylaxis of fungal infections

- The advent of well-tolerated, absorbable antifungal agents like Flu and Itra have revolutionized the attitude of medical professionals towards prophylaxis.
- Antifungal prevention is the most rapidly changing field in antifungal chemotherapy.
- Guidelines for reducing the exposure to opportunistic pathogens have recently been established.

In recent decades the incidence of opportunistic invasive fungal infections has dramatically increased [334–337]. This phenomenon is explained partially by AIDS, the increased frequency of bone marrow and organ transplants, aggressive antineoplastic therapy and better control of the complications such as haemorrhage and bacterial infections. All these changes and improvements have led to an increase in the number of patients at risk for invasive fungal infections. The difficulty clinicians had in early diagnosing and successfully treating established fungal infections has resulted in a profound interest in preventing colonization and invasion in high-risk patients.

The success of prophylaxis depends on both the host and the pathogenicity of the fungus. Different measures have to be used to prevent an airborne *Aspergillus* infection compared with an endogenous *Candida* infection preceded by colonization of mucosal surfaces. Up to now, no single agent or technique was able to prevent all fungal infections in all patient groups. In the past, topical decontamination with oral polyenes or nonabsorbable azoles was widely used. Oral polyenes were beneficial against superficial infections by *Candida*, but the results in prevention of invasive fungal infections were not overwhelming [338]. Moreover oral polyenes are not well tolerated and do not prevent invasive aspergillosis [339]. Parenteral Amph B has clearly shown activity in prevention, but its widespread use has been hampered by its high rate of side-effects and its complicated handling.

Technical measures are useful to avoid the exposure of high-risk patients to aerosolized spores of *Aspergillus*. The isolation in laminar air-flow rooms equipped with high-efficiency particulate air filters (HEPA) have reduced the incidence of invasive aspergillosis. This technique is mandatory for all bone marrow transplant recipients.

Nasal administration of Amph B may be another prophylactic technique against infections by Aspergillus. Amph B aerosols have shown high effectiveness in preventing pulmonary aspergillosis in animal models [340, 341]. Based on these positive animal data, prophylaxis with aerosolized Amph B has been proposed for human chemotherapy as well. No thorough clinical trials are yet available, but preliminary results in lung transplant patients suggest that nasal Amph B may decrease the incidence of invasive aspergillosis [342]. Prophylaxis with aerosolized Amph B in bone marrow transplant patients was well tolerated and decreased the evidence of colonization of or infection with *Aspergillus* [343]. Thus, aerosolized Amph B should be further investigated to clarify its role in prevention of pulmonary aspergillosis.

The advent of the absorbable, well-tolerated triazoles Flu and Itra has revolutionized prevention against fungal infections. For the first time absorbable agents are available which are well tolerated and easy to handle. They clearly are predestined to replace parenteral Amph B in prevention; furthermore they can be more widely applied. Most clinical studies have been done with Flu, which is intensively used for therapy of oral candidosis and secondary prevention of recurrent oral candidosis or cryptococcosis in AIDS patients. Itra, on the other hand, holds promise for treatment and prophylaxis of aspergillosis.

In a large multicenter study with AIDS patients in an advanced state of disease, Flu given prophylactically was reported to reduce the frequency of cryptococcosis, mucosal candidosis and superficial fungal infections, but it did not influence the overall mortality rate [344]. Unfortunately, the study did not investigate the rates of Flu resistance. Thus the central question remains whether the benefits of primary prophylaxis outweigh the risk of drug resistance. Flu has recently also been successful in primary prophylaxis for cryptococcosis [344a]. Flu is, of course, unable to prevent aspergillosis, which has become an increasingly recognized opportunistic fungal infection among patients with advanced AIDS. Thus generalized primary prevention against fungal infections in patients with AIDS is not recommended. Primary prophylaxis with Flu has been investigated in a variety of patient groups, including bone marrow transplant recipients [345,

346], patients undergoing intensive chemotherapy for haematological neo-plasia [332,345,347], liver transplant recipients [348], surgical patients [349] and paediatric patients with cancer [350,351].

All clinical data confirm that Flu is better tolerated than is oral Amph B (in all comparative trials) and that Flu has a good safety profile in all patient groups [345,352–354]. In all clinical trials Flu significantly reduced the incidence of fungal colonization, in particular with respect to *C. albicans*. In connection with this vital reduction, Flu was found to prevent intra-abdominal candidosis in high-risk surgical patients [349]. Colonization of non-*albicans* species (*C. glabrata* or *tropicalis*) seems, however, to be increased under Flu prophylaxis [355–357, see also Sec. 3.5]. Prevention with Flu in bone marrow transplant recipients was reported to be associated with a high proportion of fungaemia due to *C. glabrata* [346]. A case of *C. tropicalis* fungaemia has been described in a leukaemic patient receiving Flu prophylaxis [358].

Most controlled clinical studies investigating the role of Flu in prevention clearly showed a benefit superior to other preventive measures. In all studies the use of empirical Amph B, the duration of fever and the incidence of superficial infections was reduced [345,347,350,353,359].

The results regarding the efficacy of Flu on the survival and on the incidence of invasive fungal infections is still controversial. Many clinical trials have demonstrated a significant reduction of deep fungal infections [345, 351,355,360,361]. In a comparative study with clotrimazole, the chance of survival was found to be increased under Flu prophylaxis [345]. In a study with bone marrow transplant patients, Flu was found to significantly reduce invasive fungal infection and to improve survival at day 110 after transplantation [362]. Additionally, in bone marrow transplant recipients, Flu seems to be especially efficacious in preventing liver infections due to *C. albicans* [363].

However, in a study in patients undergoing intensive chemotherapy for haematologic neoplasia, the frequency of deep mycoses and the overall mortality was unaffected under prevention with Flu. It has, however to be mentioned that this study was performed in a center where aspergillosis is known to be the predominant mycosis. In none of the patients was invasive infection due to *Candida* diagnosed, but this advantage was offset by an increased number of infections caused by molds [347]. Thus, this study clearly shows that Flu does reduce the incidence of deep *Candida* infections but is unable to reduce the incidence of aspergillosis.

Itra, the triazole with a broader activity against aspergilli, represents an attractive alternative to Flu in prevention. Unfortunately, no thorough comparative clinical trials are yet available to define the role of Itra in the prevention of invasive fungal infections. The results of the few clinical trials available have been recently reviewed [337,364]. Most trials compared their results with historical controls; thus the interpretation of the findings remains vague. Itra seems to be of benefit in preventing invasive pulmonary aspergillosis in various patient groups. Based on their clinical experience, K.M. Troy and J. Cuttner [365] recommend that patients with acute leukaemia should receive Itra prevention while undergoing intensive induction chemotherapy. A problem that influences the beneficial value of Itra prevention is clearly the low oral absorption of Itra in some patients; in a long-term study with Itra in granulomatous patients, some patients clearly had Itra levels below that at which prevention is thought to be effective [366]. Thus, we need thorough clinical studies with definite dose recommendations to define the role of Itra in the field of prophylaxis.

A question still remains: At what cost do we employ antifungal prevention? For example, Flu in the doses used in neutropenic patients is more expensive than any antifungal used in prophylaxis [121, 367]. Currently no antifungal agent successfully and safely treats all fungal infections; new efficacious and cheap drugs, modalities and innovative delivery systems are needed for an effective prophylaxis against resistant species, morbidity and mortality. We have made important progress in this area, but we have not yet found the weapon to win the battle [368].

4.5   Shattered hopes

4.5.1   Genaconazole
The development of an inspiring drug had to be stopped due to potential carcinogenicity.

Six years ago the triazole genaconazole provoked high excitement among researchers and clinical mycologists [1]. Genaconazole showed broad activity, including against murine infections due to primary pathogenic fungi (histoplasmosis and coccidioidomycosis) and opportunistic fungi (cryptococcosis, candidosis and aspergillosis). The agent proved to be comparable to Flu and Amph B in prevention and early treatment of disseminated candidosis in granulocytopenic rabbits. At that time it was the best azole on the scene. Genaconazole was thoroughly investigated in phase II/III clinical trials in the United States. The first clinical results were presented at the ICAAC in 1990. Genaconazole proved to be active at a very low dose of 50 mg/day in oropharyngeal candidosis in cancer patients, and the results achieved in invasive mold infections suggested that the drug

could significantly improve treatment even in the face of severe neutropenia: 22 of 34 evaluable patients had a complete response, and 5 a partial response, of life-threatening infections, some despite profound immunosuppression [369]. Genaconazole was also clinically effective in cryptococcosis in AIDS patients and in coccidioidomycosis [370,371]. Clinicians
saw genaconazole as a real breakthrough and hoped finally to have a powerful weapon in hand to fight against molds and yeasts in immunocompromised and competent patients. Unfortunately, the development of
hepatocellular carcinomas in animals chronically treated with the drug
led to its withdrawal from development [372]. This decision meant an end
to the high expectations of clinicians and patients. The drug continued to
be available for compassionate use for some time, and there was some
discussion in the clinical world about the relevance of carcinogenicity in
long-term animal studies for a drug that was so effective in life-threatening infections not responding to available therapy. Perhaps more important was the discussion of how such drugs effective in situations where
long-term carcinogenic potential is really of no relevance (for example,
in AIDS patients) could be made available. Unfortunately, no answer to
these various discussions has been found yet.

In the meantime, Schering-Plough already has several promising new triazoles in the pipeline (see Sec. 5.2.1).

4.5.2   Saperconazole
• The development of the successor for Itra has ended, based on toxicology findings.

Saperconazole was envisaged as a successor to Itra with the same powerful antifungal efficacy over a wide spectrum and the same fungicidal
activity, but with the advantage that a parenteral formulation was feasible
[1], and the first clinical data in superficial mycoses were highly promising [373, 374]. However, as with genaconazole, saperconazole was withdrawn from development because of the appearance of tumors in laboratory animals [375].

4.5.3   Cilofungin
• Cilofungin is the first antifungal developed for human chemotherapy
  aimed at inhibiting a highly specific fungal target.

Cilofungin, a semisynthetic derivative of echinocandin B, was a specific,
non-competitive inhibitor of the 1,3-β-glucan synthetase of *Candida albicans* [1,2]. This drug was the first antifungal aimed at interfering with fun-

gal cell wall synthesis to reach clinical development. Phase II results showed satisfactory efficacy in the treatment of oesophageal candidosis in
AIDS patients and in disseminated candidosis in non-neutropenic patients.
Surprisingly, it also showed efficacy in an animal model of aspergillosis.
Unfortunately, toxicity of the vehicle necessary for its administration finally
brought an end to this gallant effort to bring something innovative and
truly fungus-specific onto the market [1].

5   Research in the antifungal field

5.1   Introduction

In recent years, biochemists have intensively studied fungal cells and have
identified several potential targets for antifungal chemotherapy, including cell wall synthesis, membrane function barriers, sterol biosynthesis,
nucleic acid synthesis, metabolic inhibition, amino acid synthesis, transport systems, macromolecular biosynthesis, adhesion and dimorphism.
Inhibition of cell wall synthesis would in theory be highly specific, since only
fungal cells build their wall with chitin and glucan. Intensive research in
this most promising field has been carried out at universities and institutes.
Several pharmaceutical companies have undertaken tremendous efforts to
discover a clinically effective drug interfering with this highly specific target, but up to now without luck. It may however be that fortune will change
and a breakthrough will occur with a drug belonging to the candin group.
Most antifungals interfere with one of the enzymatic steps involved in the
complicated synthesis of ergosterol, the Achilles' heel of the fungal cell.
Scientific knowledge about this pathway has increased enormously since
the first synthesis of a sterol biosynthesis inhibitor; the skill of chemists
in synthesizing fungus-specific inhibitors has also increased; and last but
not least, extensive clinical experience has guided both biochemists and
chemists in designing ideal inhibitors, even if only on paper. Based on this
broad experience, inhibition of sterol biosynthesis is the field in which the
greatest progress has been achieved and where the highest expectation
lies for the future.
Intensified interest in innovative, specific new approaches to antifungal
chemotherapy is evident in universities and the pharmaceutical industry;
but compared with the two targets mentioned above, the information
regarding these new targets is still in its adolescence. The most cutting-
edge scientists study the areas of genome manipulation and inhibition of
virulence factors.

5.2 Profound hopes

5.2.1 Systemic triazoles
• Three new, interesting triazole derivatives are in advanced clinical development.

The class of lanosterol $C_{14}\alpha$-demethylase inhibitors, specifically the triazoles, still promise the most profound hopes in the search for better antifungal agents. Most pharmaceutical companies working in the field of antifungal chemotherapy have chemical programs in azole synthesis.
One compound that proves the rule that "good antifungals never die" started its life 10 years ago as ICI-195739. It was characterized *in vitro* and *in vivo* and was found to have potency greater than other azoles against superficial mycoses, as well as against deep-seated mycoses caused by opportunistic or primary pathogenic fungi. The compound was also efficacious in a murine infection of *Trypanosoma cruzi* [376]. The compound was offered for licensing and disappeared for some time.
Its R-(+) enantiomer appeared in 1992 as (Z)D-0870. D-0870 has a broad antifungal spectrum including yeast, dimorphic fungi and molds [377, 378]. The drug was also inhibitory against Flu-resistant *Candida* spp. [379]. High efficacy has been demonstrated in animal models such as histoplasmosis, blastomycosis, aspergillosis, trichosporiosis, meningeal cryptococcosis and candidosis, including those caused by Flu-resistant strains such as *C. tropicalis* and *C. lusitanea* [380–387]. The efficacy of D-0870 against infections due to *C. glabrata* was found to depend on the strain. The burden in the spleen of Flu-sensitive strains could significantly be reduced, whereas no reduction was seen with Flu-resistant strains. Combinations with Amph B surprisingly demonstrated an additive effect [388]. The enantiomer was as efficacious as the racemate against Chagas disease [389]. Generally, in all animal models, the efficacy of D-0870 was superior to that of Flu. The results of some animal studies suggest that a combination of D-0870 with flucytosine may be more beneficial than each drug alone [384]. D-0870 showed good bioavailability with a half-life of 50 h [390]. Multiple dosing in HIV-positive volunteers was well tolerated; the drug had a rather longer half-life in these patient groups, namely 70 h [391].
Initial phase II results at low doses in AIDS patients with oropharyngeal candidosis were somewhat disappointing [392]. A 50-mg loading dose followed by 10 mg once daily lead at day 5 after treatment to 9 cures and 2 improvements in 11 patients. However, 4 had relapses at the 2-week follow-up visit. D-0870 was also evaluated as an alternative therapy for Flu-resistant oral candidosis. All Flu-resistant isolates appeared sensitive to

D-0870. A beneficial clinical response of oral and oesophageal candidosis was observed, but in no instance was mycological clearance achieved [393]. Zeneca has discontinued further development owing to irregular pharmacokinetics. Mochida is continuing clinical development in Japan. Voriconazole (UK-109496] has been designed as a more potent follow-up for Flu; this drug seems to be the most advanced under the new generation azoles.

The improved potency of voriconazole over Flu has been demonstrated by several *in vitro* studies, including strains with decreased susceptibility to Flu [394, 395]. Voriconazole was 124 times more potent than Flu against *C. krusei*. Voriconazole also proved to be fungicidal against *Aspergillus* spp. [395]. Furthermore, it inhibits a wide range of less common emerging pathogens like *Fusarium* spp., *Trichosporon* spp., *Penicllium marneffei* and *Acremonium* spp. [396–398].

Voriconazole was also highly potent in several animal models [399, 400]; its performance against aspergillosis in immunosuppressed animals was very encouraging [401, 401a]. Voriconazole was widely distributed throughout the body and had an oral bioavailability up to 90%, with a half-life of about 6 h; elimination of the drug was characterized by metabolic clearance [402, 403].

Voriconazole [200 mg q.d. or b.i.d.) showed clinical efficacy in 80–100% of oropharyngeal candidosis in AIDS patients; the drug was well tolerated except for a dose-related incidence of transient reversible visual disturbance [404]. Encouraging clinical responses against aspergillosis were reported at the ICAAC in 1995 [405, 406]. Clinical efficacy was seen in 75% of immunosuppressed patients with acute invasive aspergillosis (8 complete, 11 partial, 8 stable); 25% of patients failed the treatment. The majority of patients had previously been treated with Amph B or Itra without success. Voriconazole has also been evaluated in non-neutropenic patients with chronic aspergillosis. Patients received 200 mg b.i.d. for 4–24 weeks. Again, half of the patients had failed previous treatment with Amph B or Itra. At an interim analysis, 9 of 11 patients had a favorable response (2 complete, 7 partial), and 31% failed treatment. In both trials a small number of patients were withdrawn due to abnormal liver function tests. Phase III clinical trials for various infections are continuing.

After the disappointment of genaconazole, Schering-Plough continued its research and presented its newest development candidate, Sch-56592 at the ICAAC in 1995. Its *in vitro* activity proved to be superior to Flu and Amph B against a variety of primary pathogens and opportunistic fungi, including Flu-resistant strains. Some fungicidal activity was also demonstrated [407–409].

Activity in animal models was observed in systemic or vaginal candidosis [408, 410], aspergillosis [408, 410, 411], cryptococcosis [412], blastomycosis [413], histoplasmosis [414], coccidioidomycosis [415] and dermatomycosis [416]. The drug was the most powerful sterol biosynthesis inhibitor ever tested in an infection due to *Trypanosoma cruzi* [417].

Phase I studies have apparently been completed, with good tolerance up to 1 g and the prospect of once-daily dosing. The results were presented at the Second International Symposium on Recent Advances in Chemistry of Anti-Infective Agents Cambridge in 1996.

Several other triazoles are on the waiting list for development in humans. Scientists at Toyama research laboratories have detected a new water-soluble triazole, T-8581. It has a broad *in vitro* spectrum and has shown excellent activity in aspergillosis and Flu-resistant candidosis. In animals its pharmacokinetic properties were sufficient to hold out the promise of oral and once-daily dosing [418]. The researchers have concentrated their efforts on finding a drug active for aspergillosis.

Another promising azole is ER-30346, with a broad antifungal spectrum and high efficacy in murine candidosis (due to Flu-sensitive and Flu-resistant strains), aspergillosis and cryptococcosis. Good oral bioavailability has been reported in animals (rats 48%, dogs 74%), with a half-life around 31 h in dogs [419–421]. This compound was licensed to Bristol-Myers Squibb in December 1996, and a major clinical development is expected.

A series of azole derivatives carrying an *N*-acylmorpholine ring has been reported by Uriach [422]. The best of these compounds appears to be UR-9746, which showed a broad antifungal spectrum and was efficacious in murine candidosis and cryptococcosis with somewhat weaker activity in aspergillosis and histoplasmosis. It was presented as the most effective triazole in murine coccidioidomycosis; this result would mean real progress in the battle against human coccidioidomycosis, provided the animal data can be translated to excellent human data. It is, however, unclear whether this drug will ever be developed for humans, since preclinical development was suspended towards the end of 1995.

In Japan, Yoshitomi is developing another triazole, SSY-726 with beneficial effect in candidosis, cryptococcosis and aspergillosis [423]; phase II trials have been initiated in the U.K.

A further agent containing a triazole and an azolone moiety, TAK-187 has recently been presented by Takeda [424]. TAK-187 was more active *in vitro* than Flu against *C. albicans*, including Flu-resistant strains, it was also more potent against non-*albicans Candida*. The efficacy in animal models was significantly better, as Flu and Itra with ED50 values (mg/kg, oral) for TAK-187, Flu and Itra being 0.7/1.5/18 for candidosis, 1.6/100/>100 for cryptococcosis and 10/160/18 for aspergillosis in the models used. The drug is also highly efficacious in histoplasmosis. Hopefully, this compound will soon enter clinical development.

The search for azole derivatives active against deep-seated mycoses clearly continues and will remain the most promising field for success also in the near future.

5.2.2   Topical antifungals

• The choice of topical antifungals is steadily increasing.

Azole antifungals are continually being developed and brought to the market for topical use, although the high efficacy of the standard treatment is difficult to improve. Sartaconazole has recently been launched in several countries in Europe and South America [425]. Fenticonazole has been launched in the United Kingdom for treatment of vaginal thrush [426].

Lanoconazole, which was approved by the Japanese authorities in 1994, was reported to be as effective as topical Ter in the short-term treatment of tinea pedis in animal models [427]. Furthermore, it was more efficacious than bifonazole in a model of cutaneous candidosis [428], and it seems to have a wound-healing effect [429].

Flutrimazole was recently licensed for use in certain African countries. It has proven clinical efficacy, and it demonstrated anti-inflammatory properties in animal models [430–432].

The imidazole eberconazole, efficacious in tinea cruris and corporis, is nearing completion of phase III in Spain [433, 434]. Omoconazole is another topical agent for the treatment of superficial fungal infections coming to the market in Europe [435].

KP-103 was the best in a series of azolamine derivatives synthesized at Kaken with a better *in vitro* activity against *C. albicans* and *Malassezzia furfur* than other topical antifungals. The excellent therapeutic efficacy and the low relapse rate may be explained by prolonged retention of the active drug in the skin tissue [436, 437].

Butenafine, a benzylamine derivative of the allylamine developed by Kaken, was highly active in tinea corporis [438]; it was recently approved by the FDA for the treatment of athlete's foot, ringworm and other major fungal skin infections [439].

The armamentarium of topical antifungals is continuously increasing, and dermatologists have nearly unlimited choice in the battle against dermatophytic infections.

5.3   Broken hopes

• A fascinating target had to be abandoned due to lack of *in vivo* activity.

2,3-Oxidosqualene-lanosterol cyclase has long been considered an attractive antifungal target by a number of groups, including the mycologists at Hoffmann-La Roche. The mechanistically fascinating cyclization reaction, the basis of sterol biosynthesis in animals, plants and fungi, was recently reviewed by Abe and co-workers [440].

Oelschlaeger and co-workers [441–444] have reported a series of sulfur and sulfoxide analogues of episqualene, which were all very helpful in elucidating the mechanism of this cyclization, but which had very little antifungal activity, probably due to lack of penetration into the fungal cell [445]. A series of azasqualenes with good activity against the enzyme have been studied at the university of Turin [446–449]. Generally, these compounds all exhibited no overwhelming *in vitro* activity despite their good inhibitory effect on the enzyme level [450]. The group is still working in this field, designing new azasqualenes to mimic the C2, C8 and C20 carbonium ions formed during cyclization [451, 452].

At Hoffmann-La Roche in Switzerland, the antifungal research group synthesized aminoketones designed to interact with both the active site, a postulated acidic group, and the nucleophil required for stabilization of the C20 prosterol cation [453–456]. This approach successfully produced compounds strongly inhibiting 2,3-oxidosqualene-lanosterol cyclase and exhibiting a broad antifungal spectrum. The degree of the *in vitro* inhibition was comparable to that of the best antifungals on the market.

Unfortunately, the compounds were only weakly active in various animal models of fungal infections, and were ultimately abandoned. The lack of systemic activity may be due to their extremely high protein-binding capacity (>90%) and to their rapid metabolization to inactive derivatives.

In one respect, however, the program was successful. Many of the cyclase inhibitors exhibited a strong cholesterol-lowering effect in hamsters after oral application. The best agent, Ro-48-8071, lowered the LDL by about 60% in hamsters and at least by 30% in squirrel monkeys and minipigs [457]. This agent did not trigger overexpression of hepatic HMG-CoA reductase, squalene synthetase or 2,3-oxidosqualene-lanosterol cyclase itself, nor did it reduce coenzyme 10 levels. These results stand in contrast to simvastatin, an inhibitor of HMG-CoA reductase used for the treatment of cholesterolaemia. This important difference increases the attraction of the 2,3-oxidosqualene-lanosterol cyclase inhibitors for this new area.

5.4   Everlasting dreams

5.4.1   Candins: 1,3-β-glucansynthetase inhibitors
• Two candins have reached the state of clinical trials.

The dream has not died of discovering a highly fungal-specific agent targeted at inhibiting the fungal cell wall synthesis without interfering with pathways in the host. After the disappointment of cilofungin, Lilly and Merck continued their efforts to detect a more potent cell wall synthesis inhibitor suitable for clinical development. Both concentrated their labors on semisynthetic derivatives of echinocandin. In recent years many new analogues have appeared in the literature; most disappeared again, but three derivatives survived, namely LY-303.366 (Lilly), L-733.560 and L-743.82 (Merck).

All candins prevent cell.wall synthesis by blocking 1,3-β-glucansynthetase, an enzyme not present in mammalian cells. This inhibition is highly specific and leads after only a short contact to cell death [458]. These drugs have been thoroughly evaluated in vitro and in several animal models. The degree of in vivo activity was generally dependent on the mode of application; the efficacy of candins was always lower after oral application than after parenteral application.

LY-303.366 is a potent fungicidal agent against Candida spp. including azole-resistant strains. Its in vitro activity against Candida is superior to all antifungals on the market. Low to moderate activity has been observed against Aspergillus spp., but it has no effect against Cryptococcus neoformans and five other non-Candida species. LY-303.366 also exhibits activity against primary pathogenic fungi such as Histoplasma capsulatum, Coccidioides immitis and Sporotrix schenckii; however, the degree of efficacy is lower than that against Candida [459–465].

LY-303.366 is efficacious in candidosis due to both Flu-sensitive and Flu-resistant strains and in aspergillosis [459, 460, 466]. Candins have been found to exhibit in vitro and in vivo activity against Pneumocystis carinii. LY-303.366 was highly effective in Pneumocystis carinii pneumonia in animal models [467].

Single-dose oral administration of LY-303.366 in healthy volunteers was well tolerated up to 500 mg; drug-related toxicity at higher doses included abdominal pain, diarrhoea and flatulence. The drug was reliably absorbed in fasting subjects, but food reduced absorption by 35 to 75%. LY-303.366 had a long half-life (approximately 30 h) and a large distribution volume (about 10 l/kg). Multiple doses of 400 mg daily have been well tolerated [468].

LY-303.366 began phase II clinical trials in the United States in 1996; it is, however, not clear which of the three possible indications (pneumocystis, candidosis or aspergillosis) will be the first choice.

The semisynthetic pneumocandin L-733.560 exhibited high *in vitro* activity against *C. albicans* (azole-sensitive and -resistant strains), non-*albicans Candida* and *Aspergillus* spp. Moderate activity was seen in *Cryptococcus neoformans* [469–473]. Excellent responses have been observed in several animal models of candidosis, aspergillosis and *Pneumocystis carinii* infections. The drug did not influence the *Cryptococcus* burden in brain and spleen [474, 475].

This promising pneumocandin has lost its lead position and seems to have been replaced by an analogue with a greater potential. Merck announced L-743.872 as a new candidate. Development entered phase II trials at the end of 1996. The preclinical properties and the phase I data of L-743.872 were presented at the Thirty-sixth Interscience Conference on Antimicrobial Agents and Chemotherapy.

L-743.872 clearly has a broader antifungal spectrum than previous echinocandin derivatives. L-743.872 exhibits superior *in vitro* potency against *C. albicans*, including Flu- or Amph B-resistant strains [476, 477], non-*albicans Candida*, *Aspergillus* spp. and some dematiaceous fungi [476, 478–480]. It is only moderately active against *Cryptococcus neoformans*, with MIC values of 16 µg/ml. This effect is clearly lower than that observed with Amph B or Itra. L-743.872 proved efficacious against primary pathogenic fungi; the representative MIC values were 3.3 µg/ml for *Coccidioides immitis* and 0.2 µg/ml for *Histoplasma capsulatum* [477, 481]. *Fusarium* spp. and Zygomycetes were resistant [482], whereas dermatophytes responded moderately to the drug [477].

L-743.872 was found to have a synergistic effect with Flu and Amph B, the synergism being especially distinct in Flu-resistant *Candida* strains and in *Cryptococcus neoformans* [483, 484].

L-743.872 has been thoroughly studied in various animal models. The new analogue exhibited potent *in vivo* activity in murine candidosis, aspergillosis, histoplasmosis and *Pneumocystis carinii* pneumonia [485–492]. Infections due to *C. glabrata*, *C. lusitanae*, *C. parapsilosis* or *C. krusei* also responded to treatment with L-743.872, but the agent was ineffective in cryptococcosis.

L-743.872 was well tolerated, with a half-life of about 10 h after parenteral treatment [492].

Thus, two candins are in clinical development (LY-303.366 and L-743.872). Both drugs are suitable for infection due to *Candida*, *Aspergillus* or *Pneumocystis* and both have as a drawback a lack of efficacy against *Crypto-*

coccus. LY-303.366 has the advantage that oral dosing is efficacious. It is reasonable to hope that in the near future one of these highly specific drugs can be added to the armamentarium of systemic antifungals available for human use.

5.4.2   Nikkomycin Z: Chitin synthase inhibitors

- Nikkomycin Z is still alive and may finally find its way into clinical development.

Chitin synthase has been and is still a highly attractive target for antifungal research. For many years scientists at universities and in industry have studied this interesting field intensively. Chitin synthase genes have been identified in a wide range of fungi, and chitin synthesis seems to be essential for the growth of fungal cells. *C. albicans* harbors three chitin synthase genes; one, *CHS1*, has been described as essential for development of the fungus.

The research has been partially successful; researchers have detected potent fungicides for use in agriculture, but applications for human chemotherapy are not yet a reality.

The nikkomycins are chitin synthase inhibitors that have languished in the development process for years but have never reached the full development stage. Initially nikkomycin Z was found to be highly effective against murine coccidioidomycosis, but the spectrum of the drug was considered too narrow to warrant expanded development.

Recently nikkomycin Z was reported to be efficacious in pulmonary blastomycosis of the mouse. Its activity was superior to Itra and equivalent to Amph B if the reduction of infectious burden was studied [493]. Beneficial response was also observed in histoplasmosis. Nikkomycin Z inhibits the chitin synthase of *C. albicans*, but the agent is only moderately active against *C. albicans* or *C. parapsilosis* and it is ineffective against other *Candida* species [494, 495].

The reason why the interest in nikkomycin Z has never died is the fact that this drug potentiates the effect of Itra or Flu. Nikkomycin Z showed synergistic or additive effects against the majority of strains of *C. albicans*, *C. parapsilosis*, *Cryptococcus neoformans* and *Aspergillus* spp. when combined with Itra. The already high susceptibility of dimorphic fungi to nikkomycin could be significantly increased by combining nikkomycin Z with Flu [495–497]. A synergistic interaction between nikkomycin and Itra or Flu has been observed in several *Coccidioides immitis* strains. This beneficial effect seems also to be working in some animal models.

Nikkomycin Z is currently undergoing phase I trials in the United Kingdom and preclinical testing in the United States for endemic mycoses. The limited toxicology tests conducted so far suggest that nikkomycin Z is well tolerated at the doses used. Thus, after a long, lingering period, nikkomycin Z has started on its way to clinical trials.

5.4.3   Aureobasidin A, basifungin, LY-295337

• An interesting family of antifungal antibiotics with a new mechanism of action have entered phase I studies.

A large family of antifungal antibiotics isolated 6 years ago from the fermentation broth of the black fungi *Aureobasisium pullulans* are the aureobasidins, cyclic peptides containing eight amino acids and a hydroxy acid. During recent years, this family of antibiotics was thoroughly investigated; new aureobasidins have been isolated [498], and new derivatives have been synthesized by chemists at Lilly [499]. The new natural aureobasidins were more potent than aureobasidin A against *Candida* spp. [498], and the new chemical derivatives improved the knowledge of the relationship between structure and biological activity. The L-isomers were more potent antifungal agents than D-isomers. However, all analogues exhibited decreased activity against *Cryptococcus neoformans*; this difference suggests that the potential for hydrogen binding at residue 8 of aureobasidin is a key structural element for anticryptococcal activity [499].

Aureobasidin A has a broad antifungal spectrum including *Candida* spp., *Cryptococcus neoformans*, *Blastomyces dermatitidis* and *Histoplasma capsulatum* [500, 501]. *Aspergillus* isolates responded poorly to the antibiotic. The highest activity has been seen against *Candida* isolates [502].

Aureobasidin A proved highly efficacious in murine candidosis, histoplasmosis and blastomycosis [500]; however, in cryptococcosis the activity was significantly lower than expected based on *in vitro* data. *Ex vivo* experiments with *Cryptococcus neoformans* from infected liver samples indicated that the isolated fungi has a decreased susceptibility to the drug. The mechanism behind this appearance of resistance is not yet recognized, but it could lead to an understanding of the mode of action of this drug [503].

Aureobasidin seems to have entered phase I in Japan. With this fungal antibiotic interfering with a new target in the fungal cell, we could get an innovative antifungal in the armamentarium of antifungals for human use.

5.5   Disappointments

5.5.1   The pradimicins and benamicins

• The development of pradimicins and benamicins was discontinued due to toxic findings during phase I.

The pradimicins and benamicins, a growing family of antifungal antibiotics, have been around for more than 10 years. They are benzonaphthacene quinone antibiotics with D-alanine, D-serine or glycine and a saccharide side chain [1, 504, 505]. Their mechanism of action, although not definitively evaluated, has been described to involve complexing with the saccharide portions of cell surface mannoproteins in a calcium-dependent manner [504, 506]. The pradimicin derivative BMS-181184 damages the cell membrane and thereafter the microtubules [507]. This family of new antibiotics attacks a totally new target and promises to be an innovative approach for human antifungal chemotherapy.

The natural product pradimicin A had a broad spectrum of fungicidal activity and showed *in vivo* activity against a broad range of fungal infections (candidosis, cryptococcosis, aspergillosis, trichophytosis) [508]. However, its limited solubility made further development difficult. As a result, a chemical program was started at Bristol-Myers Squibb to identify water-soluble derivatives. This project was successful; several new pradimicin derivatives with higher water solubility have been detected [509].

BMS-181184 underwent thorough and intensive preclinical development. This derivative has a broad antifungal spectrum including opportunistic and primary pathogenic fungi. It is fungicidal to yeasts and to a lesser extent to filamentous fungi, but it was not fungicidal against the family of Dematiaceae. *Fusarium* spp., *Pseudoallescheria boydii*, *Malassezia furfur*, *Alternaria* and Zygomycetes respond poorly to the drug [510, 511]. BMS-181184 was highly efficacious in animal models of candidosis, cryptococcosis, aspergillosis and *Pneumocystis carinii* pneumonia [512–516]. Furthermore, BMS-181184 has been described to exert anti HIV-activity.

Late in 1995, BMS-181184 entered phase I studies, but in late 1996 its development was discontinued.

The benomicins, which were detected more or less at the same time as pradimicins, have also been subject to derivatization and to further thorough evaluation in Japan. Benanomicin A proved to be similar to the pradimicins with respect to mechanism of action and its broad fungicidal *in vitro* activity [1, 498, 517]. Benanomicin A was found to have excellent activity against *Pneumocystis carinii* pneumonia in mice, with a different mechanism of action [518]. Unfortunately, further development had to be discontinued due to cardiac toxicity.

5.6   Further in the future

5.6.1   Sterol biosynthesis inhibition: New structures and new targets
• Research in the era of ergosterol biosynthesis remains a fruitful field.

The first natural antifungal inhibiting the target of azoles was detected at the same time by Merck and Roche. Named restrictin by the former and Ro-9-1470 by the latter, this tetrahydropyran derivative with an alkenyl side chain and several congeners was isolated from the culture broth of *Penicillium* and *Aspergillus* species [519–522]. The compound was found to inhibit lanosterol C_{14}-demethylase and also showed some *in vitro* activity [520, 523]. It can be assumed that chemical programs were initiated at both institutions, but no exciting news has been forthcoming.
Abbott has put considerable effort into research to develop non-azole inhibitors of lanosterol C_{14}-demethylase. A-39806, the most potent compound from a large series of inhibitors, showed good activity on the level of the enzyme and was efficacious *in vitro* against *Candida*, *Cryptococcus* and *Aspergillus* [524, 525].
Removal of the C_4 methyl group of ergosterol precursors is essential to fulfill the requirements of a membrane sterol in fungi. Thus, the inhibition of C_4 demethylation recently reported is of great interest [526–530]. The 6-amino-22-*n*-phenylthiobenzathiazole inhibits the two demethylation steps; the drug also proved to be active *in vitro* against various *Candida* species and showed *in vivo* efficacy in murine candidosis. Although its activity was lower than that of Keto in terms of survival, complete sterilization was achieved in the surviving mice treated with the new inhibitor. These results clearly warrant further investigation and give hope that this new approach may be fruitful for human chemotherapy.

5.6.2   Cell wall active antibiotics
• New promising targets have been detected that may become successes in the future.

The glucosamine-6-phosphate needed for chitin synthesis is produced by the enzyme L-glutamine fructose-6-phosphate amidotransferase, which is the target of the dipeptide antibiotic bacilysin (also known as tetain). For many years Borowski's group (in Gdansk, Poland) has been working with this target; they have discovered a series of short peptides with a broad *in vitro* antifungal spectrum. Unfortunately, none of these compounds have shown high efficacy in animal models, and none has yet entered broader development [1, 498].

Besides the known candins, new glucan synthesis inhibitors are periodically identified during random screening. Chemical derivatization of the known candins is still going on at several institutions. Additionally, much effort has gone into molecular biology approaches (such as enzyme purification and gene cloning) to gain deeper information about the structure and mechanism of the enzyme.

Research continues on chitin synthase; chemical programs exist at various pharmaceutical companies and at universities. Furthermore, molecular biology allows increased insight into the mechanisms of cell wall synthesis. The family of nikkomycins, with their potential to be combination partners for all antifungals, is still being actively investigated.

New therapeutic targets may emerge to provide opportunities for the design of novel antifungals [498], and a breakthrough may become reality in the near future.

5.6.3   Polyenes

- The outstanding antifungal Amph B has inspired researchers to look for new polyenes from natural sources or to improve the safety profile of Amph B by derivatization.

Amph B has such outstanding antifungal activity that it is not surprising that attempts have been made to increase its therapeutic index by derivatization. The goal of such studies has been to increase solubility and decrease toxicity without losing efficacy. The name of Borowski has been the one most associated with this work [1, 531]. The first derivatives to be investigated were the *N*-acetyl derivatives, which all had decreased toxicity; however, this property was matched with reduction in activity.

Amph B methylester was the derivative with the longest life time, but its further development had finally to be discontinued due to neurotoxic side-effects [1].

Recently a series of second-generation Amph B derivatives (sterically hindered Amph B derivatives which were substituted Amadori re-arrangements produced with various sugars) have been described by the Borowski group. These compounds are water-soluble and have improved selective toxicity in animals, retaining the broad-spectrum antifungal activity of the mother compound [532].

SmithKline Beecham also has a water-soluble Amph B derivative with a better safety profile than Amph B [533] under preclinical development.

The efficacy of KY-62, another Amph B derivative, has been evaluated in murine cryptococcosis and candidosis [534].

Additionally, a semisynthetic methylpatricin derivative, SPA-753, and several amid derivatives of patricin are under preclinical evaluation as potential antifungal agents [535, 535a].

MS-8209, a derivative of Amph B, has surprisingly shown promise in the treatment of prion diseases in animal models, and the agent could, therefore, be useful in Creutzfeld-Jacob disease in humans. This claim was first made in 1992; it is unclear whether this lead has been further investigated, since no mention has appeared in the meanwhile.

Thus, work on modifying the structure of Amph B continues; however, it is uncertain whether all these efforts will ever be fruitful for human chemotherapy. Up to now, only the association of Amph B with lipid complexes or liposomes has been a success in human chemotherapy (see Sec. 4.3.2). New macrolide structures are continuously being identified, and their antifungal activities are described in the hope of finding an antibiotic with the same broad antifungal spectrum as Amph B without the drawbacks of Amph B. In recent years, new macrolide structures such as linearmycin (a linear polyene) [536], TMC-34 [537], Kanchanymycins [538], Shurimycin A [539] and RS-22A [540] have been described, but their development status is unclear.

5.6.4   Natural products

• Nature remains an unlimited source of new antifungals with innovative structures and interesting new targets.

The literature is full of new antibiotics, and a good proportion of them are antifungals. Every week one can spend a couple of hours in the library reading of inhibition zones and MICs of new substances. Some of the antibiotics mentioned stay with us a while. One reads about structure determination, activity of derivatives and structure-function studies; sometimes they are even the basis for studying a new fungal target. Others are more ephemeral, and after a mention such as "could be useful in the treatment of fungal infections", they are never heard of again. It is encouraging to be constantly reminded of the diversity of active substances that nature presents to us, and it could well be that the next significant advance in antifungal chemotherapy will have had its basis in the *Journal of Antibiotics*.

The isolation and structural elucidation of the antibiotic azoxybacilin, Ro-9-1563, an unusual amino acid structure with an azoxy moiety has recently guided researchers towards a new antifungal target. Azoxybacilin was described as efficacious against a broad spectrum of fungi; it was especially active against filamentous fungi such as *Absidia*, *Aspergillus* and dermatophytes, but it was inactive against *Cryptococcus neoformans*. First investigations in relation to its mode of action revealed that this antibiotic is antagonized by homocystein, cystein, cystathion or methionin and that it inhibits one or several steps in the sulfur-fixation pathway [541, 542]. Further in-depth studies showed that that azoxybacilin exerts its antifungal activity through inhibition of the regulation of the genes for fungal-specific sulfate assimilation. It inhibits the enhancement of transcription of the *MET4* gene, which in turn would result in partial repression of the genes required for sulfate assimilation. This is the first time that an antifungal has been detected that interferes with the regulation of gene expression, and thus isolation of this new natural product provides an approach for identifying an antifungal with a totally new mode of action [543].

5.6.5   Virulence factors
- The future of antifungal chemotherapy may lie in the field of pathogenicity.

To date all antifungals have been targeted to inhibit metabolic pathways of the fungi; none of the available drugs interfere directly with the virulence of the fungus. In the past, because basic research mainly tried to understand cell structure and to evaluate the biochemical functioning of a fungal cell, less interest was invested in understanding the pathogenicity process.

Some available antifungals have the ability to decrease the virulence of the fungal cell in addition to their primary mechanism of action. For example, fungal cells pretreated with sub-inhibitory concentrations of Amph B or azoles lose some of their virulence. Some *Candida* isolates resistant to 5-FC have decreased virulence in comparison to wild-type isolates [136]. Interest in better understanding the pathogenicity and virulence of fungal cells has continuously increased in the last years. Several virulence factors or virulence genes have been identified. The group of Kwong-Chung has studied the virulence and pathogenicity of *Cryptococcus neoformans* [544–546]. They identified at least three virulence factors: the fungus has to be able to grow at 37°C, to produce a polysaccharide capsule and to have an active phenol oxidase in order to synthesize melanin from dopa. These three virulence factors are located in three different alleles and are easily and independently changed by appropriate genetic manipulation. A single mutation in any one of these three characteristics leads to a significant reduction in virulence. Melanin also plays an important role for the pathogenicity of dematiaceous fungi. Mutants unable to synthesize melanin, which is located in the cell wall of this black fungi, lose their virulence [547]. The virulence of *C. albicans* has been found to be strongly dependent on phosphate lipase and proteinase production [548–552].

The state of the art regarding fungal virulence genes as targets for antifungal chemotherapy has recently been summarized [553]. In this review all of the above-mentioned factors are included and several others mentioned, such as the chitin synthesis gene *CHS2* and *CHS3*, the elastase gene *AFA7P*, the purine metabolism gene *ADE2*, the multiple drug resistance gene *CaMDR1* and others.

Most studies to understand the pathogenicity of fungi have been conducted at universities; only a few pharmaceutical companies have risked studying virulence factors and initiating chemical programs in this field. Two virulence factors of *C. albicans* have been intensively studied, namely phospolipase [548] and proteinase [549–555].

C. albicans secretes phospholipases, which are considered to be one of the mediators of cell penetration. It is known that other phospholipases from mammalian cells can be inhibited by lipophilic beta-blocking structures. Hoechst had a chemical synthesis program in the field of beta blocking, and as a result of this effort, several structures with antifungal activity deriving from the structure of β-hydroxyethylamine have been detected. These compounds inhibit the secretion of phospholipase and fungal growth *in vitro*. Histological examination confirmed the inhibitory effect of the beta-blocker-like structures on tissue penetration. Most of these compounds showed only weak efficacy in animal models when given alone, but in combination with Flu they were able to prevent death in mice infected with lethal inocula of *C. albicans* [554]. These β-hydroxyethylamine derivatives are lead structures for new antifungals with a totally new attack on the fungal cell.

The aspartate proteinase of *C. albicans* is the most thoroughly studied virulence factor. Its role in the pathogenicity of *Candida* species has been established in various studies [555–558], and its gene has been sequenced [559]. Furthermore, proteinase A has been crystallized [560]. Chemical synthesis programs to detect inhibitors of HIV proteases are in place at several universities and pharmaceutical companies. Unfortunately, HIV protease inhibitors are rarely active against the aspartate proteinase of *Candida* spp.

It has been known for long time that pepstatin A inhibits the production of proteinases and reduces the adherence of *Candida* cells to epithelial cells. Pepstatin A was also found to be efficacious in a model of candidosis [561]. Also, some of the antifungals on the market have been found to be potent inhibitors of the *Candida* proteinase [562]. Based on the positive results with pepstatin, several institutions started new programs to detect new *Candida*-specific protease inhibitors with higher activity at the enzymatic level combined with *in vivo* activity.

Abbott and Yamanouchi have a long-standing chemical program and have detected compounds with good inhibitory activity of the protease produced by *C. albicans* [563, 564]. In addition, new natural products with pepstatin-like structures have been isolated [565–568]. Several of these compounds showed inhibitory activity on the level of the enzyme but like pepstatin A they lacked direct inhibitory activity on the growth of fungi. None of these proteinase inhibitors has yet entered broad development, but hopefully interest in developing drugs that interfere with the pathogenicity of the fungi will increase in the future.

6   Conclusion

We have tried in this chapter to put together the most relevant information on the present state of the art of antifungal chemotherapy, including recent advances and expected advances in the field.

We can be proud of the progress that has been achieved in the field of antifungals:

- For dermatomycoses, a broad armamentarium of potent topical antifungals is available, and safe and efficacious systemic treatment with the fungicidal compound Ter is possible. The duration of treatment could be drastically reduced due to the favorable properties of Itra and Ter.
- Itraconazole has become the drug of first choice for endemic mycoses.
- Flu and Itra have increased the arsenal of drugs for opportunistic infections.
- Combination therapy with 5-FC plus Amph B still holds its traditional position in the treatment of severely compromised patients.
- New combination therapies (combining conventional antimycotics or traditional antimycotics with immunomodulators) are being evaluated.
- Antifungal maintenance therapy for opportunistic infections in AIDS patients is well established.
- New targets have been usefully exploited, and some fascinating new molecules have entered clinical development.
- New approaches interfering with host defenses or the pathogenicity of fungal cells are being investigated. Modulation of host defenses is al-

ready functional in clinical cases; however, immunomodulators are too expensive for general use.
- Prevention in patients at high risk is now possible with oral antimycotics, but prophylaxis should not yet be generally used.

Despite all these advances, the battle has as yet no clear winner; the fungus still seems to be one step ahead. Resistant strains are appearing, and new pathogenic fungi are emerging with a high potency to infect immunosuppressed patients. Fortunately, interest in mycology is increasing, and much work will be done in the future to better understand the molecular biological features of the fungus, its pathogenicity and the defense mechanisms the fungus initiates in the host.

References

1   A. Polak and P.G. Hartman: Prog. Drug Res. *37*, 181 (1991).
2   P.D. Hoeprich: Prog. Drug Res. *44*, 87,(1995).
3   P. de Keyser, M. de Backer, D.L. Massart and K.J. Westelinck: Br. J. Dermatology. *130* (Suppl. 43), 22 (1994).
4   R.J. Hay, J.M.M. Mc Gregor, J. Wuite, K.S. Ryatt, C. Ziegler and Y.M. Clayton: Br. J. Dermatol. *132* (5), 604 (1995).
5   M. Haria, H.M. Bryson and K.L. Goa: Drugs *51*, 586 (1996).
6   T.C. Jones: Br. J. Dermatol. *132* (5), 683 (1995).
7   U. Budimulja, K. Kuswadji, S. Bramano, J. Basuki, L.S. Judanarso and S. Untung: Br. J. Dermatology. *130* (Suppl. 43), 29 (1994).
8   N.S. Ryder, in: J.W. Rippon and R.A. Fromtling (eds.): Cutaneous Antifungal Agents, Dekker, New York 1993, p. 127.
9   C.A. Needham, A.J. Bangs, K. Atkin and D.P. O'Sullivan: Br. J. Dermatol. *133* (Suppl. 45), 27 (1995).
9a B.H.C. Stricker, M.M. van Riemsdijk, M.C.J.M. Sturkenboom, and J.P. Ottervanger: Br. J. Clin. Pharmacol. *42* (3), 313 (1996).
10 F. Schatz, M. Bräutigam, E. Obrowolski, I. Effendy, H. Haberl, H. Mensing, G. Eidinger and A. Stütz: Clin. Exp. Dermatol. *20*, 377 (1995).
11 M.J.D. Goodfield, L. Andrew and E.G.V. Evans: Br. Med. J. *304* (6835), 1151 (1992).
12 N.H. Shear and A.K. Gupta: Arch. Dermatol. *131*, 937 (1995).
13 M. Bräutigam, S. Nolting, R. E. Schöpf and G. Weidinger: Br. Med. Journal *311* (7010), 919 (1995).
13a G.F. Schiraldi, S. Lo Cicero, M.D. Colombo, D. Rossato, M. Ferrarese and E. Soresi: Br. J. Dermatol. *134* (Suppl. 46), 25 (1996).
14 T.J. Zhu: J. Clin. Dermatol. 23 (4), 198 (1994).
15 P. De Doncker, J. Decroix, G.E. Piérard, D. Roelant, R. Woestenborghs, P. Jacqmin, F. Odds, A. Heremans, P. Dock and D. Roseeuw: Arch. Dermatol. *132*, 34 (1996).
16 A. Farag, M. Taha and S. Halim: Br. J. Dermatol. *131* (5), 684 (1994).
17 C.S. Munro, J.L. Rees and S. Shuster: Acta Derm. Venereol. 72 (2), 13 (1992).
18 C.K. Wong and Y.L. Cho: Br. J. Dermatol. *133* (2), 329–331 (1995).
19 W. Bergman and F.F.H. Rutten: Ned. Tijdschr. Geneeskd. *138* (47), 2346 (1994).

20   A. Polak: J. Eur. Acad. Dermatol. Veneréol. *4* (Suppl. 1), S11 (1995).

21   M. Haria and H.M. Bryson: Drugs *49*, 103 (1995).

22   Y. Clayton: Poster at the Dermatology 2000, Vienna (1993).

23   C. Marcireau, M. Guilloton and F. Karst: Antimicrob. Agents Chemother. *33*, 1228 (1989).

24   A. Polak, in: J. Ryley (ed.): Handbook of Experimental Pharmacology, Chemotherapy of Fungal Disease *96*,Springer-Verlag, Berlin 1990, p. 153.

24a   J.W. Rippon and R. Fromtling (eds.): Cutaneous Antifungal Agents 1, Marcel Dekker, New York 1993.

25   W. Melchinger, A. Polak and J. Müller: Mycoses *33*, 393 (1988).

26   A. Polak: Mycoses *36*, 101 (1993).

27   H. Mensing, A. Polak, M. Zaug, R. Reckers-Czaschka and E. Schöpf: Dermatology 2000, Vienna, Abstract 800 (1993).

28   M. Zaug: J. Eur. Acad. Dermat. Venereól. (Suppl. 1), S23 (1995).

29   A. Polak: J. Eur. Acad. Dermat. Venereól. 4 (Suppl. 1), S11 (1995).

30   A. Polak: Mycoses *36*, 43 (1993).

31   J. Laurahanta, M . Zaug, A. Polak and D. Reinel: JAMA Southeast Asia *9* (Suppl. 4), 23 (1993).

32   M. Zaug: Eighth International Mycological Symposium of the Polish Dermatological Society, Bydgoszcz, Poland,. Abstract 15 (1994).

33   M. Feuilhade, R. Baran, S. Goettmann, P. Pietrini, C.Viguié, G. Badillet and C. Larnier: Clinical Dermatology 2000, Vancouver, Abstract 375 (1996).

34   S. Dole, C. Larnier and A. Chicoye: Clinical Dermatology 2000, Vancouver, Abstract 309 (1996).

35   I. Rekacewicz, J.C. Guillaume, F. Benkhraba, A. Archimbaud,M. Baspeyras, F. Boitier, M. Bussiere, A. Coin, M.C. Di Crezenzo, J. Duvalet al.: Ann. Dermatol. Vénéréol. *117*, 709 (1990).

36   J.E. Sansom, J.L. Burton and J.P. Leeming: Br. J. Dermatol. *132* (4), 650 (1995).

37   J. Faergemann, T.C. Jones, O. Hettler and Y. Loria: Br. J. Dermatol. *134* (Suppl. 46), 12 (1996).

38   S.E. Reef, M.M. McNeil, J.D. Sobel and R. Pinner: Infect. Dis. Clin. Practice *4* (1), 36 (1995).

39   C.M. Perry, R. Whittington and D. McTavish: Drugs *49* (6), 984 (1995).

40   T.W. Austin, M. Steben, M.Powell, B. Romanowski, D.W. Mergan, G.E. Garber and L.J. Margesson: Can. J. Infect. Dis. *7* (2), 110 (1996).

41   S. Faro: Infect. Dis. Obstet. Gynecol. *1*, 202 (1994).

42   I.W. Fong: Genitourn. Med. *68* (6), 374 (1992).

43   E.S. Mahgoub, in: G.L. Mandell, R.G. Douglas and J.E.J. Bennett (eds.): Agents of Mycetoma in principles and practice of infectious diseases, New York 1990, p. 1977.

44   A.G.M. Buiting, L.G. Visser, R.M.Y. Barge and J.W. van't Wout: Ned. Tijdschr. Geneesk. *137*, 1513 (1993).

45   J.P. Nozais, M.A. Canel, A. Atry and M. Danis: Bull. Soc. Pathol. Exot. *88*, 103 (1995).

46   S. Menon and J.C.W. Edwards: Br. J. Rheumatol. *33*, 292 (1994).

47   H.C. Gugnani, B.C. Ezenanolue, M. Khalil, C.D. Amoah, E.U. Ajuiu and A. Oyewo: Mycoses *38*, 485–488 (1995).

48   A. Polak: J. Chemother. 2 (4), 211 (1990).

49   A. Polak, in: Recent Progress in Antifungal Chemotherapy, H. Yamaguchi, G.S. Kobayashi and H. Takahashim (eds.), Chap. 7, Marcel Dekker New York (1991), p. 77.

50   D. Borelli: Rev. Infect. Dis. *9* (Suppl. 1), S57 (1987).
51   G. Moulin, Th. Cognat, E. Ferrier and H. Iligier: J. Dermatol. Paris *14*, 54 (1989)
52   M.A.H. Bayles: Chemotherapy *38* (Suppl. 1), 27 (1992).
52a   P. Esterre, C.K. Inzan, E.R. Ramarcel, A. Andriantsimahavandy, M. Ratsioharana, J.L. Pecarrere and P. Roig: Br. J. Dermatol. *134* (Suppl. 46), 33 (1996).
52b   P. Mayser, K. Gründer, S. Quadripur, F.M. Koehn, W.B. Schill and G.S. de Hoog: Hautarzt *47* (9), 693 (1996).
53   C.A. Kauffman: Clin. Infect. Dis. *21*, 981 (1995).
54   C.A. Kauffman: Clin. Infect. Dis. *22* (Suppl. 2), S148–153 (1996).
55   P.K. Sharkey Mathis, C.A. Kauffman, J.R. Graybill, D.A. Stevens, J.S. Hostettler and G. Cloud: Am. J. Med. *95* (3), 279 (1993).
56   C.A. Kauffman, P.G. Pappas, D.S. McKinsey, R.A. Greenfield, J.R. Perfect, G.A. Cloud, C.J. Thomas and W.E. Dismuskes: Clin. Infect. Dis. *22* (1), 46 (1996).
57   I. Marinova, V. Szabadosova, O. Brandeburova and V. Krcmery: Chemotherapy *40* (4), 287 (1994).
58   P. Kien, E. Garey, A. Brow, F, Edwards and D. Armstrong: Clin. Infect. Dis. *14*, 841 (1992).
59   D.K. Braun and C.A. Kauffman: Mycoses *35* (11–12), 305 (1992).
60   B. Neumeister, P Bartmann, G. Gaedicke and R. Marre: Mycoses *35* (5–6), 115 (1992).
61   A. Goldschmied-Reouven, J. Friedman and C. Block: J. Mycol. Méd. *3* (2), 99 (1993).
62   E. Anaissie, P. Nelson, M. Beremand, D. Kontoyiannis and M G. Rinaldi, in: Current topics in medical mycology, M. Borgers, R. Hay, M.G. Rinaldi (eds.) *4*, 231 (1992).
63   G.P. Melcher, D.A. McGough, A.W. Fothergill, C. Norris and M.G. Rinaldi: J. Clin. Microbiol. *13* (6), 1461 (1993).
64   L.K. Ammari, J.M. Puck and K.L. McGowan: Clin. Infect. Dis. *16* (1), 148–150 (1993).
64a   E. Cofranesco, C. Boschetti, M.A. Viviani, C. Bargiggia, A.M. Tortorano, M. Cortellaro and C. Zanussi: Haematologia *77* (3), 280 (1992).
65   M. Nucci, N. Spector, S. Lucena, P.C. Bacha, W. Pulcheri, A. Lamosa, A. Derossi, M.J. Caiuby, J. Macieria and H.P. Oliveira: Eur. J. Clin. Microbiol. Infect. Dis. *11* (12), 1160 (1992).
65a   T.J. Walsh, B. de Pauw, E. Anaissie and P. Martino: J. Med. Vet. Mycol. *32* (Suppl. 1), 33 (1994).
66   R.T. Spielberger, M.J. Felleroni, A.J. Coene and R.A. Larson: Clin. Infect. Dis. *16* (4), 528 (1993).
67   G.P. Giacoia: South. Med. J. *85* (12), 1247 (1992).
68   D.J. Fisher, C. Christy, P. Spafford, M. Maniscalco, D.J. Hardy and P.S. Graman: Ped. Infect. Dis. J. *12* (2), 151 (1993).
69   M.G. Sidarous, M. O'Reilly, C.E. Cherubin: Clin. Cardiol. *17* (4), 215 (1994).
70   J.O. Lopes, S.H. Alves, J.P. Benevenga, A.C. Rosa and V.C. Gomez: Rev. med. trop. São Paulo *36* (2), 121 (1194).
71   J.R. Perfect, W.A. Schell and M.G. Rinaldi: J. Med. Vet. Mycol. *31*, 175 (1993).
72   J.M. Still, K. Orle and E.J. Law: Burns *20* (5), 467–468 (1994).
73   S.M.H. Qadri and M.E. Ellis: J. Nat. Med. Assoc. *84* (5), 449 (1992).
74   T. Sirisantha: Japanese J. Med. Mycol. *37* (1), 5 (1996).
75   V. Sirisantha and T. Sirisantha: Pediatr. Infect. Dis. J. *14* (11), 935 (1995).
76   W.M. Tsui, K.F. Ma and D.N.C. Tsang: Histopathology *20* (4), 287 (1992).
77   S. Remadi, C. Lotfi, V. Finci, A. Ismail, D. Rogiano, P. Vassilakos and T.A. Seemayer: Acta Cytol. *39* (4), 798 (1995).
78   K.H. Keddy, K.P. Klugman: Southern African J. Epidemiol. Infection *9* (2), 51 (1994).

79   S. Yamada, T. Maruaka, K. Nagai, N. Tsumura, T. Yamada, Y. Sakata, K. Tominaga, T. Motohiro, H. Kato. K. Makimura and H. Yamagichi: Scan. J. Infect. Dis. *27* (1), 85 (1995),

80   S. Hirasaki, T. Ijichi, S. Araki, H. Gotoh and M. Nakagawa: Internal Medicine (Tokyo), *31* (5), 622 (1992).

81   A. Kunova, S. Spanik, T. Kllar, J. Trupl and V. Kremery: Chemotherapy *42* (2),157 (1996).

82   S.F. Welbel, M.M. McNeil, A. Pramanik, R. Silberman, A.D. Oberle, G. Midgley, S. Crow and W.R. Jarvis: Pediatr. Infect. Dis. J. *13* (2), 104 (1994).

83   R. Mesnard, T. Lamy, C. Dauria and P. Y. le Pryse: Acta Haematol. *87*,78 (1992).

83a   M.V.M. Stolk-Engelaar and N.J.M. Cox: Eur. J. Clin. Microbiol. Infect. Dis. 12 (2), 142 (1992).

84   T.A. Ruxin, W.D. Steck, T.N. Helm, W.F. Bergfeld and B.J. Bolwell: Arch. Dermatol. *132* (4), 382 (1996).

85   M. Alvarez, B.L. Ponga, C. Rayon, J.G. Gala, M.C.R. Porto, M. Gonzales, J.V. Martinez-Suarez and J.L. Roderiguez-Tudela: J. Clin. Microbiol. *33* (12), 3290 (1995).

86   P. Bourbeau, D.A. McGough, H. Fraser, N. Shah and M.G. Rinaldi: J. Clin Microbiol. *30* (1),3019 (1992).

87   A. Gautheret, F. Dromer, J.H. Bourhis and A. Andremont: Clin. Infect. Dis. *20* (4), 1063 (1995)

88   F. Jakobs, B. Byl, N. Bourgeois, J. Coremans-Pelsener, S. Florquin, G. Depre, J. van der Stadt, M. Adler, M. Gelin and J.P. Thys: Mycoses *35* (11–12), 301 (1992).

89   S.P. Abbott, L. Sigler, R. McAller, D.A. Mcgough, M.G. Rinaldi and G. Mizell: J. Clin. Microbiol. 33 (10), 2692 (1995).

90   C.A. Benne, C. Neeleman, C. Bruin, B.S. Hoog and A. De Fleer: Eur. J. Clin. Microbiol. Infect. Dis. *12* (2), 118 (1993).

91   W. Wanachiwanawin, M. Thianprasit, S. Fucharoen, A. Chaiprasert, N.S.N. Ayudhya, N. Sirthanaraktul, and A. Piankijagum: Trans. Roy. Soc. Trop. Med. Hyg. *87* (3), 296 (1993).

92   S. Hood and D.W. Denning: J. Antimicrob. Chemother. *37* (Suppl. B), 71 (1996).

93   M. Petoello-Montovani, A. Casadevall, T.R. Kollmann, A. Rubinstein and H. Goldstein: Lancet *339*, 21 (1992).

94   B.K. Carroll, S. Cohen, J. Whisenant, D.Riley, and P Beatty: Ninety-fourth Meeting of the American Society of Microbiology, Abstract 606 (1994).

95   W.G. Powderly, G.S. Kobayashi, G.P. Herzig and G. Medoff: Am. J. Med. *84*, 826 (1988).

96   S.L. Kelly, D.C. Lamb, D. Kelly, N.J. Manning, J. Loeffler, H. Hebart, U. Schuhmacher and H. Einsele: FEBS Lett. *400* (1), 80 (1997).

97   J. Bolard and P. Veni: J. Liposome Res. *3* (3), 409 (1993).

98   S.C. Hartsel, C. Hatch and W. Ayenew: J. Liposome Res. *3* (3), 377 (1993).

99   W.H. Beggs: Ninety-fourth Meeting of the American Society of Microbiology, Abstract 19 (1994).

100   P.D. Hoeprich: Clin. Infect. Dis. *14* (Suppl. 1), S114 (1992).

101   J.E. Edwards Jr. and S.G. Giller: Clin. Infect. Dis. *14* (Suppl. 1), S106 (1992).

101a   J.S. Conklin, M.Kwing and W.M. Wasan: Pharm Res. *13* (9 Suppl.), S117 (1996).

102   M.M. Zaman, S. Burney, D. Landman and J.M. Quale: Clin. Infect. Dis. *22* (2), 378 (1996).

103   M.F. Fernandez-Miera, M. Farinas, M.J. Del C Hazas Feo and P. Sanroma Mendizabal: Medicina Clinica *102* (11), 434 (1994).

104   M.P. Nagata, C.A. Gentry and E.M. Hampton: Ann. Pharmacother. *30*, 811 (1996).

105 G.A. Sarosi and P.C. Johnson: Clin. Infect. Dis. *14* (Suppl. 1), S60 (1992).

106 H. Albrecht, H.J. Stellbrink, J. Petersen, A. Patzak, H. Jaeger and H. Greten: Dtsch. Med. Wochenschr. *119* (18), 657 (1994).

107 V.R. Singh, D.K. Smith, J. Lawrence, P.C. Kelly, A.R. Thomas, B. Spitz and G.A. Sarosi: Clin. Infect. Dis. *23* (3), 563 (1996).

108 B. Dupont, D.W. Denning, D. Marriot, A. Sugar, M.A. Viviani and T. Sirisanthana: J. Med. Vet. Mycol. *32* (Suppl. 1), 65 (1994).

109 F. de Lalla, G. Pellizer, A. Vaglia, V. Manfrin, M. Franzetti, P. Fabris and C. Stecca: Clin. Infect. Dis. *20* (2), 263 (1995).

110 D.W. Denning: Clin. Infect. Dis. *23*, 608 (1996).

111 G. Lopez-Berestein, R.L. Hopfer, R. Mehta, K. Mehta, M.P. Sullivan and M. Keating: J. Infect. Dis. *151*, 704 (1985).

112 V. Joly, P. Aubry, A. Ndayiragide, I. Carriere, E. Kawa, N. Mlika-Cabanne, JP. Aboulker, JP. Coulaud, B. Larouze and P. Yeni: Clin. Infect. Dis. *23*, 556 (1996).

113 P. Joli, JC. Joly, R. Farinotti, L. Saint Julien, M. Cheron, C. Carbon and P Yeni: Antimicrob. Agents Chemother. *38* (2), 177 (1994).

114 A. Ayestaran, R.M. Lopez, J.B. Estibalez, L. Pou, A. Julia, A. Lopez, B. Pascual: Antimicrob. Agents. Chemother. *40* (3), 609 (1996).

115 P. Villani, M.B. Regazzi, R. Maserati, P. Viale, F. Alberici and I. Buggia: Pharm. World Sci. *16* (5 Suppl. G), G30 (1994).

116 K.M. Wasan, M.G. Rosenblum, L. Chung and G. Lopez-Berestein: Antimicrob. Agents Chemother. *38* (2), 223 (1994).

117 E.W.M. van Etten, M.T. ten Kate, L.E.T. Stearne and I.A.J.M. Bakker Woudenberg: Antimicrob. Agents Chemother. *39* (9), 1954 (1995).

118 D. Chitnavis, J. Maddon and T.J. Littlewood: Blood *86* (Suppl. 1), 510A (1995).

119 M.L. Andria, M.D. Povronik, J.P. Lynch, M.L. Auber and C.I. Beall: Proc. Am. Soc. Clin. Oncol. *15*, 334 (1996).

120 T.M. Sievers, B.M. Kubak and A. Wong-Beringer: J. Antimicrob. Chemother. *38* (3), 333 (1996).

120a P. Villani, M.B. Regazzi, R. Maserati, P. Viale, F. Alberici and R. Giacchino: Drug Res. *46* (4), 445 (1996).

121 J.W. Hiemenz and T.J. Walsh: Clin. Infect Dis. *22* (Suppl2), S133 (1996).

122 E. Anaissie, V. Paetznick, J. Adler-Moore, G.P. Bodey: Eur. Clin. Microbiol. Infect. Dis. *10*, 665 (1991).

123 H. Schneemann: Krankenhauspharmazie *4*, 161–71 (1992).

124 J. Graybill: Clin. Infect. Dis. *22* (Suppl2), S166 (1996).

125 S. de Marie, R. Janknegt and I.A.J.M. Bakker Woudenberg: J. Antimicrob. Chem. *33*, 907 (1994).

126 J. Adler-Moore, G. Fujii, M.J.A. Lee, A. Satorius, A. Bailey and R. Proffitt : J. Liposome Res. *3*, 151(1993).

127 J. Adler-Moore and R.T. Proffitt: J. Liposome Res. *3* (3), 429 (1993).

128 J. Adler-Moore: Bone Marrow Transplantation *14* (Suppl. 5), S3 (1994).

129 V. Heinemann, B. Kähny, A. Debus, K. Wachholz and U. Jehn: Bone Marrow Transplantation *14* (Suppl. 5), S8 (1994).

130 W. Krüger, M. Stockschläder, B. Rüssman, C. Berger, M. Hofknecht, I. Sobottka, B. Kohlschütter, G. Kröger, M. Horstmann, H. Kabisch and R.A. Zander: Br. J. Haematol. *91* (3), 684 (1995).

131 F. Meunier, H.G. Prentice and O. Ringden: J. Antimicrob. Chem. *28* (Suppl. B), 83 (1991).

132   O. Ringden, E. Andström, M. Remberger, B.M. Svahn and J. Tollemar: Bone Marrow Transplantation *14* (Suppl. 5), S10–14 (1994).

133   R.A. Bowden, M. Cays, T. Gooley, R.D. Mamelok and J.A. Van Burik: J. Infect. Dis. *173*, 1208 (1996).

134   B.A. Opppenheim, R. Herbrecht and S. Kusne: Clin. Infect. Dis. *21* (5),1145 (1995).

135   P.K. Sharkley, J.R. Graybill, E.S. Johnsen, S.G. Hausrath, R.B. Pollard, A.Kolokathis, D. Mildvan, P. Havard, R.H.K. Eng, T.F. Patterson et al.: Clin. Infect. Dis. *22* (2), 315 (1996).

136   O. Ringden, F. Meunier, J. Tollemar, P. Ricci, S. Tura, E. Kuse, M.A. Viviani, N.C. Gorin, J. Klastersky, P. Fenaux et al.: J. Antimicrob. Chemother. *28* (Suppl. B), 73 (1991).

137   W. Mills, R. Chopra, D.C. Linch and A.H. Goldstone: Br. J. Haematol. *86* (4), 754 (1994).

138   V. Monforte, C. Murio, A. Roman, G. Gavalda, C. Bravo, M. Montana, A. Pahissa and F. Morell: Eur. Resp. J. *8* (Suppl. 19), 129s (1995).

139   P.C. Gokhale, N.A. Kshirsagar, M.U. Khan, S.K. Pandya, R.H. Merchant and K.P. Mehta: J. Antimicrob. Chemother. *33* (4), 889 (1994).

140   M. Viviani, G. Rizzardini, A.M. Tortorano, M. Fasan, A. Capetti and A.M. Roverselli: Infection *22* (2), 137–142 (1994).

141   T.T.C. Ng and D.W. Denning: Arch. Intern. Med. *155* (10), 1093 (1995).

142   A. Wong-Behringer, P.M. Behringer and J.P. Rho: Formulary *31* (3),169 (1996).

143   J. Lister: Blood *84* (Suppl. 1), 306A (1994).

144   M.D. Strasser, R.J. Kennedey and R.D. Adam: Arch. Intern. Med. *156* (3), 337 (1996).

145   J.W. Hiemenz, J. Lister, E.J. Anaissie, M.H. White, M. Dinubile, G. Horowith and L. Lee: Blood *86* (Suppl. 1), 849A (1995).

146   J. Mehta, R. Powles, S. Sinhal, B. Jameson and J. Treleaven: Eur. J. *31* (Suppl. 5), S255 (1995).

147   M.G. Tierny, A.M. Runet, W.M. McLean, B.W. Toye and G.E. Garber: Can. J. Hosp. Pharm. *47* (4), 171–175 (1994).

148   A.Polak and H. Scholer: Rev. Inst. Pasteur *13*, 233 (1980).

149   A. Polak: J. Antimicrob. Chemother. *26* (4), 465 (1990).

150   J.P. Greenstein, C.E. Carter, H.W. Chalkley and F.M. Lezuthardt: J. Natl. Cancer Inst. *7*, 9 (1946).

151   B.E. Harris, R.B. Diasio, B.W. Manning and T.W. Federle: Antimicrob. Agents Chemother. *29*, 44 (1986),

152   A. Polak: Handbook of Experimental Pharmacology vol. 96, Chemotherapy of Fungal Dis., chap. 6, Springer-Verlag Berlin (1990), p. 153.

153   H.J. Scholer and A.Polak: Antimicrob. Drug Resistance, chap. 14, Academic Press New York (1984), p. 393.

154   S. Weber and A. Polak: Mycoses *35*, 163 (1992).

155   W.L. Whelan and P. Magee: J. Bacteriol. *145*, 896 (1981).

156   M.O. Fasoli, D. Kerridge and J.F. Ryley: J. Med. Vet. Mycol. *28*, 27 (1990).

157   A. Polak: Mycoses *35*, 9 (1992).

158   C.A. Kaufmann and P.T. Frame: Antimicrob. Agents Chemother. *11*, 244 (1997).

159   A.M. Stamm, R.B. Diasio, W.E. Dismuskes, S. Shadomy, G.A. Cloud, C.A. Bowles, G.H. Karam and A. Espinel-Ingroff: Am. J. Med. *83*, 236 (1987).

160   T.J. Walsh: Clin. Infect. Dis. *15* (6), 1003–1018 (1992).

161   M. White, C. Cirrinicione, A. Blevins and D. Armstrong: J. Infect. Dis. *165*, 960 (1992).

162   H. Vanden Bosche and P. Marichal, in: Recent Progress in Antifungal Chemother-

apy, H. Yamaguchi, G.S. Kobayashi and H. Takahashim (eds.), chap. 3, Marcel Dekker New York (1991), p. 25.

163   C.A. Hitchcock and P.J. Wittle, in: Cutaneous Antifungal Agents, J.W. Rippon and R. Fromtling (eds.), chap. 15, Marcel Dekker New York (1993), p. 183.

164   C.A. Lyman and T.J. Walsh: Drugs *44* (1), 9 (1992).

165   J.A. Como and W.E. Dismuskes: N. Eng. J. Med. *330* (4), 263 (1993).

166   J.C. Fleishaker, L.K. Pewarson. P.G. Pearson, L.C. Wienkers and G.R. Peters: Phar. Res. *12* (9 Suppl.), S373 (1995).

167   T.J. Walsh, M. Rubin, J. Hathorn, J. Gress and M. Thaler: Arch. Intern. Med. *151*,765 (1991).

168   B.F. Dupont, F. Dromer and L. Improvisi: J. Mycol. Méd. *6* (Suppl. 2), 12 (1996).

169   B.S. Zingman: J. Mycol. Méd. *6* (Suppl. 2), 3 (1996).

170   M. Tumbarello, G.Caldarola, E. Tacconelli, G. Morace, B. Posteraro, R. Cauda and L. Ortona: J. Antimicrob. Chemother. *38* (4), 691 (1996).

171   M. Ruhnke, A. Eigler, I. Teenegen, B. Geisler, E. Engelmann and M. Trautmann: J. Clin. Microbiol. *32*, 2093 (1994).

172   E.M. Johnson and D.W. Warnock: J. Antimicrob. Chemother. *36*, 751 (1995).

173   M. McCullough and S. Hume: J. Med. Vet. Mycol. *33*, 33 (1995).

174   F. Barchiesi, R.J. Hollis, D.A. McGough, G. Scalise, M.G. Rinaldi and M.A. Pfaller: Clin. Infect. Dis. *20* (3), 634 (1995).

175   J. Berenguer, T.M. Diaz-Guerra, B. Ruiz Diez, J.C.L.B. de Quiros, J.L. Rodriguez-Tudela and J.V. Martinez-Suarez: J. Clin. Microbiol. *34* (6), 1542 (1996).

176   F. Barchiesi, R.J. Hollis, M. Del Poeta, D.A. McGough, G. Scalise, M.G. Rinaldi and M.A. Pfaller: Clin. Infect. Dis. *21* (3), 561 (1995).

177   D.A. Goff, S.L. Koletar, W.J. Buesching, J. Barnishan and R.J. Fass: Clin. Infect. Dis. *20* (1), 77 (1995).

178   A. Kunova, J. Trupl, S. Spanik, L. Drgona, J.Sufliarsky, J.Lacka, V.Studena, E. Kukuckova, T: Kollar, P. Pichna, E. Oracova and V. Jkrcmery: Chemotherapy *41*, 39 (1995).

179   M.F. Price, M.T. LaRocco and L.O. Gentry: Antimicrob. Agents Chemother. *38* (6), 1422 (1994).

180   M.H. Nguyen, V.L. Yu, A.J. Morris, D.R. Snydman, M.L. Mguyen, J.E. Peacock and M.A. Rinaldi: Abstr. Gen. Meet. Am. Assoc. Microbiol. 95, 106 (1995).

181   D.C. Lamb, A. Corran, B.C. Baldwin, J. Kwong-Chung and S.L. Kelly: FEBS Lett. *368* (2), 326 (1995).

182   D. Sanglard, K. Kuchler, F. Ischer, J.I. Pagani, M. Monod and J. Bille: Antimicrob. Agents Chemother. *39* (11), 2378 (1995).

183   T. Parkinson, D.J. Falconer and C.A. Hitchcock: Antimicrob. Agents Chemother. *39* (8), 1696 (1995).

184   P. Marchial, J. Gorrens, M.C. Coene, L. Le Jeune and H. Vanden Bossche: Mycoses *38*, 111 (1995).

185   K. Vankateswarlu, D.W. Denning, N.J. Manning and S.L. Kelly: FEMS Microbiol. Lett. *131* (3), 337 (1995).

186   H. Vanden Bossche, P. Marchial and F. Odds: Trends Microbiol *2*, 393 (1994).

187   X. He, R.N. Tiballi, L.T. Zarins, S.F. Bradley, J.A. Sangeorzan and C.A. Kauffman: Antimicrob. Agents Chemother. *38* (10), 2495 (1994).

188   E.M. Johnson, G.D. Kathleen, A. Azeleey and D.W. Warnock: J. Antimicrob. Chemother. *36*, 787 (1995).

189   M.O. Gearthart: Ann. Pharmacother *28* (19), 1177 (1994).

190   W. Inman, G. Pearce and L. Wilton: Eur. J. Clin. Pharmacol. *46* (2), 115 (1994).

191   T.J. Pursley, I.K. Blomquist, J. Abraham, H.F. Andersen and J.A. Bartley: Clin. Infect. Dis. *22* (2), 336 (1996).

192   M. Zervos and F. Meunier: Omt. J. Antimicrob. Agents *3*, 147 (1994).

193   N.C. Karyotakis and E.J. Anaissie: Curr. Opin. Infect. Dis. *7*, 658 (1994).

194   D.P. Niclau, H.M. Crowe, C.H. Nightingale and R. Quintiliani: Ann. Pharmacother. *29* (10), 994 (1995).

195   R.M. Cadle, G.J. Zenon, M.C. Rodriguez Barradas and R.J. Hamill: Ann. Pharmacother. *29* (2), 191 (1994).

196   K.L. Kunze, L.C. Wienkers, K.E. Thummel and W.F. Trager: Drug Metab. Dispos. *24* (4), 414 (1996).

197   D.J. Black, K.L. Kunze, L.C. Wienkers, B.E. Gidal, T.L. Seaton, N.D. McDonnell, J.S. Evans, J.E. Bauwens and W.F. Trager: Drug. Metab. Disp. *24* (4), 422 (1996).

198   K.L. Kunze and W.F. Trager: Drug. Metab. Dispos. *24* (4), 429 (1996).

199   A. Plettenberg, A. Stoehr, G. Hoeffken, C. Bergs, B. Tschechne and M. Ruhnke: Infection *22* (2), 118 (1994).

200   G. Barbaro, G. Barbarini, W. Calderon, B. Grisiorio, P. Alcini and G. Di Lorenz: Gastroenterology *111* (5), 1169 (1996).

201   M. Akova, H.E. Akalm, O. Uzum, M. Hyran, G. Tekuman and E. Kansu: Clin. Infect. Dis. *18* (3), 298 (1994).

202   D.E. Lake, J. Kunzweiler, M. Beer, D.N. Buell and M.Z. Islam: Chemotherapy *42*, 308 (1996).

202a G. Barbaro, G. Barbarini, W. Calderon, B. Griserio, P. Alcini and G. Di Lorenzo: Gut *39* (Suppl. 3), A35 (1996).

203   L. Laine and L. Rabeneck: Aliment. Pharmacol. Ther. *9* (5), 553 (1995).

204   A. Wildfeuer, H. Laufen, R.A. Yeates and T. Zimmermann: Mycoses *39* (1), 123 (1996).

205   F. Parente, S. Ardizzone, M. Cernuschi, S. Antinori, R. Esposito and M. Moroni: Am. J. Gastroenterol. *89* (3), 416 (1994).

206   L. Rabeneck and L. Laine: Arch. Intern. Med. *154* (23), 2705 (1994).

207   J.L. Pagani, J.P. Chave, A Iten, C. Durussel, J. Bille and M.P. Glauser: Schweiz. Med. Wochenschr. *126* (9 Suppl. 74 Pt 2), 49S (1996).

208   L. Bernstein, W. Hsu, J. Schliozberg and S Iqbal: *76* (1), 83 (1996).

209   S.G. Revankar, W. Kirkpatrick, R.K. McAtee, O.P. Dib, A.W. Fothergill, S.W. Redding, M.G. Rinaldi and T.F. Patterson: J. Infect. Dis. *174*, 821 (1996).

210   J.H. Rex, J.E. Bennettt, A.M. Sugar, P.G. Pappas, C.M. van der Horst, J.E. Edwards, R.G. Washburn, W.M. Scheld, A.W. Karchmer, A.P. Dine et al.: N. Eng. J. Med. *331* (20), 1325 (1994).

211   P. Kujath, K. Lerch, P. Kochendorfer and C. Boos: Infection *21* (6), 376 (1993).

212   B.E. de Pauw, J.M.M. Raemaekers, J.P. Donnelly, B.J. Kullberg and F.G.M. Meis: Annales of Hematology *70* (2), 83 (1995).

212a E. Anaissie, R.O. Darouiche, D. Abi Said, O. Uzon, J. Mera, L.O. Gentry, T. Williams, D.P. Kontoyiannis, C.L. Karl and G.P. Bodey: Clin. Infect. Dis. *23* (5), 964 (1996).

213   D. Armstrong: Clin. Infect. Dis. *16* (1), 1 (1993).

214   E. Presterl and W. Graninger: Eur. J. Clin. Microbiol. Infect. Dis. *13* (4), 347 (1994).

215   C. Fasano, J. O'Keeffe and D. Gibbs: Eur. J. Clin. Microbiol. Infect. Dis. *13* (4), 351 (1994).

216   H. Bilgen, F. Ozek, V. Korten, B. Ener and D. Molbay: Infection *23* (6), 394 (1995).

217   N. Gurses and A.G. Kalayci: Clin. Infect. Dis. *23* (3), 645 (1996).

218   T.J. Walsh, P.O. Whitcomber, S.G. Revankar and P.A. Pizzo: Cancer *76* (11), 2357 (1995).

219 A. del Palacio, M.S. Cuetera, M. Ferro, E. Perez Blazquez, J.A. Lopez Sana and M.P. Roiz: Mycoses *36*, 193 (1993).

220 M.E. Akler, H. Vellend, D.M. McNeely, S.L. Walmsley and W.L. Gold: Clin. Infect. Dis. *20* (3), 657 (1995).

221 L.G. Jacobs, E.A. Skidmore, K. Freeman, D. Lipschultz and N. Fox: Clin. Infect. Dis. *22* (1), 30 (1996).

222 P. Fan-Havard, C. O'Donovan, S.M. Smith, M. Bamberger and R.H. K. Eng: Clin. Infect. Dis. *21* (4), 960 (1995).

223 H.S. Leu and C.T. Huang: Clin. Infect. Dis. *20* (5),1152 (1995).

224 S.H. Ansari, M.H. Levin and S Lipshitz: J. Urol. *154* (5), 1870 (1995).

225 F.Menichetti, M.Fiorio, A. Tosti, G. Gatti, M.B. Pasticci, F. Miletich, M. Marroni, D. Bassetti and S. Pauluzzi: Clin. Infect. Dis. *22* (5),838 (1996).

226 S.D. Nightingale: Arch. Intern. Med. *155* (5), 538 (1995).

227 M.C. Meyohas, J.L. Meynard, D. Bollens, P. Roux, A.M. Deluol, J.L. Poirot, W. Rozenbaum, C. Meyaud and J. Frottier: J. Infect. *33* (1), 7 (1996).

228 J.A. Newton, P.Olson, S.A.Tasker, W.D. Bone, M.T. Nguyen and E.C. Oldfield: Clin. Infect. Dis. *17* (3), 563 (1993).

229 J.P. Viard, C. Hennequin, N. Fortineau, N. Pertuiset, C. Rothschild and H. Zylberberg: Lancet *346* (8967),118 (1995).

230 F. Dromer, S. Mathoulin, B. Dupont, O. Burgiere, L. Letenneur and the French Cryptococcosi Group: Clin. Infect. Dis. *22* (Suppl. 2), S154 (1996).

231 W.W.Yew, P.C. Wong, C.F. Wong, J. Lee and C. H. Chau: Drugs. Exp. Clin. Res. *22* (1), 25 (1996).

232 E.J. Anaissie, D.P. Kontoyiannis, V. Huls, S.E. Vartvarian, C. Karl, R. Prince, J. Bosso and G.P. Bodey: J. Infect. Dis. *172* (2), 599 (1995).

233 D.A. Stevens: N. Engl. J. Med. *332* (16), 1077 (1996).

234 G.P. Pappas, R.W. Bradsher, S.W. Chapman, C.A. Kauffman, A. Dine, G.A. Cloud and W.A. Dismuskes: Clin. Infect. Dis. *20* (2), 267 (1995).

234a D. McKinsey, C.A. Kauffman, P.G. Cloud, W.M. Girard, P. K. Sharkey, R.J. Hamill, C. Thomas and W.E. Dismuskes: Clin. Infect. Dis. *23* (5), 996 (1996).

235 S. Norris, J. Wheat, D. McKinsey, D. Lancaster, B. Katz and J. Black: Am. J. Med. *96* (6), 504 (1994).

236 H. Vanden Bossche, D.W. R. Mackenzie, G. Cauwenbourg (eds.): Aspergillus and Aspergillosis, Plenum Press New York (1988).

236a Mycoses *37* (Suppl. 2), (1994).

237 J.M. Poirier, F. Berlioz, F. Isnard and G. Cheymol: Therapy *50* (Suppl.), 492 (1995).

238 M. Schaffner-Korting, H. Korting, W. Rittler and W. Obermüller: Infection *23* (5), 292 (1995).

239 S.K. Hann, J.B. Kim, S. Im, K.H. Kann and Y.K. Park: Br. J. Dermatol. *129* (4),500 (1993).

240 F. Moreno, T.C. Hardin, M.G. Rinaldi and J.R. Graybill: J. Am. Med. Assoc. *269* (12), 1508 (1993).

214 J. Drayton, G. Dickinson abd M.G. Rinaldi: Clin. Infect. Dis. *18* (2), 266 (1994).

242 J. Ahonen, K.T. Alkkola and P.J. Neuvonen: Therapie *50* (Suppl.), 190 (1995).

243 J. Ahonen, K.T. Alkkola and P.J. Neuvonen: Therapie *50* (Suppl.), 421 (1995).

244 R.H.B. Meyboom, K. de Jonge, H. Veentjer, J.A.M. Dekens-Konter and G.H.P. de Koning: Ned.Tijdschr.Geneeskd. *138* (47), 2353 (1994).

245 P.J. Neuvonen and K.M. Jalava: Clin. Pharmacol. Ther. *60* (1), 54 (1996).

246 P. Honig, D. Wortham, R. Hull, K. Zamani, J. Smith and L. Cantilena: Clin. Pharmacol. Ther. *55* (29), 165 (1994).

247   L. de Repentigny, J. Ratelle and the HIV Itraconazole Ketoconazole Project Group: Chemotherapy *42*, 374 (1996).

248   M. Eichel, G. Just-Nübling, E.B. Helm and W. Stille: Mycoses *39* (Suppl. 1), 102 (1996).

249   T. Inamatsu, T. Mori, K. Watanabe, A. Ita and H. Ikemoto: Chemotherapy *38* (Suppl. 1), 56 (1992).

250   J.W. van t'Wout: Chemotherapy *38* (Suppl. 1), 23 (1992).

251   J. de Gans, P. Portegies, G. Tiessens, J.K. Eeftinck-Schattenkerk and C.J. van Boxtel-Patton: AIDS *6*, 185 (1992).

252   M.A. Viviani, A.M. Tortorano, R. Woenstenberghs and R. Cauwenbergh: Mykosen *30*, 233 (1988).

253   M.A. Viviani, A.M. Tortorano, A. Pagano, G.M. Vigevani, G. Gubertini, S. Cristina, M.L. Assaisso, F. Suter, C. Farina, B. Minettiet al.: J. Am. Acad. Dermatol. *23*, 587 (1990).

254   D.W. Dismuskes and D.A. Stevens: Rev. Infect. Dis. *12*, 1147 (1990).

255   T.S. Jennings and T.C. Harding: Ann. Pharmacother. *27* (10), 1206 (1993).

256   J.J. Keating, T. Rogers, M. Petrou, J.D. Cartledge, D. Woodrow and M. Nelson: J. Clin. Pathol. *47* (9), 805 (1994).

257   B. Lebeau, H. Pelloux, C. Pinel, M. Michalllet, J.P. Gout, C. Pison, P. Delormas, J.P. Bru, J.P. Brion, P. Ambroise-Thomas and R. Grillot: Mycoses *37* (5-6), 171 (1994).

258   D.W. Denning, J.Y. Lee, J.S. Hodtetler, P. Pappas, C.A. Kauffman, D.H. Dewsnup, J.N. Galgiani, J.R. Graybill, A.M. Sugar, A. Catanzaroet al.: Am. J. Med. *97*, 135 (1994).

259   M. Jorgensen, A. Glanville, M. Rowland, J. Mundy, P. MacDonald and A. Keogh: Aust. N.Z. J. Med *24* (4), 452 (1994).

260   S.M. Hakim, L.J.R. Milne, C. Fox, I.M. Nawroz, G. Webb and G.T. Vaugham: Br. J. Clin. Pract. *47* (6), 312 (1993).

261   C. Sanchez, E. Mauri, D. Dalmau, S. Quintana, A. Aparico and J. Garau: Clin. Infect. Dis. *21* (6), 1485 (1995).

262   G.P.M. Mannes, S. van der Heide, W.M.C. van Aalderen and J. Gerritsen: Eur. Resp. J. *6* (Suppl. 17), 217S (1993).

263   I. Huttegger, M. Brandauer and J. Riedler: Atemwegs Lungenkrankh. 21 (9), 471 (1995).

264   J.R. Graybill, in: Chemotherapy of Fungal Therapy, J.F. Ryley (ed.), Springer Verlag, Berlin (1990), chap. 19, p. 455.

264a P.K. Sharkey, J.R. Graybill, M.G. Rinaldi, D.A. Stevens, R.M. Tucker, J.D. Peterie, P.D. Hoeprich et al.: J. Am. Acad. Dermatol. *23*, 577 (1990).

265   A. del Palacio, C. Gomez-Hernando, F. Revenga, E. Carabias, A. Gonzalez, M.S. Cuetara and E.M. Johnson: Clin. Exp. Dermatol. *21* (3), 241 (1996).

266   J. Gene, A. Azon-Masoliver, J. Guarro, F. Ballester, I. Pujol, M. Llovera and C. Ferrer: J.Clin. Microbiol. *33* (10), 2774 (1995).

267   D.I. Wittle and S. Kominos: Clin. Infect. Dis. *21* (4), 1068 (1995).

268   T.J. Babinchak, E.B. Rotheram and M. Slifkin: Clin. Infect. Dis. *21* (3), 772 (1995).

269   S.M. Kralovic and J.C. Rhodes: J. Infect. *31* (2), 107 (1995).

270   J. Wheat, R. Hafner, A.H. Korzun, M.T. Limjoco, P. Spencer, R.A. Larsen, F.M. Hecht and W. Powderly: Am. J. Med. *98* (4), 336 (1995).

271   J. Wheat, R. Hafner, M. Wulfsohn, P. Spencer, K. Squires, W. Powderly, B. Wong, M. Rinaldi, M. Saag, R. Hamill et al.: Ann. J. Med *118*, 610 (1993).

272   W.E. Dismuskes, R.W. Bradsher, G.C. Cloud, C.A. Kauffman, R.B. George, D.A. Stevens, W.M. Girard, M.S. Saag and C. Bowles Patton: Am. J. Med. *93*, 489 (1992).

273 R.Negroni, O. Palmierei, F. Koren, I.N. Tiraboschi, R.L. Galimberti: Rev. Infect Dis. *9* (Suppl.), S47 (1987).
274 P.K. Sharkey-Mathis, C.A. Kauffman, J.R. Graybill, D.A. Stevens, J.S. Hostetler, G. Cloud and W.E. Dismukes: Am. J. Med. *95*, 279 (1993).
275 G. Medoff, M. Comfort, G.S. Kobayashi: Proc. Assoc. Exp. Biol. Med. *138*, 571–574 (1971).
276 A. Polak: Chemotherapy *28*, 461 (1982).
277 A. Polak: Chemotherapy *33*, 381 (1987).
278 W.E. Dismuskes, in: Diagnosis and Therapy of Systemic Fungal Infections, K. Holmberg and R. Meyer (eds.) chap. 10, Raven Press New York (1989).
279 T.J.Walsh, J. van Cutsem, A. Polak and J.R. Graybill: J. Med. Veterin. Mycol. *30* (Suppl. 1), 225–240 (1992).
280 M. Thaler, J. Bacher, T. O'Leary: J. Infect. Dis. *158*, 80 (1988).
281 C. Lovannitti, R. Negroni, J. Bava, J. Finquelievivh and M. Kral: Mycoses *38* (11–12), 449 (1995).
282 A. Schaffner and P.G. Frick: J. Infect. Dis. *151*, 902-910 (1985).
283 A. Schaffner, personal communication.
284 A.M. Sugar, C.A. Hitchcock, P.F. Troke and M. Picard: Antimicrob. Agents Chemother. *39* (3), 598 (1995).
285 E.J. Anaissie, R. Hachem, N.C. Karyotakis, A. Gokaslan, M.C. Dignani and L.C. Stephans: Antimicrob. Agents Chemother. *38* (11), 2451 (1994).
286 J.E. Bennett, W.E. Dismuskes, R.J. Duma, G. Medoff, M.A. Sande, H. Gallis, J. Leonard, B.T. Fields, M. Bradshaw, H. Haywood et al.: N. Engl. J. Med. *301* (3), 127 (1979).
287 W.E. Dismuskes, G. Cloud, H.A. Gallis, T.M. Kerkering, G. Medoff, P.C. Craven, L.G. Kaplowitz, J.F. Fisher, C.R. Gregg, C.A. Bowles et al.: N. Engl. J. Med. *317* (6), 334 (1987).
288 R. Allendoerfer, A.J. Marquis, M.G. Rinaldi and J.R. Graybill: Antimicrob. Agents Chemother. *35*, 726 (1991).
289 P. Francis and T.J. Walsh: Clin. Infect. Dis. *15* (6), 1003 (1992).
290 W.E. Dismuskes: Clin. Infect. Dis. *17* (Suppl. 2), S507 (1993).
291 M White, C. Cirrincione, A. Blevins and D. Armstrong: J. Infect. Dis. *165*, 960 (1992).
292 R.A. Larsen, S.A. Bozzette, B.E. Jones, D. Haghighat, M.A. Leal, D.Forthal, M. Bauer, J.G. Tilles, J.A. McCutchan and J.M. Leedom: Clin. Infect. Dis. *19*, 741 (1994).
293 M.A. Viviani: J. Antimicrob. Chemother. *35*, 241 (1995).
294 G. Just-Nübling, C. Lauenberger, E.B. Helm, S. Falk and W. Stille: Forschg. Praxis *9* (106), VI (1990).
295 P. Cottagnoud, M. Rossi, J. Ross and K. Neftle: Infect. Dis. Clin. Practice *4* (6), 456 (1995).
296 V Chotmongkol and S. Jitipimolmard: Trop. Med. Public Health *26* (2), 381 (1995).
297 S.G. Filler and J.E. Edwards: Curr. Clin. Topics Infect. Dis. *15*, 1 (1995).
298 P.E. Verweij, J.P. Donnelly, B.J. Kullberg, J.F.G.M. Meis and P.E. de Pauw: Infection *22* (2), 81 (1994).
299 H.M. Gilbert, E.D. Peters, S.J. Lang and B.J. Hartman: Clin. Infect. Dis *22* (2), 348 (1996).
300 I.K.P. Cheng, G.X. Fang, T.M. Chan and M.K. Chan: Quart. J. Med. *71*, 265, 407 (1989).
301 A. Slingeneyer, B. Laroche, F. Stec, B. Canaud, J.J. Beraud and C. Mion: Perit. Dial. Bulletin *4* (Suppl. 1), 60 (1984).
302 B. Dupont and E. Drouhet: J. Inf. Dis. *152*, 577 (1985).
303 P.A. Burch, J.E. Karp and J. Merz: J. Clin. Oncol. *5*, 1985 (1987).

304   T. Walsh and P.A Pizzo, in: Holmberg, R.D. and Meyer (eds.): Diagnosis and Therapy of Systemic Fungal Infections, Raven Press, New York 1989, p. 47.

305   R. Negroni, A.M. Robles and A. Arechiavala: Rev. Argentina de Micologia *18* (1), 2 (1995).

306   T.J. Walsh, J. Van Cutsem, A. Polak and J.R. Graybill: J. Med.Vet. Mycol. *30* (Suppl. 1), 225 (1992).

307   P. Pucetti, A. Menacci, E. Cenci, R. Spaccapelo, P. Mosci and K.H. Enssle: J. Infect. Dis. 269 (6), 1325 (1994).

308   J.E. Lutz, K.V. Clemons, W.C. Darbonne, J.T. Curnutte and D.A. Stevens: Clin. Infect, Dis. *23* (4), 899 (1996).

309   A. Polak: Mycoses *34*, 109 (1991).

310   J.L. Herrmann, N. Dubois, M. Fourgeaud, D. Basset and P.H. Lagrange: J. Antimicrob. Chemother. *34* (6), 1051 (1994).

311   J.E. Lutz, K.V. Clemons and D.A. Stevens: Clin. Infect. Dis. *23* (4), 899 (1996).

312   V.Joly, L. Saint Julien, C. Carbon and P. Yeni: J. Infect. Dis. *170* (5), 1331 (1994).

313   A. Polak: Mycoses *34*, 205 (1991).

314   D. Arenberg, E. Nanarro, E. Roilides, V. Thomas, J. Peter, J.W. Lee, P.S. Francis, P.A. Pizzo and T.J. Walsh: Ann.Meet. Am. Soc. Microbiol., Abstract F-90, p. 423 (1990).

315   E. Brummer, F. Nassar and D.A. Stevens: Antimicrob. Agents Chemother. *38* (9), 2158 (1994).

316   F. Nassar, E. Brummer and D.A. Stevens: Cell. Immunol. *164* (1), 113 (1995).

317   C.R. Vitt, J.M. Fidler, D. Ando, R.J. Zimmermann and S.L. Aukerman: J. Infect. Dis. *169* (2), 369 (1994).

318   E.G. Playford and R. Wells: Aust. N. Z. J. Med. *26* (4), 620 (1996).

319   C.J. Clancy, L.E. Diaz and M.H. Nguyen: Clin. Infect. Dis. *23* (4), 899 (1996).

320   T. Himura, T. Hirayama, M. Banzai, T. Oda, N. Saito and M. Numazaki: Jpn. J. Antibiot. *47* (4), 428 (1994).

321   C. Hennequin, M. Benkerrou, J.L. Gaillard, S. Blanche and S. Fraitag: Clin. Infect. Dis. *18* (3), 490 (1994).

322   M.E. Grauer, C. Bokemeyer, W. Bautsch, M. Freund and H. Limk: Infection *22* (4), 55 (1994).

323   G.P. Bodey, E. Anaissie, J. Gutterman and S.Vadhan Raj: Clin. Infect. Dis. *17* (4), 705 (1993).

324   R.T. Spiegerlberger, M.J. Falleroni, A.J. Coene and R.A. Larsen: Clin. Infect. Dis. *16* (4), 528 (1993).

325   G. Schiller, C. O'Neill, J. Neumunaitis, D. Ando and J. O'Byrne: Blood *82* (Suppl. 1) 517a (1993).

326   P.A. Pizzo, K.J. Robichaud, F. Gill and F.G. Witebsky: Am.J. Med. *72*, 101 (1982).

327   EORTC International Antimicrob. Therapy Cooperative Group: Am J.Med. *86*, 668 (1989).

328   G. Plum, C. Scheid, C. Franzen, H. Schutt-Gerowitt, H. Seifert and P. Dias Wickramanayake: Zbl. Bakteriol. *284* (2), 361 (1996).

329   E.A. Blumberg and A.C. Reboli: Clin. Infect. Dis. *22* (3), 462 (1996).

330   C. Viscoli, E. Castagnola, M.T. van Lint, C. Moroni, A. Garaventa, M.R. Rossi, R. Fanci, F. Menichetti, D. Caselli, M. Diacchino and M. Congiu: Eur. J. Cancer *32* (5), 814 (1996).

331   M. Fukuda, H. Hirashima, R. Kurane, T. Abe, K.Sampi and K. Tominaga: Jpn. J. Antibiot. *47* (8), 1065 (1994).

332   A. Schaffner: Baillieres Clin. Infect. Dis. *1*, 449 (1994).

333 I.S. Faser and D.W. Denning: Blood Rev. 7, 208 (1993).
334 G. Bodey, G. Bueltmann, E Duguid, D. Gibbs, H. Hanak, M. Hotchi, G. Mall, P. Martino, F. Meunier, S. Milliken et al.: Eur. J. Clin. Microbiol. Infect. Dis. 11, 99 (1992).
335 B. Pfaffenbach, K. Donhuijsen, J. Pahnke, R.J. Adamek, M. Wegener and D. Ricken: Med. Klin. 89, 229 (1994).
336 N. Funai, Y. Shimamato, O. K. Tokunaga, W. Sugihara and M Yamaguchi: Acta Haematol. 93, 25 (1995).
337 U. Schuler, M Mölle and G. Ehninger: Mycoses 38 (Suppl. 1), 45 (1995).
338 Working Party of the British Society for Antimicrob. Chemotherapy: J. Antimicrob. Chemother. 32, 5 (1993).
339 F. Meunier: Int. J. Antimicrob. Agents 4, 73 (1994).
340 A.D. Allen, K.N. Sorensen, M.J. Nejdl, C. Durrant and R.T. Proffit: J. Antimicrob. Chemother. 34, 1001 (1994).
341 C. Cicigna, E.M. Bernard, M.H. White, W.P. Tong, D.S. Gordon and D. Armstrong: Abstr. Gen. Meet. Am. Soc. Microbiol. 95, 108 (1995).
342 A. Roman, J. Gavalda, C. Bravo, M. Montane, M. Monforte, V. Monforte, C. Murio, N. Martin, I. Calco, A. Ferrer, A. Pahissa and F. Morell: Eur. Resp. J. 7 (Suppl. 18), 249S (1994).
343 D. Maharaj, M.L. Guerra, R. Smith and P. Cassileth: Blood 82 (Suppl. 1), 636a (1993).
344 W.G. Powderly, D.M. Finkelstein, J. Feinberg, P. Frame, W. He, Ch van der Horst, S.L. Koletar, M.E. Eyster, S.A. Spector and S.A. Bozette: N. Engl. J. Med. 332 (11), 700 (1995).
344a N. Singh, M.J. Barnish, S.Berman, B.S. Bender, M.M. Wagener, M.G. Rinaldi and V.L. Yu: Clin. Infect. Dis. 23 (6), 1282 (1996).
345 M.E. Ellis, F.H. Clink, P. Ernst, M.A. Halim. A. Padmos, D. Spencer, M. Kalin, S.M. Hussain-Qadri, J. Burnie and W. Greer: Eur. J. Clin. Microbiol. Infect. Dis. 13, 3 (1994).
346 J.R. Wingard, W.G. Merz, M.G. Rinaldi, C.B. Miller, J.E. Karp and R. Saral: Antimicrob. Agents Chemother. 37 (9), 1847 (1993).
347 A. Schaffner and M Schaffner: J. Infect. Dis. 172, 1035 (1995).
348 C. Lumbreras, V. Cuervas-Mons, P. Jara, A. del Palacio, V.S. Furion, C. Barrios, E. Moreno, A.R. Noriega and C.V. Paya: J. Infect. Dis. 174 (3), 583 (1996).
349 P. Eggimann, P. Francoli, J. Bille, R. Schneider, G. Chapuis and R. Chiolero: Schweiz. Med. Wochenschr. 124 (33 Suppl. 63), 11 (1994).
350 J. Feusner, P. Robinson, N. Seibel, G. Reaman, M. Waskerwitz and C. Thompson: Proc. Am. Soc. Clin. Oncol. 13 (30), 444 (1994).
351 J. Cap, A. Mojezesova, E. Kyserova, E. Bubanska, K. Hatiar, J. Trupl and V. Krcmery: Chemotherapy 39, 438 (1993).
352 G.P. Bodey, E.J. Anaissie, L.S. Elting, E. Estey, S. O,Brien and H. Kantarjian: Cancer 73 (8), 2099 (1994).
353 P.H. Chandrasekar and C.M. Gatny: Chemotherapy 40, 136 (1994).
354 F. Menichetti, A. Del Favero, P. Martino, G. Bucaneve, A. Micozzi and D. D'Antonio: Ann. Intern. Med. 120 (11), 913 (1994).
355 M.E. Ellis, S.M. Hussain Qadri, D. Spence, M.A. Halim, P. Ernst and H. Clink: J. Antimicrob. Chemother. 33 (6), 1223 (1994).
356 R. Inci, N. Aksoy, E. Tumbay, A. Cevik and A.R. Moral: Br. J. Anaesth. 74 (Suppl. 1), 116 (1995).
357 P.H. Chandraskar and C.M. Gatny: J. Antimicrob. Chemother. 33 (2), 309 (1994).
358 A.J. Barnes, A.M. Wardley, B.A. Oppenheimer, G.R. Morgenstern, J.H. Scarffe, D.W. Warnock and E.M. Johnson: J. Infect. Dis. 33 (1), 43 (1996).
359 M.A. White: Curent Opinion Infect. Dis. 6, 737 (1993).

360 J. Hamacher, A. Spiliopoulos and L.P. Nicod: Schweiz. Med. Wochenschr. *126* (10 Suppl. 75), 85 (1996).

361 K. Yamac, E. Senol and R. Haznedar: Postgrad.Med. J. *71* (835), 284 (1995).

362 M.A. Slavin, B. Osborne, R. Adams, M.J. Levenstein, H.G. Schoch, A.R. Feldman, J.D. Meyers and R.A. Bowden: J. Infect. Dis. *171* (6), 1545 (1995).

363 J. van Burik, R.A. Bowden and G.B. McDonald: Gastroenterology *110* (4 Suppl. 1), A 1350 (1996).

364 A. Glasmacher, E. Molitor, J. Mezger and G. Marklein: Mycoses *39*, 249 (1996).

365 K.M. Troy and J. Cuttner: Blood *82* (10 Suppl. 1), 549 A (1993).

366 R. Mouy, F. Veber, S. Blanche, J. Donadieu, R. Brauner, J.C. Levron, C. Griscelli and A. Fischer: J. Pediatr. *125* (6), 998 (1994).

367 S.L. Prestona and L.L. Briceland: Am. J. Health Syst. Pharm. *52* (2), 164 (1995).

368 O. Uzon and E.J. Anaissie: Blood *86* (6), 2063 (1995).

369 E.J. Anaissie, D.P. Kontoyiannis, S. Vartivarian, H.M. Kantarjian, S. O'Brien, S.A. Giralt, B.S. Andersson, C. Karl, R.E. Champlin and G.P. Bodey: Clin. Infect. Dis. *17*, 1022 (1993).

370 B.L. Lee, A.M. Padula, M.G. Täuber, H.F. Chambers and M.A. Sande: J. Acq. Imm. Def. Syn. *5*, 600 (1992).

371 J.S. Hostetler, A. Catanzaro, D.A. Stevens, J. R. Graybill, P.K. Sharkey, R. A. Larsen, R.M. Tucker, A.D. Al-Haidary, M.G. Rinaldi, G.A. Cloud and J.N. Galgiani: J. Med. Vet. Mycol. *32*, 105 (1994).

372 D. Loebenberg, A. Cacciapuoti, R. Parmegiani, E.L. Moss, F. Menzel, B. Antonacci, C. Norris, T. Yarosh-Tomaine, R.S. Hare and G.H. Miller: Antimicrob. Agents Chemother. *36*, 498 (1992).

373 L. Franco, I. Gomez and A. Restrepo: Int. J. Dermatol. *31*, 725 (1992).

374 H. Zienicke and H.C. Korting: Mycoses *36*, 131 (1993).

375 Drugs of the Future *20*, 1300 (1995).

376 K. Lazardi, J.A. Urbina and W. de Souza: Antimicrob. Agents Chemother. *35*, 736 (1991).

377 M.A. Pfaller, M.J. Bale, B. Buschelman and P. Rhomberg: Diagn. Microbiol. Infect. Dis. *19* (2), 75 (1994).

378 C.B. Moore, D. Lane and D.W. Denning: J. Antimicrob. Agents Chemother. *32* (6), 831 (1993).

379 H.M. Wardle, D. Law, C.B. Moore, C. Mason and D.W. Denning: Antimicrob. Agents Chemother. *39* (4), 868 (1995).

380 K.V. Clemens, L.H. Hanson and D.A. Stevens: Antimicrob. Agents Chemother. *37* (5), 1177 (1993).

381 K.V. Clemens and D.A. Stevens: Antimicrob. Agents Chemother. *39* (3), 778 (1995).

382 N.C. Karyotaki, M.C. Dignani, R. Hachem and E.J. Anaissie: Antimicrob. Agents Chemother. *39* (2), 571 (1995).

383 L.K. Najvar, P. James, M.F. Luther and J.R. Graybill: J. Antimicrob. Chemother. *38* (4), 671 (1996).

384 J.R. Graybill, L.K. Najvar, J.D. Holmberg and M.F. Luther: Antimicrob. Agents Chemother. *39* (4), 924 (1995).

385 A.L. Correa, G. Velez, M. Albert, M. Luther, M.G. Rinaldi and J.R. Graybill: J. Med. Vet. Mycol. *33*, 367 (1995).

386 K.V. Clemens, M. Martinez, M.E. Homola and D.A. Stevens: J. Med. Vet. Mycol. *34*, 241 (1996).

387 D.W. Denning, L.Hall, M. Jackson and S. Hollis: Antimicrob. Agents Chemother. *39* (5), 1809 (1995).

388 B.A. Altinson, R. Bacanegra, A.L. Colombo and J.R. Graybill: Antimicrob. Agents Chemother. *38* (7), 1604 (1994).

389 J.A. Urbina, G. Payares, J. Molina, C. Sanjona, A. Liendo, K. Lazardi, M.M. Piras, R. Piras, N. Perez, P. Wincker and J.F. Ryley: Science *273*,969 (1996).

390 J. Burggraaf, J. Van Rooy, R.A. Yates and A.F. Cohen: Br. J. Clin. Pharmacol. *39* (5), 562P (1995).

391 S. de Wit, R.P. O'Doherty, R.P. Smith, R. Yates and N. Clumeck: 35th Interscience Conference on Antimicrobial Agents and Chemotherapy Abstract Book, F97 (1995).

392 D. De Wit, B. Dupont, J.D. Carttledge, D.A. Hawkins, D.W. Denning and N. Clumeck: Derwent Conferences Fast Track *2* (14), 177 (1994).

393 J.D. Carttledge, D.W. Denning, D. B. Dupont, S. de Wit and D.A. Hawkins: Derwent Conferences Fast Track *2* (14), 182 (1994).

394 P. Belanger, H. Sanati, R. Fratti, A.Ibrahim and M. Ghannoum: Abstr. Gen. Meet. Am. Soc.Microbiol. (96 Meet), 86 (1996).

395 A.L. Barry and S.D. Brown: Antimicrob. Agents Chemother. *40* (8), 1948 (1996).

396 G.W. Pve, G.P. Oliver and P.F. Troke: 35th Interscience Conference on Antimicrobial Agents and Chemotherapy Abstract Book, F72 (1995).

397 F. Barchiesi, M. Restrepo, D.A. McGough and M.G. Rinaldi: 35th Interscience Conference on Antimicrobial Agents and Chemotherapy Abstract Book, F71 (1995).

398 35th Interscience Conference on Antimicrobial Agents and Chemotherapy Abstract Book, F81–F85 (1995).

399 C.A. Hitchcock, R.J. Andrews, B.G.H. Lewis and P.F. Troke: 35th Interscience Conference on Antimicrobial Agents and Chemotherapy Abstract Book, F74 (1995).

400 C.A. Hitchcock, R.J. Andrews, B.G.H. Lewis and P.F. Troke: 35th Interscience Conference on Antimicrobial Agents and Chemotherapy Abstract Book, F75 (1995).

401 D. George, P. Miniter and V.T. Andriole: Clin. Infect. Dis. *21* (3), 774 (1995).

401a M.V. Martin, J. Yeats and C.A. Hitchcock: Antimicrob. Agents Chemother. *41* (1), 13 (1997).).

402 B.E. Patterson and P.E. Coates: 35th Interscience Conference on Antimicrobial Agents and Chemotherapy Abstract Book, F78 (1995).

403 B.E. Patterson,S. Roffey, S.G. Jezequel and B. Jones: 35th Interscience Conference on Antimicrobial Agents and Chemotherapy Abstract Book, F79 (1995).

404 P.F. Troke, K.W. Brammer, C.A. Hitchcock, S. Yonren and N. Sarantis: 35th Interscience Conference on Antimicrobial Agents and Chemotherapy Abstract Book, F73 (1995).

405 D. Denning, A.del Favero, E. Gluckman, D. Norfolk, M Ruhnke, S. Yonren, P.F. Troke and N. Sarantis: 35th Interscience Conference on Antimicrobial Agents and Chemotherapy Abstract Book, F80 (1995).

406 B. Dupont, D.W. Denning, H. Lode, S. Yonren, P.F. Troke and N. Sarantis: 35th Interscience Conference on Antimicrobial Agents and Chemotherapy Abstract Book, F81 (1995).

407 J.R. Perfect and W.A. Schell: 35th Interscience Conference on Antimicrobial Agents and Chemotherapy Abstract Book, F64 (1995).

408 A.M. Sugar and X.P. Liu: 36th Interscience Conference on Antimicrobial Agents and Chemotherapy Abstract Book, F65 (1996).

409 36th Interscience Conference on Antimicrobial Agents and Chemotherapy Abstract Book, F62, F63 (1996).

410 A. Cacciapuota, R. Parmegiani, D. Loebenberg, B. Antonacci, E.L. Moss, F. Menzel,

C. Norris, R.S. Hare and G.H. Miller: 36th Interscience Conference on Antimicrobial Agents and Chemotherapy Abstract Book, F66 (1996).

411 B. Dupont, L Improvisi and F. Dromer: 36th Interscience Conference on Antimicrobial Agents and Chemotherapy Abstract Book, F93 (1996).

412 J.R. Perfect, G.M. Cox, R.K. Dodge and W.A. Schell: Antimicrob. Agents Chemother. *40* (8), 1919 (1996).

413 A.M. Sugar and X.P. Liu: Antimicrob. Agents Chemother. *40* (5), 1314 (1996).

414 J. Wheat, C. Bick, P. Connolly, M. Smedema, M. Durkin, S. Kohler and D. Loebenberg: 36th Interscience Conference on Antimicrobial Agents and Chemotherapy Abstract Book, F101 (1996).

415 J.E. Lutz, K.V. Clemens and D. A. Stevens: 36th Interscience Conference on Antimicrobial Agents and Chemotherapy Abstract Book, F100 (1996).

416 R. Parmegiani, A. Cacciapuota, D. Loebenberg, B. Antonacci, C. Norris, T. Yarosh-Tomaine, M. Michalski, R.S. Hare and G.H. Miller: 36th Interscience Conference on Antimicrobial Agents and Chemotherapy Abstract Book, F67 (1996).

417 J.A. Urbina, G. Payares, C. Sanoja, L.M. Contreras, A. Liend, M.M. Piras and R. Piras: 36th Interscience Conference on Antimicrobial Agents and Chemotherapy Abstract Book, F102 (1996).

418 A. Yotsuji, K. Shimizu, H. Nishida, NR. Hori, N. Ishii, S. Yamamoto, H. Watanabe, H. Imaizumi and H. Narita: Derwent Conference Fast Track *3* (16), NCE 95-1640 (1995).

419 K. Hata, J. Kimura, H. Miki, T. Toyosawa, M. Moriyama and K. Katsu: Antimicrob. Agents Chemother. *40* (10), 2243 (1996).

420 K. Hata, J. Kimura, H. Miki, T. Toyosawa, M. Moriyama and K. Katsu: Antimicrob. Agents Chemother. *40* (10), 2237 (1996).

421 36th Interscience Conference on Antimicrobial Agents and Chemotherapy Abstract Book, F91–F94 (1996).

422 35th Interscience Conference on Antimicrobial Agents and Chemotherapy Abstract Book, F84–89 (1995).

423 36th Interscience Conference on Antimicrobial Agents and Chemotherapy Abstract Book, F75–F77 (1996).

424 K. Itoh, K. Okonogi, A. Tasaka, R. Hyashi, N. Tamura, N. Tsuchimori, T. Kitazaki, Y. Mataushita and J. Obita: 36th Interscience Conference on Antimicrobial Agents and Chemotherapy Abstract Book, F74 (1996).

425 Arzneim. Forsch. *42* (5a), 691-773 (1992).

426 Scrip 2021, 21 (1995).

427 Y. Niwano, T. Tabuchi, K. Kanai, H. Hamaguchi, H. Yamaguchi and K. Uchida: Antimicrob. Agents Chemother. *39*, 2353 (1995).

428 Y. Niwano, A. Seo, K. Kanai, H. Hamaguchi, K. Uchida and H. Yamaguchi: Antimicrob. Agents Chemother. *38* (9), 2204 (1994).

429 Y. Niwano, H. Koga, K. Kanai, H. Hamaguchi and H. Yamaguchi: Arzneim. Forsch. *46* (2), 218 (1996).

430 R&D Focus Drug News *4* (22), 2 (1995).

431 O. Binet, J. Soto-Melo, J. Delgadillo, I. Izquierdo and J. Forn: Mycoses *37*, 455 (1994).

432 M. Merlos, M.L. Vericat, J. Garcia-Rafanell and J. Forn: Inflamm. Res. *45* (1), 20 (1995).

433 E. Font, A. del Palacio, S. Cuetera, A. Rodriguez-Noriega, S. Lopez, L. Iglesias and C.I. Wassermann: Meth. Find. Exp. Clin. Pharmacol. *17* (Suppl. 1), Abs CO 54 (1995).

434 R&D Focus Drug News *5* (30), 4 (1996).

435 R&D Focus/Lotus Notes, Dec 9, 1996.

436 Derwent Conference Fast-Track *4* (16) (1996).
437 36th Interscience Conference on Antimicrobial Agents and Chemotherapy Abstract Book, F78–F80 (1996).
438 36th Interscience Conference on Antimicrobial Agents and Chemotherapy Abstract Book, LM34 (1996).
439 Scrip 2177, 17 (1996).
440 I. Abe, M. Rohmer and G.D. Prestwich: Chem Rev. *93*, 2189 (1993).
441 Y.F. Yeng, A.C. Oelschlager, N.H. Georgopapadakou, P.G. Hartman, F. Scheliga: J. Am. Chem. Soc. *117*, 670 (1995).
442 Y.F. Yeng, A.C. Oelschlager and P.G. Hartman: J. Org. Chem. *59*, 5803 (1994).
443 Y.F. Yeng, D.S. Dodd, A.C. Oelschlager and P.G. Hartman: Tetrahedron *51*, 5255 (1994).
444 I. Abe, W. Liu, A.C. Oelschlafer and G.D. Prestwich: J. Am. Chem. Soc. *118*, 9180 (1990).
445 D.S. Dodd, A.C. Oelschlager, N.H. Georgopapadakou, A. Polak and P.G. Hartman: J. Org. Chem. *57*, 7226 (1992).
446 G. Balliano, P. Milla, M. Ceruti, L. Carrrano, F. Viola, P. Brusa and L. Cattel: Antimicrob. Agents Chemother. *38*, 1904 (1994).
447 M. Ceruti, G. Balliano, F. Viola, G. Grosa, F. Rocco and L. Cattel: Eur. J. Med. Chem. *22*, 199 (1987).
448 M. Ceruti, G. Balliano, F. Viola, G. Grosa, F. Rocco and L. Cattel: J. Med. Chem *35*, 3050 (1992).
449 M. Ceruti, F. Rocco, F. Viola, G. Balliano, G. Grosa and F. Dioso: Eur. J. Med. Chem. *28*, 675 (1987).
450 D. Airaudi, M. Ceruti, C. Bianca and V.F. Marchisio: Mycoses *39*, 51 (1996).
451 F. Viola, P. Brusa, G. Balliano, M. Ceruti, O. Boutaud, F. Schuber and L. Cattel: Biochem. Pharmacol. *50*, 787 (1995).
452 L. Cattel, M. Ceruti, G. Balliano, F. Viola, G. Grosa, F. Rocco and P. Brusa: Lipids *30*, 235 (1995).
453 S. Jolidon, A. Polak, P.G. Hartman and P. Guerry, in: Recent Advances in the Chemistry of Anti-Infective Agents, H.P. Bentley and R. Pondsford (eds.), Royal Society of Chemistry, Cambridge (1993), p. 223.
454 S. Jolidon, A. Polak, P. Guerry and P.G. Hartman: Biochem. Soc. Trans. *18*, 47 (1990).
455 S. Jolidon, A. Polak, P. Guerry and P.G. Hartman: Pestic. Sci. *31*, 588 (1991).
456 S. Jolidon, A. Polak, P. Guerry and P.G. Hartman, in: Molecular Aspects of Chemotherapy, D. Shugar, W. Rode and E. Borowsky (eds.), Springer Berlin (1991), p. 143.
457 O.H. Morand, J. Aebi, H. Dehmlow, Y. Ji, N. Gains, H. Lengsfeld and J. Himber: J. Lipid Res. *38*, 148 (1997).
458 K. Bartizal, T. Scott, G.K. Abruzzo, C.J. Gill, C. Pacholok, L. Lynch and H. Kropp: Antimicrob. Agents Chemother. *39* (5), 1070 (1995).
459 D. Zeckner, T. Butler, C. Boylan, B. Boyll, P. Watson and W. Current: 36th Interscience Conference on Antimicrobial Agents and Chemotherapy Abstract Book, F 98 (1996).
460 W.E. Dismuskes: Derwent Conference Fast-Track *4* (6), NCE-96-0636 (1996).
461 R. Rennie, C. Sand and S. Smith: 36th Interscience Conference on Antimicrobial Agents and Chemotherapy Abstract Book, F45 (1996).
462 D.A. Stevens, M. Martinez and M.J. Devine: 36th Interscience Conference on Antimicrobial Agents and Chemotherapy Abstract Book, F46 (1996).
463 B. Hoban, A. Kabani, J. Karlowsky, M. Friesen, G. Harding, M. Turik and G. Zhanel:

36th Interscience Conference on Antimicrobial Agents and Chemotherapy Abstract Book, F 47 (1996).

464 G. Harding, J. Karlowsky, T. Balko, D. Hoban, A. Kabani, S. Zelenitsky, M. Turik and G.G. Zhanel: 36th Interscience Conference on Antimicrobial Agents and Chemotherapy Abstract Book, F49 (1996).

465 33rd Interscience Conference on Antimicrobial Agents and Chemotherapy Abstract Book, Abstracts 358–368 (1993).

466 P. Raab, D. Zeckner, B. Boyll, C. Boylan and W. Current: 36th Interscience Conference on Antimicrobial Agents and Chemotherapy Abstract Book, F167 (1996).

467 M.S. Barlett, W.L. Current, M. Goheen, C.J. Boylan, C.H. Lee, M.M. Shaw, S.F. Queener and J.W. Smith: Antimicrob. Agents Chemother. 40 (8), 1811 (1996).

468 R. Lucas, K. Desante, B. Hatcher, J. Hemingway, R. Lachno, S. Brooks and M. Turik: 36th Interscience Conference on Antimicrobial Agents and Chemotherapy Abstract Book, F50 (1996).

469 J.V. Martinez-Suarez and J.L. Rodriguez-Tudela: Antimicrob. Agents Chemother. 40 (5), 1277 (1996).

470 M.B. Kurtz, C. Douglas, J. Marrinan, K. Nollstadt, J. Onishi, S. Dreikorn, J. Milligan, J. Thompson, J.M. Balkovec, F.A. Bouffard et al.: Antimicrob. Agents Chemother. 38 (12), 2750 (1994).

471 P.W. Nelson and J.H. Rex: 35th Interscience Conference on Antimicrobial Agents and Chemotherapy Abstract Book, F99 (1995).

472 J.A. Vazquez, M.E. Lynch and J.D. Sobel: Abstr. Gen. Meet. Am. Soc. Microbiol. 95, 105 (1995).

473 K. Bartizal, T. Scott, G.K. Abruzz, C.J. Gill, C. Pacholok, L. Lynch and H. Kropp: Antimicrob. Agents Chemother. 39 (5), 1070 (1995).

474 K.H. Nollstadt, M.A. Powles, H. Fujioka, M. Aikawa and D.M. Schatz: Antimicrob. Agents Chemother. 38 (10), 2258 (1994).

475 G.K. Abruzzo, A.M. Flattery, C.J. Gill, J.G. Smith, V.B. Kropp and K. Bartizal: Antimicrob. Agents Chemother. 39 (5), 1077 (1995).

476 P.W. Nelson, M. Lozano-Chiu and J.H. Rex: 36th Interscience Conference on Antimicrobial Agents and Chemotherapy Abstract Book, F28 (1996).

477 A.W. Fothergill, D.A. Sutton and M.G. Rinaldi: 36th Interscience Conference on Antimicrobial Agents and Chemotherapy Abstract Book, F29 (1996).

478 J.A. Vazquez, D. Boikov, M.E. Lynch and J.D. Sobel: 36th Interscience Conference on Antimicrobial Agents and Chemotherapy Abstract Book, F30 (1996).

479 M. Del Poeta, W.A. Schelll and J.R. Perfect: 36th Interscience Conference on Antimicrobial Agents and Chemotherapy Abstract Book, F33 (1996).

480 J.A. Vazquez, M.T. Arganoza, P. Steffan and R. Arkins: 36th Interscience Conference on Antimicrobial Agents and Chemotherapy Abstract Book, F35 (1996).

481 A. Espinel-Ingroff: 36th Interscience Conference on Antimicrobial Agents and Chemotherapy Abstract Book, F31 (1996).

482 N.X. Chiu, I. Weitzman and P. Della Latta: 36th Interscience Conference on Antimicrobial Agents and Chemotherapy Abstract Book, F34 (1996).

483 K. Bartizal, A. Flattery, F.L. Lynch, C. Pacholok, C.J. Gill, H. Rosen, P. Scott and H. Kropp: 36th Interscience Conference on Antimicrobial Agents and Chemotherapy Abstract Book, F32 (1996).

484 S.P. Franzot and A. Casadevall: 36th Interscience Conference on Antimicrobial Agents and Chemotherapy Abstract Book, F 36 (1996).

485 G.K. Abruzzo, A.M. Flattery, C.J. Gill, L. Kong, J.G. Smith, V.B. Pikounis, H. Kropp,

H. Rosen and K. Bartizal: 36th Interscience Conference on Antimicrobial Agents and Chemotherapy Abstract Book, F37 (1996).

486 L. Najvar, A. Fothergill, M. Luther and J. Graybill: 36th Interscience Conference on Antimicrobial Agents and Chemotherapy Abstract Book, F38 (1996).

487 E.M. Bernard, T. Ishimaru and D. Armstrong: 36th Interscience Conference on Antimicrobial Agents and Chemotherapy Abstract Book, F39 (1996).

488 A.M. Flattery, G.K. Abruzzo, J.G. Smith, C.J. Gill, H. Rosen, H. Kropp and K. Bartizal: 36th Interscience Conference on Antimicrobial Agents and Chemotherapy Abstract Book, F40 (1996).

489 J.G. Smith, G.K. Abruzzo, C.J. Gill, A.M. Flattery, L. Kong, H. Rosen, H. Kropp and K. Bartizal: 36th Interscience Conference on Antimicrobial Agents and Chemotherapy Abstract Book, F41 (1996).

490 M.A. Powels, J. Anderson, P. Liberator and D.H. Schmatz: 36th Interscience Conference on Antimicrobial Agents and Chemotherapy Abstract Book, F 42 (1996).

491 L. Najvar, J.R. Graybill, E. Montalbo, F. Barchiesi and M. Luther: 36th Interscience Conference on Antimicrobial Agents and Chemotherapy Abstract Book, F43 (1996).

492 R&D Focus Drugs News 5 (39), 9 (1996).

493 K.V. Clemons and D.A. Stevens: Clin. Infect. Dis. 23 (4), 874 (1996).

494 T. Chapman, O. Kinsman and J. Houston: Antimicrob. Agents Chemother. 36, 1909 (1992).

495 R.K. Li, A.W. Fothergill and M.G. Rinaldi: 36th Interscience Conference on Antimicrobial Agents and Chemotherapy Abstract Book, F189 (1996).

496 M.E. Flores and R.F. Hector: 36th Interscience Conference on Antimicrobial Agents and Chemotherapy Abstract Book, F190 (1996).

497 Derwent Conference Fast Track 4 (16), NCE 96 1427, 1497 (1996).

498 N. Awazu, K. Ikai, J. Nishimura, S. Mizutani, K. Takesago: J. Antibiot. 48 (6), 525 (1995).

499 M.J. Rodriguez, M.J. Zweifel, J.D. Farmer, R.S. Gordee, R.J. Loncharich: J. Antibiot. 49 (4), 386 (1996).

500 32nd Interscience Conference on Antimicrobial Agents and Chemotherapy Abstract Book, Abstracts 496, 497, 498 (1992).

501 K. Takesako, H. Kuroda, T. Inoue, F. Haruna, Y. Yoshikawa, I. Kato: J. Antibiot. 46 (9), 1414 (1993).

502 A.I. Aller, M.E. Mazuelos, M.D. Morilla and O. Montero: Chemotherapy 41 (4), 276 (1995).

503 L. Green, B. Petersen, P. Raab, D. Zeckner, W.L. Current and J. A. Radding: 34th Interscience Conference on Antimicrobial Agents and Chemotherapy Abstract Book, F165 (1994).

504 N.H. Georgopapadakou and J.S. Tkacz: Trends Microbiol. 3 (3), 98 (1995).

505 T. Tsuno, H. Yamamoto, Y. Narita, K. Suzuki, T. Hasegawa, S. Kakinuma, K. Saitoh, T. Furumai and T. Oki: J. Antibiot. 46 (3), 420 (1993).

506 T. Ueki, K. Numata, Y. Sawada, M. Nishio, H. Ohkuma, S. Toda, H. Kamachi, Y. Fukagawa and T. Oki: J. Antibiot. 46 (3), 455 (1993).

507 Derwent Conference Fast Track 4 (16), NCE-96-1499-1500 (1996).

508 T. Takauchi, T. Hara, H. Naganawa, M. Okada, M. Hamada, H. Umezawa, S. Gomi, M. Sezaki, S. Kondo: J. Antibiot. 41, 807 (1988).

509 Annual Drug Data Report 16 (7), 670 (1994).

510 J.C. Fung-Tomc, B. Minassian, E. Huczko, B. Kolek, D.P. Bonner and R.E. Kessler: Antimicrob. Agents Chemother. 39 (2), 295 (1995).

511 H.M. Wardle, D. Law and D.W. Denning: Antimicrob. Agents Chemother. *40* (9), 2229 (1996).

512 T. Oki, M. Kakushima, M. Hirano, A. Takahashi, A. Ohta, S. Masuyoshi, M. Hatori, H. Kamei: J. Antibiot. *45* (9), 1512 (1992).

513 C.E. Gonzalez, D.Shetty, N. Giri, W. Love, K. Kligys, C. Lyman, J. Bacher, T.J. Walsh: 36th Interscience Conference on Antimicrobial Agents and Chemotherapy Abstract Book, F181 (1996).

514 C.E. Gonzalez, D.Shetty, N. Giri, W. Love, K. Kligys, T. Sein C. Lyman, J. Bacher, T.J. Walsh: 36th Interscience Conference on Antimicrobial Agents and Chemotherapy Abstract Book, F182 (1996).

515 M. Restrepo, L. Najvar, R. Bocanegra, M. Luther and J. Graybill: 36th Interscience Conference on Antimicrobial Agents and Chemotherapy Abstract Book, F183 (1996).

516 H. Yang, R.L. Drain, J.M. Clark: 34th Interscience Conference on Antimicrobial Agents and Chemotherapy Abstract Book, F173 (1994).

517 M. Watanabe, S. Gomi, H. Tohyama, K Ohtsuka, S. Shibahara, S. Inouye, H. Kobayashi, S. Suzuki, S. Kondo, T. Takeuchi and H. Yamaguchi: J. Antibiot. *49* (4), 366 (1996).

518 A. Yasuoka, S. Oka, K. Komuro, H. Shimizu, K. Kitada, Y. Nakamura, S. Shibahara, T. Takeuchi, S. Kondo K. Shimada: Antimicrob. Agents Chemother. *39* (3), 720 (1995).

519 O.D. Hensens, C.F. Wichmann, L.M. Liesch, F.L. Van Middlesworth, K.E. Wilson and R.E. Schwartz: Tetrahedron *47*, 3915 (1991).

520 R.E. Schwartz, C. Dufresne, J.E. Flor, A.J. Kempf, K.E. Wilson, T. Lam, J. Onishi, J. Milligan, R.A. Fromtling, G.K. Abruzzo, R. Jenkins, K. Glazomitski, G. Bills, L. Zitano, S. Del Val Mochales, M.N. Omstead: J. Antibiot. *44* (5), 463 (1991).

521 S. Matsukuma, T. Ohtsuka, H. Kotaki, H. Shirai, T. Sano, K. Watanabe, N. Nakayama, Y. Itezono, M. Fujiu, N. Shimma, K. Yokose, T. Okuda: J. Antibiot. *45*, 151 (1992).

522 Y. Aoki, F. Yoshihara, M. Kondoh, Y. Nakamura, N. Nakayama and M. Arisawa: Antimicrob. Agents Chemother. *37*, 2662 (1993).

523 Y. Aoki, T. Yamazaki, M. Kondoh, J. Sudoh, N. Nakajama, Y. Sekine, H. Shimada and M. Arisawa: J. Antibiotics *45*, 180 (1992).

524 J.O. Capobianco, C.C. Doran, R.C. Goldman and B. De: J. Antimicrob. Chemother. *30*, 781 (1992).

525 D. Zakula, J.O. Capocianco and R.C. Goldman: 35th Interscience Conference on Antimicrobial Agents and Chemotherapy Abstract Book, F105 (1995).

526 T. Kuchta, C. Leka, P. Farkas, H. Budjakova, E. Belajova, N.J. Russell, K. Hata, J. Kimura, H. Miki, T. Toyosawa, T. Nakamura, K. Katsu: Antimicrob. Agents Chemother. *39*, 1538 (1995).

527 H. Bujdakova, T. Kuchta, E. Sidoova and A. Gvozdajakova: FEMS Microbiol. Lett. *112*, 329 (1993).

528 H. Bujdakova and M. Muckova: Int. J. Antimicrob. Agents *4*, 303 (1994).

529 T. Kuchta, K. Bartkova and R. Kubinec: Biochem. Biophys. Res. Comm. *189*, 85 (1992).

530 T. Kuchta, H. Bujdakova and E. Sidoova: Folia Microbiol. *34*, 504 (1998).

531 F. Mignini, B. Cybulska, F. Santacroce, I. Covelli and E. Borowski: Abstr. Gen. Meet. Am. Soc. Microbiol. *94*, 608 (1994).

532 E. Borowski, J. Grybowska, J. Gumieniak, P. Sowinski, B. Cybulska, T. Zieniawa, F. Mignini, F. Santacroce, J. Bolard: Abstr. Gen. Meet. Am. Soc. Microbiol. *95*, 105 (1995).

533 L.K. Najvar, M.F. Luther and J.R. Graybill: J. Antimicrob. Chemother. *36* (6), 1005 (1995).

534 L.K. Najvar, J. Fothergill, J.R. Graybill and S. Regen: 35th Interscience Conference on Antimicrobial Agents and Chemotherapy Abstract Book, F110 (1995).

535 A. Bonabello, M.R. Galmozzi, G. Buffa and T. Bruzzese: Twelfth Int. Congress of Pharmacology, Poster 12.2.23 (1994).

535a T. Bruzzese, C. Rimaroli, A. Bonabello, E Ferrari and M. Signorini: Eur. J. Med. Chem. *31* (2), 962 (1996).

536 S. Sakuda, U. Guce-Bigol, M. Itoh, T. Nishiura and Y. Yamada: Tetrahedron Lett. *36* (16), 2777 (1995).

537 J. Kohno, M. Nishio, K. Kawano, S. Suzuki and S. Komatsubara: J. Antibiot. *48* (10), 1173 (1995).

538 H.P. Fiedler, M. Nega, C. Pfefferle, I. Groth, C. Kempter, H. Stephan, J.W. Metzger: J. Antibiot. *49* (8), 758 (1996).

539 S. Kumazawa, Y. Asami, K. Awane, H. Ohtani, C. Fukuchi, T. Mikawa and T. Hayase: J. Antibiot. *47* (6), 688 (1994).

540 M. Ubukata, N. Shiraishi, K. Kobinata, T. Kudo, Y. Yamaguchi, H. Osada, Y. Shen and K. Isono: J. Antibiot. *48* (4), 289 (1995).

541 M. Fujiu, S. Sawairi, H. Shimada, H. Tanaka, Y. Aoki, T. Okuda and K. Yokose: J. Antibiot. *47*, 833 (1994).

542 Y. Aoki, M. Kondoh, M Nakamura, T. Fujii, T. Yamazaki, H. Shimada and M. Arisawa: J. Antibiot *47*, 909 (1994).

543 Y. Aoki, M. Yamamoto, S.M. Hosseini-Mazinani, N. Koshikawa, K. Sugimoto and M. Arisawa: Antimicrob. Agents Chemother. *40*, 127 (1996).

544 K.J. Kwong-Chung, I. Polacheck and T.J. Popkin: J. Bacteriol. *150* (3), 1414 (1982).

545 J.C. Rhodes, I. Polacheck and K.J. Kwong-Chung: Infect. Immun. *36*, 1175 (1982).

546 K.J. Kwong-Chung and J.C. Rhodes: Infect. Immun. *51* (1), 218 (1986).

547 A. Polak: Mycoses *33* (5), 215 (1989).

548 K. Barrett-Bee, Y. Hayes, R.C. Wilson and J.F. Ryley: J. Gen. Microbiol. *131*, 1217 (1985).

549 K.J. Kwon-Chung, C. Lehman, C. Good and P.T. Magee: Infect. Immun. *49*, 571 (1985).

550 M. Monod, G. Togni, B. Hube and D. Songland: Mol. Microbiol. *13*, 157 (1994).

551 R. Rüchel: Biochim. Biophys. Acta *559*, 99 (1981).

552 D.R. Davies: Annu. Rev. Biophys. Chem. *19*, 189 (1990).

553 J.R. Perfect: Antimicrob. Agents Chemother. *40* (7), 1577 (1996).

554 H. Hänel, R. Kirsch, H.L. Schmidts and K. Kottmann: Mycoses *38* (7/8), 251 (1995).

555 F. De Bernardis, R. Lorenzini, B. Verticchio, L. Agatensi and. A. Cassone: J. Clin. Microb. *27* (119), 2598 (1989).

556 F. De Bernardis, L. Agatensi, I.K. Ross, G. Emerson R. Lorenzini, P.A. Sullivan and A. Cassone: J. Infect. Dis. *161*, 1276 (1990).

557 G. Togni, D. Songland and M. Monod: J. Med. Vet. Mycol. *32*, 257 (1994).

558 I.K. Ross, F. De Bernardis, G.W. Emerson, A. Cassone and P.A. Sullivan: J. Gen. Microb. *136*, 687 (1990).

559 B. Hube, C.J. Turver, F.C. Odds, H. Eifert, G.J. Boulnois, H. Köchel and R. Rüchel: J. Med. Vet. Mycol. *29*, 129 (1991).

560 M. Badasso, S.P. Wood, C. Anuilar, J.B. Cooper, T.L. Blundell and T. Dreyer: J. Mol. Biol. *232* (2), 701 (1993).

561 R. Rüchel, B. Ritter and M. Schaffrinski: Zbl. Bakt. *273*, 391 (1990).

562 L. Angiolella, F. De Bernardis, C. Bromuro, F. Mondollo, T. Ceddia and A. Cassone: J. Chemother. *2* (1), 55 (1990).

563 Hirayama, Matayuki, Ichara, Masoto, Abe, Kenji: Jpn Kokai Tokkyo Koho 8 pp (1993).

564 Hirayama, Matayuki, Ichara, Masoto, Abe, Kenji: Jpn Kokai Tokkyo Koho 18 pp (1993).

565 T. Sato, K. Nagai, M. Shibazaki, K. Abe, Y. Takebayashi and B. Lumanau: J. Antibiot. *47* (5), 566 (1994).

566 T. Sato, M. Shibazaki, H. Yamaguchi, K. Abe, H. Matsumoto and M. Shimizu: J. Antibiot. *47* (5), 588 (1994).

567 J. Bolonick and A.S. Delk: World Drug Alert Antimicrob. 10 Nov., 36 (1994).

568 World Drug Alert Antimicrob. 17 Aug., 28 (1995).

Index Vol. 49

The references of the Subject Index are given in the language of the respective contribution.
Die Stichworte des Sachregisters sind in der jeweiligen Sprache der einzelnen Beiträge aufgeführt.
Les termes repris dans la Table des Matières sont donnés selon la langue dans laquelle l'ouvrage est écrit.

Index of titles
Verzeichnis der Titel
Index des titres
Vol. 1–49 (1959–1997)

Author and paper index
Autoren- und Artikelindex
Index des auteurs et des articles
Vol. 1–49 (1959–1997)

Experience with bitoscanate in hook-worm disease and trichuriasis in Mexico *19*, 23 (1975)	F. Biagi
Analysis of symptoms and signs related with intestinal parasitosis in 5,215 cases *19*, 10 (1975)	F. Biagi R. López J. Viso
Untersuchungen zur Biochemie und Pharmacologie der Thymoleptika *11*, 121 (1968) The role of adipose tissue in the distribution and storage of drugs *28*, 273 (1984)	M. H. Bickel
The β-adrenergic-blocking agents, pharmacology, and structure-activity relationships *10*, 46 (1966)	J. H. Biel B. K. B. Lum
Prostaglandins *17*, 410 (1973)	J. S. Bindra R. Bindra
In vitro models for the study of antibiotic activities *31*, 349 (1987)	J. Blaser S. H. Zinner
The red blood cell membrane as a model for targets of drug action *17*, 59 (1973)	L. Bolis
Epidemiology and public health. Importance of intestinal nematode infections in Latin America *19*, 28 (1975)	D. Botero
Clinical importance of cardiovascular drug interactions *25*, 133 (1981) Serum electrolyte abnormalities caused by drugs *30*, 9 (1986)	D. Craig Brater
Update of cardiovascular drug interactions *29*, 9 (1985)	D. Craig Brater Michael R. Vasko
Some practical problems of the epidemiology of leprosy in the Indian context *18*, 25 (1974)	S. G. Browne
Brain neurotransmitters and the development and maintenance of experimental hypertension *30*, 127 (1986)	Jerry J. Buccafusco Henry E. Brezenoff

Pharmacology and toxicology of axoplasmic transport 28, 53 (1984)	Fred Samson Ralph L. Smith J. Alejandro Donoso
Clinical experience with bitoscanate 19, 96 (1975)	M. R. Samuel
Tetanus: Situational clinical trials and therapeutics 19, 367 (1975)	R. K. M. Sanders M. L. Peacock B. Martyn B. D. Shende
Epidemiological studies on cholera in non-endemic regions with special reference to the problem of carrier state during epidemic and non-epidemic period 19, 594 (1975)	M. V. Sant W. N. Gatlewar S. K. Bhindey
Epidemiological and biochemical studies in filariasis in four villages near Bombay 18, 269 (1974)	M. V. Sant W. N. Gatlewar T. U. K. Menon
Hookworm anaemia and intestinal mal-absorption associated with hookworm infestation 19, 108 (1975)	A. K. Saraya B. N. Tandon
The effects of structural alteration on the anti-inflammatory properties of hydrocortisone 5, 11 (1963)	L. H. Sarett A. A. Patchett S. Steelman
The impact of natural product research on drug discovery 23, 51 (1979)	L. H. Sarett
Aldose reductase inhibitors: Recent developments 40, 99 (1993)	Reinhard Sarges Peter J. Oates
Anti-filariasis campaign: Its history and future prospects 18, 259 (1974)	M. Sasa
Barbiturates and the $GABA_A$ receptor complex 34, 261 (1990)	Paul A. Saunders I. K. Ho
Platelets and atherosclerosis 29, 49 (1985)	Robert N. Saunders
Immuno-diagnosis of helminthic infections 19, 119 (1975)	T. Sawada K. Sato K. Takei

The problem of diphtheria as seen in Bombay *19*, 452 (1975)	M. M. Wagle R. R. Sanzgiri Y. K. Amdekar
Drug nephrotoxicity – The significance of cellular mechanisms *41*, 51 (1993)	Robert J. Walker J. Paul Fawcett
Nicotine: An addictive substance or a therapeutic agent? *33*, 9 (1989)	David M. Warburton
Cell-wall antigens of *Vibrio cholerae* and their implication in cholera immunity *19*, 612 (1975)	Y. Watanabe R. Ganguly
Steroidogenic capacity in the adrenal cortex and its regulation *34*, 359 (1990)	Michael R. Watermann Evan R. Simpson
Antigen-specific T-cell factors and drug research *32*, 9 (1988)	David R. Webb
Where is immunology taking us? *20*, 573 (1976) Immunology in drug research *28*, 233 (1984)	W. J. Wechter Barbara E. Loughman
Natriuretic hormones *34*, 231 (1990)	W. J. Wechter Elaine J. Benaksas
The effects of NSAIDs and E-prosta-glandins on bone: A two signal hypothesis for the maintenance of skeletal bone *39*, 351 (1992)	William J. Wechter
Metabolic activation of chemical carcinogens *26*, 143 (1982)	E. K. Weisburger
A pharmacological approach to allergy *3*, 409 (1961) Adverse reactions of sugar polymers in animals and man *23*, 27 (1979) Biogenic amines and drug research *28*, 9 (1984)	G. B. West
A new approach to the medical interpretation of shock *14*, 196 (1970)	G. B. West M. S. Starr